CAMBRIDGE LIBRARY COLLECTION

Books of enduring scholarly value

History of Medicine

It is sobering to realise that as recently as the year in which On the Origin of Species was published, learned opinion was that diseases such as typhus and cholera were spread by a 'miasma', and suggestions that doctors should wash their hands before examining patients were greeted with mockery by the profession. The Cambridge Library Collection reissues milestone publications in the history of Western medicine as well as studies of other medical traditions. Its coverage ranges from Galen on anatomical procedures to Florence Nightingale's common-sense advice to nurses, and includes early research into genetics and mental health, colonial reports on tropical diseases, documents on public health and military medicine, and publications on spa culture and medicinal plants.

The Works, Literary, Moral, and Medical, of Thomas Percival, M.D.

A physician and medical reformer enthused by the scientific and cultural progress of the Enlightenment as it took hold in Britain, Thomas Percival (1740–1804) wrote on many topics, including public health and demography. His influential publication on medical ethics is considered the first modern formulation. In 1807, his son Edward published this four-volume collection of his father's diverse work. Some of the items here had never been published before, including a selection of Percival's private correspondence and a biographical account written by Edward. Volume 2 contains essays on moral and literary subjects, notably a Socratic discourse on truth as well as miscellaneous observations on the influence of habit and association. Also included are a memoir of the philanthropist Thomas Butterworth Bayley and the text of Percival's *Medical Ethics* (1803), which has been reissued separately in this series along with his *Essays Medical and Experimental* (revised edition, 1772–3).

Cambridge University Press has long been a pioneer in the reissuing of out-of-print titles from its own backlist, producing digital reprints of books that are still sought after by scholars and students but could not be reprinted economically using traditional technology. The Cambridge Library Collection extends this activity to a wider range of books which are still of importance to researchers and professionals, either for the source material they contain, or as landmarks in the history of their academic discipline.

Drawing from the world-renowned collections in the Cambridge University Library and other partner libraries, and guided by the advice of experts in each subject area, Cambridge University Press is using state-of-the-art scanning machines in its own Printing House to capture the content of each book selected for inclusion. The files are processed to give a consistently clear, crisp image, and the books finished to the high quality standard for which the Press is recognised around the world. The latest print-on-demand technology ensures that the books will remain available indefinitely, and that orders for single or multiple copies can quickly be supplied.

The Cambridge Library Collection brings back to life books of enduring scholarly value (including out-of-copyright works originally issued by other publishers) across a wide range of disciplines in the humanities and social sciences and in science and technology.

The Works,
Literary, Moral, and Medical,
of Thomas Percival, M.D.

To which are Prefixed,
Memoirs of His Life and Writings,
and a Selection from
His Literary Correspondence

VOLUME 2

THOMAS PERCIVAL

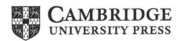
CAMBRIDGE
UNIVERSITY PRESS

CAMBRIDGE
UNIVERSITY PRESS

University Printing House, Cambridge, CB2 8BS, United Kingdom

Published in the United States of America by Cambridge University Press, New York

Cambridge University Press is part of the University of Cambridge.
It furthers the University's mission by disseminating knowledge in the pursuit of
education, learning and research at the highest international levels of excellence.

www.cambridge.org
Information on this title: www.cambridge.org/9781108067348

© in this compilation Cambridge University Press 2014

This edition first published 1807
This digitally printed version 2014

ISBN 978-1-108-06734-8 Paperback

THE

WORKS

OF

THOMAS PERCIVAL, M.D.

IN FOUR VOLUMES.

THE

WORKS,

LITERARY, MORAL,

AND

MEDICAL,

OF

THOMAS PERCIVAL, M.D.

F. R. S. AND A. S.—F. R. S. AND R. M. S. EDIN.

LATE PRES. OF THE LIT. AND PHIL. SOC. AT MANCHESTER; MEMBER OF
THE ROYAL SOCIETIES OF PARIS AND OF LYONS, OF THE MEDICAL
SOCIETIES OF LONDON, AND OF AIX EN PROVENCE, OF THE
AMERIC. ACAD. OF ARTS, &c, AND OF THE AMERIC.
PHIL. SOC. AT PHILADELPHIA.

TO WHICH ARE PREFIXED,

MEMOIRS of his LIFE and WRITINGS,

AND A SELECTION FROM HIS

LITERARY CORRESPONDENCE.

A NEW EDITION.

———

VOL. II.

PRINTED BY RICHARD CRUTTWELL, ST. JAMES's-STREET, BATH;
FOR J. JOHNSON, ST. PAUL's CHURCH-YARD, LONDON.

1807.

TABLE OF CONTENTS.

———

MORAL and LITERARY DISSERTATIONS.

6 CONTENTS.

MORAL AND LITERARY

DISSERTATIONS:

CHIEFLY INTENDED

AS THE SEQUEL

TO

A FATHER'S INSTRUCTIONS.

" REM TIBI SOCRATICÆ POTERUNT OSTENDERE CHARTÆ.

" ——— QUO VIRTUS, QUO FERAT ERROR."   HOR.

TO THE RIGHT REVEREND

RICHARD WATSON, D. D. F. R. S.

LORD BISHOP OF LANDAFF,

&c. &c. &c.

MY LORD,

PERMIT me again to offer this volume of Moral and Literary Differtations to your Lordfhip's acceptance and patronage. The work has been much enlarged; and I fhall think myfelf happy if it continue to be honoured with your indulgence and approbation. I feel a lively fenfe of the value of your friendfhip; and venerate thofe diftinguifhed talents and virtues which you have fo uniformly and affiduoufly exerted in the promotion of fcience, religion, and liberty. With every affectionate wifh for

A 2

your Lordſhip's health, felicity, and the ſtill further extenſion of your uſefulneſs, and with the moſt cordial reſpect and attachment,

I have the honour to be,

My LORD,

Your Lordſhip's much obliged,

And moſt faithful humble ſervant,

THOMAS PERCIVAL.

THE PREFACE.

—◄◄◄◆►►►—

IN offering to the public a miscellaneous work like
the following, it may be proper to give a brief
account of the different parts of which it is composed.
The SOCRATIC DISCOURSE was written several
years ago, for the use of the author's own family;
and a few printed copies of it were distributed amongst
his friends. The approbation with which it has been
honoured by some of the most judicious of them, has
abated his diffidence concerning it; and the desire of
rendering his private labours of utility to mankind
has induced him to commit it again to the press. It
forms the first part of a plan which he has long had
in contemplation, of teaching his elder children the
most important barnches of ethics, viz. VERACITY,
FAITHFULNESS, JUSTICE, and BENEVOLENCE, in a
systematic and *experimental* manner, by EXAMPLES.
But various causes have hitherto prevented, and will
probably continue to prevent, the completion of his
design. He cordially wishes, therefore, that some
moralist of more leisure and superior abilities, into

whofe hands this little piece may fall, would execute
in its full extent what is here fo partially and imperfectly attempted.

To promote the love of truth, and to excite an
averfion to duplicity and falfehood, are objects which
merit the moft ferious attention in the bufinefs of
education: and as the minds of children at an early
age are incapable of difcerning the diftinctions and
fubordinations of moral duty, the rules prefcribed to
them fhould be abfolute and without exception. But
in the more advanced period of youth, obfervation
and reading will neceffarily point out many deviations
from thefe rules, not only in the converfation and
conduct of their friends, but in the moft applauded
actions which hiftory records: and when fuch reflections fuggeft themfelves, it is a proof that the
powers of the underftanding are unfolded; and that
it will be feafonable to graft rational knowledge on
the love of virtue. For to obviate error is the firft
ftep towards rectitude; and the abufe of reafon in our
moral judgments too frequently terminates in depravity of principle.

The author has in general given his authorities for
the facts which he has related, that hiftoric truth
may be diftinguifhed from the fictions, introduced for
the fake of illuftration: but in the ftory of the King
of Navarre, afterwards Henry IV. of France, they
have been unavoidably intermingled. On this point
M. Boulard, an advocate of confiderable rank at Paris,
who has tranflated the prefent work into very elegant

French, thus expreſſes himſelf: *On a vu qu'il dit dans ſa préface qu'il a ajouté quelques faits de ſon invention, à ce qu'il a raconté de Henri IV. Je penſe qu'il auroit été plus convenable de ne pas mêler des fictions à l'hiſtoire.* But the author does not recollect any hiſtorical fact, which fully exemplifies the caſe in queſtion: and the reference to Sully's Memoirs will ſhew the preciſe boundary between truth and fiction.

It is well known to the learned, that Socrates gave riſe to a new mode of inſtruction in the ſchools of philoſophy; and that Plato and Xenophon, by recording the moral converſations of their amiable maſter, excited a taſte for dialogue, which has prevailed through all ſucceeding ages. The mode of exemplification purſued in the preſent work has neceſſarily occaſioned ſome deviation from each of theſe great originals; who are indeed themſelves ſo different as to agree only in one common outline. But the author has copied both in many particulars, eſpecially in the adoption of real characters for the *dramatis perſonæ*, or ſpeakers in his diſcourſe. How far he has done juſtice to the talents or opinions of Philocles, it is not for him to determine. But if the ſentiments imputed to his late honoured friend be ſuch as he would not have avowed, let it be remembered, that Plato alſo wrote what Socrates diſclaimed;*

---

* The LYSIS. When Socrates heard this dialogue of Plato read, in which he ſupported the principal character, " Gods!'" he exclaimed, " how this young man makes me ſay what I never " thought!"

and that the author alone is anfwerable for whatever he has delivered.

The Essays on the Influence, of Habit and Association; on Inconsistency of Expecta- tion in Literary Pursuits; on the Advan- tages of a Taste for the general Beauties of Nature and of Art; on the Alliance of Na- tural History and Philosophy with Poetry; and on the Intellectual and Moral Conduct of Experimental Pursuits; have been read be- fore the Literary and Philosophical Society of Manchefter, and honoured with a place in their journals. But in thefe feveral compofitions the dis- cerning reader will perceive evident traits of paternal inftruction: and that both in the choice of the fub- jects, and in the method of difcuffing them, he has had in view the interefts of thofe in whofe improve- ment he is moft nearly and tenderly concerned. They will therefore, he trufts, be deemed no improper fequel to the Socratic Discourse.

The compofition of a Tribute to the Memory of Charles de Polier, Esq; devolved upon him as the friend of the deceafed, and officially as Presi- dent of the very refpectable fociety which appointed this record of his merit. It was written under the impreffion of heart-felt forrow, and on that account may perhaps be fufpected of exhibiting a picture too ftrong in its lineaments, and too glowing in its co- lours. But time, which calms every emotion, and reftores the due authority of judgment over imagi-

nation, has made no change in the author's sentiments concerning the character he has drawn; and
the infertion of it in this work, whilft it gratifies the
feelings of his mind, is perfectly confonant to the
general defign which he has in view: for it offers
a moft inftructive model to young men, who are animated with the laudable ambition of uniting liberal
and polite manners with the more folid attainments
of learning and virtue.

The APPENDIX contains fuch remarks and illustrations, as further reflection or reading have fuggefted
fince thefe Differtations were written. The author
is fully apprized of the peculiar delicacy and difficulty of the moral topics which he has attempted to
inveftigate; and trufts, that he fhall always be difpofed to acknowledge and to rectify any errors into
which he may have fallen. For he deems a return
to truth and reafon more honourable than the poffes-
fion even of infallible judgment; and fincerely adopts
the fentiment of a celebrated writer, " that the man
" who is free from miftakes can pretend to no praife,
" except what is derived from the juftnefs of his un-
" derftanding; but that he who corrects his miftakes,
" difplays at once the juftnefs of his underftanding,
" and the candour of his heart."

MANCHESTER, *September* 20, 1788.

A

SOCRATIC DISCOURSE

ON

TRUTH.

——<<<◇>>>——

INTER SILVAS ACADEMI QUÆRERE VERUM.

HOR.

.

A

SOCRATIC DISCOURSE

ON

TRUTH.

TO

T. B. P.

YOU have often been a witnefs, my dear Son, of
the pleafure experienced by me in the recollection of the Academical years which I paffed at
——, in the purfuit of general fcience, before I engaged in my profeffional ftudies at the univerfity of
——: and you have no lefs frequently heard me
exprefs the higheft veneration for the profound learning and exalted character of Philocles, under whofe
tuition the charms of knowledge firft attracted my
regard. I have lately revifited thofe fcenes fo delightful to my youth; but, leaving to your conception the emotions which I felt, I fhall relate to you
a SOCRATIC CONVERSATION that occurred there
in my prefence, between Philocles and your kinfman
Sophron. This amiable youth, who is likely to reflect a luftre on the facred office, to which, I truft,

he will ere long be called, had been reciting to his profeſſor an academical compoſition on the importance of TRUTH, and on the folly, infamy, and baſeneſs of LYING and DECEIT: and, when he laid down the book, Philocles expreſſed an earneſt wiſh, that ſuch ſentiments might ever influence the heart, and direct the conduct of his pupil. But general rules, continued he, are inſufficient for our government in the diverſified and complicated occurrences of life: and, if we be ambitious of acting with wiſdom, honour, and virtue, it is neceſſary that we ſhould make ourſelves acquainted with the various branches and ſubordinations of each moral duty. Let us, therefore, take a particular view of TRUTH, and of her inſeparable companion FAITHFULNESS. You are no novice in theſe ſubjects; and Euphronius, I am perſuaded, will be pleaſed to hear you exerciſed in the diſcuſſion of them.

I preſume you will concur with me in opinion, that MORAL TRUTH is the *conformity of our expreſſions to our thoughts;* and FAITHFULNESS, *that of our actions to our expreſſions:* And that LYING or FALSEHOOD *is generally a mean, ſelfiſh, or malevolent, and always an unjuſtifiable, endeavour to deceive another, by ſignifying or aſſerting that to be truth or fact, which is known or believed to be otherwiſe; and by making promiſes, without any intention to perform them.*

But if we believe our aſſertions or ſigns to be true, and they ſhould afterwards prove to be falſe, tell me, Sophron, are we then guilty of lying?

No, replied Sophron; we shall have committed only an error or mistake: for under such circumstances we must have been deceived ourselves, and could have had no design of imposing upon others?

But is every breach of promise a lie, continued Philocles?

I should think not, answered Sophron, if the promise were made with sincerity, and the violation of it be unavoidable.

Your distinction is just, said Philocles; and there are also certain conditions, obvious to the general sense of mankind, understood or implied in almost every promise, on which the performance must depend. Whang-to, emperor of China, who governed his people like a father, and regarded his own elevation and power as trusts delegated for their good, had a daughter who was his only child, and the darling of his old age. He promised her in marriage to Oufanquey, the son of his favourite mandarine; and that he would bequeath to him all his dominions as her dowry. Oufan-quey was at that time a youth of the most promising abilities and dispositions; but the prospect of royalty, and the adulation of a court, soon corrupted his heart. He became haughty, insolent, and cruel; and the people anticipated, with horror, the tyranny which they must endure under his government. By the institutions of the Chinese, the great officers of state may remonstrate to the emperor, when his decrees are injurious to the public interest; and this privilege has often tended to abate the rigour of defpotifm. Whang-to heard, with grief and aftonifhment, the complaints of his mandarines againft Oufan-quey. He fummoned him into his prefence; and being fatisfied with the proofs of his demerit, he addreffed the officers of ftate in the following terms: " I engaged my daughter in marriage, " and promifed the inheritance of my dominions, to " Oufan-quey, a youth who was wife, humane, and " juft. In departing from virtue, he has cancelled " thefe obligations, and forfeited his title to both." Then turning to Oufan-quey, he faid, " I command " you to retire from my court, and to pafs the re- " mainder of your days in the moft diftant province " of my empire."

But is it not deemed peculiarly honourable, Sophron, to perform a promife, when paffion or felf-intereft ftrongly incites us to the violation of it?

Nothing raifes our admiration higher, faid Sophron; and I beg leave to relate to you a ftory, which places this truth in a very ftriking point of view. A Spanifh cavalier, without any reafonable provocation, affaffinated a Moorifh gentleman, and inftantly fled from juftice. He was vigoroufly pur-fued; but availing himfelf of a fudden turn in the road, he leaped, unperceived, over a garden wall. The proprietor, who was alfo a Moor, happened to be at that time walking in the garden; and the Spaniard fell upon his knees before him, acquainted him with his cafe, and in the moft pathetic manner implored concealment. The Moor liftened to him

by good men, who cannot however reasonably or conscientiously fulfil them. When JESUS had washed the feet of several of his disciples, he came to Simon Peter : *And Peter said unto him, Lord, dost thou wash my feet? JESUS answered and said, what I do thou knowest not now ; but thou shalt know hereafter. Peter said unto him, thou shalt never wash my feet! JESUS answered him, if I wash thee not, thou hast no part with me. Simon Peter said unto him, Lord, not my feet only, but also my hands and my head.** Nor can even vows, however solemn, be binding, when the object of them is the commission of a crime: for though appeals to the Deity are sacred pledges of our sincerity, they make no change in the nature or legality of actions; and it would be the grossest superstition to suppose, that the violation of GOD's ordinances can either be honourable or acceptable to Him.† David, in revenge for an insult offered him by Nabal, vowed that he would put to the sword every male of his family. But his wrath was afterwards appeased; and he became so sensible of the injustice of his design, that he said, *Blessed be the LORD who has kept his servant from evil.*‡ It should seem, that the Roman emperor Trajan thought it might be criminal in his officers, under certain circumstances, to maintain the allegiance which they had sworn to him.‖ On the appointment of Suberanus to be captain of the royal guard,

---

* John, chap. xiii.   † See Appendix, sect. ii.

‡ 1 Sam. xxv. 22.   ‖ See Appendix, sect. iii.

he prefented him with a fword, as the badge of his
fealty, faying, " Let this be drawn in my defence, if
" I rule according to equity; but if otherwife, it may
" be employed againft me."*

The conclufion concerning the obfervance of promifes may be extended to Veracity, notwithftanding
the extravagant declaration of one of the Fathers,
" that he would not violate truth, though he were
" fure to gain heaven by it." Whenever, from the
concurrence of extraordinary circumftances, the practice of one virtue is rendered incompatible with the
performance of another of much higher obligation, it
is evident that the inferior muft yield to the fuperior
duty. An example will elucidate and evince the
juftnefs of this obfervation.

After the horrid maffacre of the Huguenots in
France, which began on St. Bartholomew's day 1572,
the King of Navarre was very rigoroufly guarded, by
the order of the Queen-mother, Catherine de Medicis.
But one day, when he was hunting near Senlis,
during the heat of the chafe, he feized a favourable
opportunity of making his efcape; and galloping
through the woods, with a few faithful friends,
amongft whom was young Rofny, afterwards Duke
of Sully, he croffed the Seine at Poiffy,† and fled to
the caftle of a nobleman, who was a zealous though
fecret Proteftant, and ftrongly attached to his intereft.
Troops of horfe were foon difpatched different ways

* Pliny.
† See Sully's Memoirs; and alfo the Preface to this Work.

in purfuit of him. One of thefe detachments ftopped
at the gates of the caftle, where Henry was then re-
frefhing himfelf; and the captain demanded permiffion to fearch for him, fhewing the royal mandate to
bring the head of Henry, and to put his attendants
to the fword. Refiftance was evidently vain; and
compliance would have been a breach of hofpitality,
friendfhip, and humanity; at the fame time that it
muft have proved fatal to the interefts of the reformed
religion, and to the whole body of Proteftants in
France, who had no other protector than the King of
Navarre. The nobleman therefore, without hefitation, and with an undaunted countenance, inftantly
faid, " Wafte not your time, fir, in fruitlefs fearches.
" The King of Navarre, with his friends, paffed this
" way about two hours ago; and if you fet fpurs to
" your horfe, you will overtake him before the night
" approaches." The captain and his troop, fatisfied
with this anfwer, rode off at full fpeed; and the King
was then left at liberty to provide for his fafety, by
difguifing himfelf, and taking a different route.

Under fuch circumftances as you have defcribed,
all mankind, obferved Sophron, would condemn a
ftrict adherence to TRUTH.* But what do you
think of the conduct of the Portuguefe flave, whofe

* " Infani fapiens nomen ferat, æquus iniqui,
" Ultra quam fatis eft virtutem fi petat ipfam."
Hor. Ep. VI. lib. i. ver. 15.

" That which being done admits of a rational juftification, is the
" effence, or general character, of a MORAL DUTY."——Dialogue
concerning Happinefs, by James Harris, efq; p. 175.

breach of veracity, and even perjury, is extolled by
Abbé Raynal, in his Hiſtory of the European Set-
tlements?   This negro, who had fled into the woods
to enjoy the liberty which was his natural right,
having learned that his old maſter was arreſted, and
likely to be condemned for a capital crime, came into
the court of juſtice; aſſumed the guilt of the faɛt;
ſuffered himſelf to be impriſoned; brought falſe,
though judicial proofs of his crime; and was executed
inſtead of his beloved maſter.

The diſapprobation of falſehood, in this inſtance,
anſwered Philocles, is ſuppreſſed for a while, by our
admiration of the affeɛtion, gratitude, generoſity, and
greatneſs of mind, diſplayed by the negro.   We
lament the bondage of ſuch a hero; and regret that
his exalted virtues were not diſplayed on a more
important and honourable occaſion.   But when theſe
firſt emotions are over, and we diſpaſſionately refleɛt
on the conduɛt of the ſlave, we muſt condemn it as

"" The right to truth may be forfeited in particular caſes, as by one
" who hath formed a deſign to kill another, and if not hindered, will
" probably accompliſh his wicked purpoſe.   Neither the perſon
" whoſe life is aimed at ſhould he ſave himſelf by a lie, nor
" any one who ſhould tell an officious lie for him, will be guilty
" of the leaſt injuſtice to him whom by this means they keep from
" perperrating the miſchief intended.   Inſtead of a wrong, it is a
" kindneſs."——Grove's Moral Philoſophy, vol. ii. p. 415.

"" Adhering to the *ordinary* rules of duty, in theſe *extraordinary*
" caſes, may ſometimes occaſion greater evils to our country, or to
" mankind, than all the virtues any one mortal can exert, will
" repair."——Hutcheſon's Moral Philoſophy, vol. ii. 4to. p. 117.
See a farther diſcuſſion of this ſubjeɛt in the Appendix, ſeɛt. iv,
Conſult alſo Geneſis, chap. xii.

an unjuftifiable facrifice of truth, of his own life, and of the duty which he owed to fociety.* The divine command, *Thou fhalt not bear falfe witnefs* AGAINST *thy neighbour*, cannot furely be fuppofed to imply that we may bear *falfe witnefs in his* FAVOUR; becaufe this would be to forbid private injury, and to authorize public wrongs. Judicial teftimony, in the prefent circumftances of the moral world, is effential to the well-being of fociety; and to leffen the general credibility of it, by introducing into courts of law falfehood and perjury, is a high crime againft the ftate, and feverely punifhed in all countries which have emerged from barbarifm. Befides, the good of the community requires that juftice fhould be executed on the offender himfelf, to prevent him from committing other crimes: and it would give encouragement to vice, if an innocent perfon, perhaps. tired of life, or influenced by enthufiaftic notions of honour, friendfhip, or love, might fuffer for another who is guilty.

The certainty of punifhment, even in mifdemeanors, is ftrongly urged by the Marquis de Beccaria, the great advocate for judicial lenity; and he thinks the forgivenefs of the injured party himfelf fhould not interrupt the execution of juftice. "This may be an "act of good-nature and humanity," he obferves, "but it is contrary to the good of the public. For "although a private citizen may difpenfe with fatis- "faction for his private injury, he cannot remove the

* See Appendix, fect. iv.

" neceffity of public example. The right of punifhing
" belongs not to any individual in particular, but to
" the fociety in general, or the fovereign who repre-
" fents that fociety; and a man may renounce his
" own portion of this right, but he cannot give up
" that of others."

The conduct of the negro, faid Sophron, however
erroneous it might be in point of wifdom, or unjuftifiable with refpect to its morality, was perfectly generous and difinterefted.   But the fame elegant writer
who records this fact has related another example of
the violation of truth, from motives purely *felfifh*,
which I cannot condemn, though I know not how to
juftify.   I will endeavour to recollect, and to repeat
the ftory.   A Britifh ferjeant was taken prifoner by
the favages in America, who prepared themfelves to
put him to death, with all the barbarity which their
fkill in torture could invent.   Shocked with the view
of the horrid fufferings which awaited him, he thus
addreffed the Indians: " Mighty warriors, your pre-
" parations are vain, for my body is invulnerable;
" and if you will fet me at liberty, I will teach you
" how to become fo.   Think not that I impofe upon
" you by falfe pretenfions.   I am willing that you
" fhould try upon me an experiment, which may
" fatisfy your doubts.   Let the chief who holds my
" hanger now ftrike with all his force.   I equally
" defy the fharpnefs of the inftrument, and the
" ftrength of his arms."   Whilft he was faying thefe
words, he bent his head, and laid bare his neck.   The

Indian eagerly advanced, and by one furious blow
fevered the head from the body. Thus the poor
ferjeant, by his prefence of mind, exchanged lingering
tortures for an eafy and inftantaneous death.

Euphronius here remarked, that the ftory is of
doubtful authority, by the confeffion of the Abbé
himfelf. But admitting the truth of it, continued
he, for the fake of argument, what moralift can be
fo rigid as not to deem the conduct of the ferjeant at
leaft excufable? Perhaps no man, in fimilar circumftances, would have acted differently, if he poffeffed
fufficient compofure to devife, or addrefs to practife,
fuch an expedient. The cafe is not analogous to that
of martyrdom for religion. The horrid fufferings to
be endured in this inftance could anfwer no good end;
and fociety received not the leaft injury, either immediate or remote, by the evafion of them.

Recollecting an hiftorical fact of unqueftionable
truth, and ftrictly applicable to the point in debate, I
requefted permiffion to relate it. When Columbus
and his crew were caft away on an ifland, more
than thirty leagues from Hifpaniola, nothing remained
to them in profpect, but to end their miferable days
with naked favages, far from their country and their
friends. To add to thefe calamities, the natives
began foon to murmur at the refidence of the Spaniards amongft them; the fupport of whom became
burdenfome to men ignorant of agriculture, and un-
accuftomed to exertion or induftry. They brought
in provifions with reluctance, furnifhed them fpa-

ringly, and even threatened entirely to withhold
them. Such a refolution muft have occafioned inevitable deftruction to the Spaniards; but Columbus
prevented it by a happy device, that revived all the
admiration and reverence with which the Indians firft
regarded thefe ftrangers. By his fkill in aftronomy
he knew there was fhortly to be a total eclipfe of the
moon. On the day before it happened, he affembled
the principal perfons of the diftrict, and after re-
proaching them for their defection from thofe whom
they had lately revered, he told them that the Spaniards were fervants of the Great Spirit, who dwells
in heaven: that, offended at their refufal to fupport
the objects of his peculiar favour, the Deity was
preparing to punifh their crime with exemplary feverity; and that the moon fhould be darkened that very
night, and affume a bloody hue, as a fign of the
Divine wrath, and an emblem of the vengeance ready
to fall on them. To this marvellous prediction fome
of the barbarians liftened with carelefs indifference;
others, with credulous aftonifhment: but when the
moon began gradually to withdraw her light, and at
length appeared of a red colour, all were ftruck with
terror. They ran with confternation to their houfes,
and returning to Columbus loaded with provifions,
threw them inftantly at his feet, conjuring him to in-
tercede with the Great Spirit, to avert the deftruction
with which they were threatened. Columbus, feeming to be moved by their entreaties, promifed to
comply with their defire. The eclipfe went off, the

moon recovered its fplendour; and from that time the Spaniards were not only furnifhed profufely with provifions, but treated with the moft fuperftitious attention.* This folemn deceit of Columbus may be juftified by the rights of neceffity. Shipwrecked on a diftant coaft, in the profecution of an enterprize, which in his mind appears to have originated from honourable and ufeful views, and deftitute of every means of fupplying himfelf and his affociates with fuftenance, he had a claim to the protection, affiftance, and fupport of the people who were fpectators of his calamity: and it was a happy fertility of genius, which fuggefted to him an expedient far preferable to the force of arms. But I feel a fecret wifh that this truly great man had mixed lefs of falfity with his artifice. He might have reprehended the Indians for their want of hofpitality, alarmed their fears by his prediction, and excited their wonder and reverence by its fulfilment, without denouncing in fuch unguarded terms the immediate vengeance of Heaven. Truth is fo important, and of fo delicate a nature, that every poffible precaution fhould be employed to extenuate its violation, although the facrifice be made to duties which fuperfede its obligation.

Philocles very obligingly thanked me for recalling to his memory fo pertinent a fact. He then turned to his pupil, and afked him what he thought of the maxim, which fome perfons have adopted, "that "faith is not to be kept with rogues or traitors."

* See Robertfon's Hiftory of America, vol. i. book ii.

I think the maxim, replied Sophron, falſe in itſelf, and highly injurious to ſociety. For, independent of the licentiouſneſs and cruelty to which it might give riſe, a man owes to his own honour and peace of mind, except on very extraordinary occaſions, the ſtrict performance of his promiſe. And this opinion ſeems to have influenced the conduct of the great Viſcount Turenne, and of Sir Richard Herbert. The former was attacked one night by robbers near Paris, who ſtripped him of his money, watch, and rings. He engaged to give them a hundred *louis d'ors*, if they would return him a ring, of little intrinſic worth, but on which he ſet a particular value. The highwaymen complied; and one of them had the bold-neſs to go to his houſe the ſucceeding day, and in the midſt of a large company to demand, in a whiſper, the performance of his promiſe. The Viſcount gave orders for the money to be paid; and ſuffered the villain to eſcape, before he related the adventure.*

Sir Richard Herbert, being ſent by Edward the Fourth to reduce certain rebels in North-Wales, laid ſiege to Harlech caſtle, in Merionethſhire; a fortreſs ſo ſtrong, that he deſpaired of taking it but by block-ade and famine. The captain of it offered to ſurrender, on condition that Sir Richard *would do what he could to ſave his life*. The condition was accepted; and Sir Richard brought the commander to the King, requeſting his Majeſty to grant him a pardon, as the expectation of this favour had induced him to yield

* See Ramſay's Life of Turenne.

up an important caftle, which he might have defended.
Edward replied to Sir Richard Herbert, " That as
" he had no power by his commiffion to pardon
" any one, he might therefore, after the reprefenta-
" tion hereof to his Sovereign, deliver him up to
" juftice." Sir Richard Herbert anfwered, " He
" had not yet done *the beft he could for him;* and
" therefore moft humbly defired his highnefs to do
" one of two things; either to put him again
" in the caftle where he had been, and command
" fome other to take him out; or, if his highnefs
" would not do fo, to take his life for the captain's,
" that being the laft proof he could give, that he had
" ufed his utmoft endeavour to fulfil his promife."
The King, finding himfelf fo much urged, pardoned
the captain, but beftowed on Sir Richard Herbert no
" other reward for his fervice."*

Thefe gentlemen, faid Philocles, difplayed a delicate fenfe of honour; and though I am dubious,
whether the conduct of Monfieur Turenne has the
fanction of the great Roman cafuift,† yet, according
to my judgment, both he and Sir Richard Herbert
acted conformably to the laws of reafon and rectitude.
For every *lawful* promife, made by one poffeffing
prefence of mind, and the free ufe of reafon, no event
or confideration fucceeding, which an unbiaffed under-

---

* See the Life of Lord Herbert of Cherbury.

† " Si prædonibus pactum pro capite pretium non attuleris, nulla
" fraus eft, ne fi juratus quidem id non feceris."——Cic. de Off.
lib. iii. cap. 29.

ftanding would deem fufficient to render it *unlawful,* ought to be religioufly obferved.* But promifes, extorted by fear, and that clearly contravene our duty to fociety, are void in themfelves. Thus an engagement made with fincerity, under the ftrong impreffions of terror, to a highwayman or murderer, not to bear teftimony againft him, can be of no validity; becaufe there fubfifts an antecedent claim of the community, which cannot be difpenfed with by any of its members. I have fuppofed the engagement to be fincere; for if entered into with a previous defign of violation, a breach of truth and faithfulnefs is in fome degree committed, notwithftanding its injuftice or illegality.

But when you deliver to another as a certain truth what you believe to be falfe, are you guilty of lying, fhould it afterwards prove to be true?

Yes, anfwered Sophron; becaufe my intention is to deceive, and to make a fuppofed falfehood pafs for truth. Chian-fu was an officer in the guards of the emperor of Japan. He had formed a tender connection with one of the ladies of the court, and was on the point of marriage, when a formidable infurrection in a diftant ifland of the empire, occafioned by the tyranny and cruel exactions of the government, obliged him to leave the capital without delay, to affume his poft in the royal army. The war was protracted through various caufes; and he bore with great impatience fo long an abfence from his miftrefs.

* See Grove's Moral Philofophy..

By the influence of a bribe, he obtained permiſſion from the commander in chief to return to Jeddo for a few weeks, during which time he hoped to celebrate his nuptials. But dreading leſt the emperor ſhould reſent his deſertion of the army at ſo critical a conjuncture, he pretended that he brought tidings from the general, of an important advantage gained over the enemy, which was likely ſoon to be ſucceeded by a complete victory. Theſe accounts were founded on probability, not on truth; his falſehoods, however, procured him the moſt favourable reception at court. He married the lady; and after a week ſpent in feſtivity, prepared for his departure to join the army. An expreſs at this time arrived, with the news of the entire defeat of the inſurgents; but no mention was made of any previous diſpatches by Chian-fu. The emperor ſuſpected that he had been guilty of deceit. He was ſtrictly examined, confeſſed his crime, and the motives of it; and was condemned to ſuffer immediate death. For lying is a capital offence, by the laws of Japan.

If truth, reſumed Philocles, be an agreement between our words and thoughts, are you under an obligation to expreſs all your thoughts?

No, ſaid Sophron, prudence often forbids it; and it is no violation of truth to conceal thoſe thoughts, or that knowledge, with which another has no right to be acquainted. On a particular occaſion, the Jews demanded of JESUS, *What ſign ſheweſt thou unto us?* *JESUS anſwered and ſaid, Deſtroy this temple, and*

*in three days I will raife it up.   Then faid the Jews,
Forty and fix years was this temple in building, and
wilt thou rear it up in three days?   But he fpake of
the temple of his body.   When therefore he was arifen
from the dead, his difciples remembered that he had
faid this unto them.**

Sometimes, when improper or treacherous questions are afked, filence would be no lefs dangerous
than an explicit declaration of our fentiments.   In
thefe cafes we fhall be juftified in the ufe of fuch
evafions as do not contradict the truth.   When the
chief priefts and fcribes inquired of our Saviour, whether it was lawful to pay tribute unto Cæfar?   *He
perceived their craftinefs, and faid unto them, Why
tempt ye me?   Shew me a penny: whofe image and
fuperfcription hath it?   They anfwered and faid, Cæfar's.
And he faid unto them, Render unto Cæfar the things
which be Cæfar's, and unto* GOD *the things which be*
GOD's.   *And they could not take hold of his words
before the people: and they marvelled at his anfwers,
and held their peace.*

Under the reign of the cruel and bigoted queen
Mary, the princefs Elizabeth, her fifter, fuffered a
variety of perfecutions on account of her fteady attachment to the Proteftant religion.   It is faid fhe
was one day interrogated concerning the LORD's-
Supper, and that fhe returned the following prudent
and evafive anfwer:

" CHRIST was the word that fpake it;
" He took the bread and brake it;

* John ii. 18.

" And what the word did make it,
" That I believe and take it."*

Philocles expreſſed much ſatisfaction in the judicious diſtinction which his pupil had made, and obſerved, that the conduct of the princeſs Elizabeth is
fully juſtified by the example of the apoſtle Paul, in
circumſtances not very diſſimilar. The Athenians had
a law, which rendered it capital to promulgate any
new divinities.† And when Paul preached to them
JESUS and the RESURRECTION, he was accuſed of
having broken this law, and of being a ſetter forth of
ſtrange gods; and was carried before the Areopagus, a
court of judicature, which took cognizance of all
criminal matters, and was in a particular manner
charged with the care of the eſtabliſhed religion. An
impoſtor, in ſuch a ſituation, would have retracted
his doctrine, to ſave his life; and an enthuſiaſt
would have ſacrificed his life, without attempting to
ſave it by innocent means. But the Apoſtle wiſely
avoided both extremes; and availing himſelf of an
inſcription, " TO THE UNKNOWN GOD," which he
had ſeen upon an altar in the city, he pleaded in his
own defence, *Whom ye ignorantly worſhip, him declare
I unto you.* By this preſence of mind he evaded the
law, and eſcaped condemnation, without departing
from the truth of the Goſpel, or violating the honour
of GOD.‡

* Walpole's Cat. of Royal and Noble Authors.

† Socrates ſuffered under this law.

‡ Vide Acts xvii. 23. Alſo Lord Lyttelton's Obſervations on the
Converſion and Apoſtleſhip of St. Pau'.

Though I am no general admirer, continued Philocles, of the maxims of morality delivered by Lord
Chefterfield, yet I think his remarks on the prefent
fubject peculiarly worthy of attention. " The pru-
" dence and neceffity," fays the noble author, " of
" frequently concealing the truth, infenfibly feduces
" people to violate it. It is the only art of mean
" capacities, and the only refuge of mean fpirits.
" Whereas concealing the truth upon proper occa-
" fions is as prudent and as innocent, as telling a lie
" upon any occafion is infamous and foolifh.. I will
" ftate you a cafe in your own department. Suppofe
" you are employed at a foreign court, and that the
" minifter of that court is abfurd or impertinent
" enough to afk you what your inftructions are; will
" you tell him a lie, which, as foon as found out, and
" found out it certainly will be, muft deftroy your
" credit, blaft your character, and render you ufelefs
" there? No. Will you tell him the truth then,
" and betray your truft? As certainly, No. But
" you will anfwer with firmnefs, That you are fur-
" prized at fuch a queftion; that you are perfuaded
" he does not expect an anfwer to it; but that at all
" events he certainly will not have one. Such an
" anfwer will give him confidence in you; he will
" conceive an opinion of your veracity, of which
" opinion you may afterwards make very honeft and
" fair advantages."

Philocles proceeded to interrogate his pupil, whether falfity, when in jeft, is to be deemed a lie? But

Sophron declined the queſtion, as too nice for his deciſion, and deſired to hear the ſentiments of Philocles, who delivered them in the following terms. Wit and irony, raillery and humour, are often deviations from the ſtrict rules of veracity: but they are allowed by common conſent; and, under proper reſtrictions, they contribute to enliven converſation, and to improve our manners. But jocularity is certainly culpable, and may be deemed a ſpecies of lying, when it is intended to deceive without any good end in view; and eſpecially with the ungenerous one of diverting ourſelves at the painful expence of another. The practice alſo may lead to more criminal falſehoods; and it is related with honour of Ariſtides, that he held truth to be ſo ſacred, *ut ne joco quidem mentiretur*.

Some jocular lies have produced the moſt ſerious and affecting conſequences; of which I will give you an example or two, in the youthful frolics of Hilario, a nobleman who now looks back with ſorrow and regret on the ſufferings occaſioned by his levity. When he was a ſtudent at Cambridge, he went at midnight crying *fire! fire!* to the chamber door of one of the fellows of ———, a gentleman univerſally admired for his literary and poetical abilities, but who was of a timid and melancholy diſpoſition. The gentleman, awaked out of a ſound ſleep, and attentive only to the firſt ſuggeſtions of fear, leaped through the window at the hazard of loſing his life by the fall. Not long after this tranſaction, Hilario went up to London; and dining in a mixed company

of perfons of fafhion, he happened to fit near a grave
old gentleman, who took the firft opportunity of
making particular inquiries concerning a youth, then
at Cambridge, whom he knew to be intimately acquainted with this nobleman. Hilario inftantly fuf-
pedted that the ferious Don was a rich uncle of his
friend, and determined that he would give fuch an
account of the nephew, as fhould occafion a folemn
letter of reproof, over which he hoped to regale himfelf on his return to college. He therefore jocularly
faid, that his companion was a fine jolly fellow, always forming connedtions with the girls; that he
loved to rattle the dice; and that he had lately loft
his next quarter's allowance, which would lower his
courage at play for fome time to come. From the
alteration which he perceived in the ftranger's countenance, he was affured of the fuccefs of his *hum*, an
abfurd term given to this fhameful kind of lie: and
when he got back to Cambridge, he haftened to the
apartment of his friend, to enjoy the laughter which
he fhould raife at his expence. But how was he
fhocked to find him in the delirium of a fever, occafioned by a billet, which had been delivered the preceding day, purporting, " That Lucinda had juft
" beftcwed her hand upon a perfon much more de-
" ferving of her affedtions, than he had been repre-
" fented to her father by Hilario, his affociate in
" pleafure, extravagance, and profligacy."

By fuch thoughtlefs and unjuftifiable violations of
truth, Hilario was often wounding his own peace of

mind, and involving his connections in diftrefs. He
was, however, at length compelled to correct this
criminal habit, through the horror which he felt on
having given rife to a fatal duel between two bro-
thers, by jocularly infinuating to one of them, that
he was rivalled in the affections of his miftrefs by
the other.

It would be happy, faid I, if we could afcertain
the reftrictions under which thefe fallies of frolic and
jocularity may be indulged with innocence. One
general rule may, I think, be admitted, that the entertainment which we thus create to ourfelves, fhould
be fuch only as will be a future fubject of mirth even
to thofe who are the prefent fufferers by it. But to
ufe the words of an excellent moralift, " as every
" action may produce effects, over which human power
" has no influence, and which human fagacity cannot
" forefee; we fhould not lightly venture to the verge
" of evil, nor ftrike at others, though with a reed,
" left, like the rod of Mofes, it become a ferpent in
" our hands."*

Philocles now purfued the fubject, by inquiring
into the nature of EQUIVOCATION; which Sophron
defined to be a mean expedient to avoid the declaration
of truth, without verbally telling a lie. An equivocation, faid he, confifts of fuch expreffions as admit of
more than one meaning. The fpeaker ufes them in one
fenfe, and defigns that the hearer fhould underftand
them in another. Cicero mentions a certain perfon,

* Dr. Hawkfworth.

who made a truce with the enemy for thirty days, and treacherously evaded his agreement by laying waste the country during the nights; alleging, that the truce was for so many *days*, not nights.* Such an equivocation as this has all the guilt and infamy of a lie; but I do not feel myself inclined to condemn the duplicity practised by a gentleman on the following occasion. He was returning home from the assizes at York, and was attacked on the road by a highwayman, to whom he delivered a small purse of money. The robber told him that he should not be satisfied with a few guineas, and sternly demanded he sum which he knew he had received, and then carried about him. The gentleman, with great apparent terror, drew out of his pocket a leathern bag, and giving it to the highwayman, said, " *Take what you want*, but spare my life." The robber eagerly received it, and was transported with the value of his acquisition. He rode off with it through bye lanes, till he arrived at a place of security. There he stopped to examine his booty, which to his astonishment he found to consist only of a quantity of halfpence, together with a copy of the dying speech and earnest exhortations of a malefactor, who had been executed the preceding day for robbery.

Can you acquit me, Philocles, said I, of the criminality of equivocation, when in the exercise of my professional duties, I study, by cheerful looks and ambiguous words, to remove from my patients the

---

* Vid. Cicero de Officiis, lib. i. cap. 13.

horrors of defpair, to mitigate the apprehenfions of danger, and to deceive them into hope; that by adminiftering a cordial to the drooping fpirit, I may fmooth the bed of death, or revive even expiring life? For there are maladies which rob the philofopher of fortitude, and the Chriftian of confolation.

From my heart I acquit you, anfwered Philocles, with his wonted humanity. You do a kindnefs, not a wrong, to the perfon whom you thus deceive; and may reafonably prefuppofe his future approbation of that conduct, which meets with the prefent acquies-cence of all his friends. The amiable and elegant Pliny, who had the niceft fenfe of honour, recites with applaufe, in a letter to Nepos, a ftory, which may perhaps contribute to fatisfy your mind, and remove your fcruples.

The hufband of the celebrated Arria, Cæcinna Pætus, was very dangeroufly ill. Her fon was alfo fick at the fame time, and died. He was a youth of uncommon accomplifhments, and fondly beloved by his parents. Arria prepared and conducted his fu-neral in fuch a manner, that her hufband remained entirely ignorant of the mournful event which occa-fioned that folemnity. Pætus often inquired with anxiety about his fon; to whom fhe cheerfully replied, that he had flept well, and was better. But if her tears, too long reftrained, were burfting forth, fhe inftantly retired to give vent to her grief; and when again compofed, fhe returned to Pætus with dry eyes and a placid countenance, quitting, as it were, all the tender feelings of the mother at the threshold of her husband's chamber.*

But addressing himself to Sophron, is it not a species of equivocation, and a breach of faithfulness, continued Philocles, when we do not perform our promises, according to the plain and obvious meaning of them?

Without doubt it is, answered Sophron. The moralist whom I before quoted, relates, that ten Romans, who had been taken in the battle of Cannæ, were sent by Hannibal to the senate, to propose an exchange of prisoners. Before they set out, each of them engaged, by an oath, to return to the camp of the Carthaginians, if the embassy should prove ineffectual. The senate rejected the offers of Hannibal, and nine of the prisoners honourably rendered themselves up to him: but the tenth refused to return, on pretence that he had already discharged himself of his oath. For it seems that he went back to the camp of the Carthaginians soon after he quitted it, to fetch some necessaries, which he had designedly left behind, that he might be able to plead his having complied literally with the terms of his engagement. But the senate disdained the deceit, and commanded the artful wretch to be sent bound to Hannibal.

Mental and other private reservations neither absolve nor even extenuate the guilt of lying. When the unfortunate Mary, queen of Scotland, was married to the dauphin of France, the king, his father,

* Plin. Epist. XVI. lib. iii.

folemnly ratified every article infifted upon by the
Scotch parliament, for preferving the independence
of their nation, and for fecuring the fucceffion of the
crown to the houfe of Hamilton. But Mary by his
perfuafion had antecedently and privately fubfcribed
three deeds, by which fhe configned the kingdom of
Scotland, on failure of her own iffue, to his family;
declaring all her promifes to the contrary to be void.*
The remark of Bifhop Taylor may be adopted, as
the beft comment on tranfactions of this infamous
nature. If the words be a *lie* without *refervation*,
they are fo with it: for this does not alter the words
themfelves, nor the meaning of the words, nor the
purpofe of him who delivers them.†

But in what light are we to regard the ftratagems,
falfehoods, and acts of deceit, which have been employed in war, and often with applaufe, both in ancient and modern times?

In reply to this interefting queftion, Philocles obferved, that war is feldom founded in juftice; and
that therefore we cannot be furprized that it fhould
occafion, amongft thofe who wage it, a fufpenfion of
the common laws of morality. The fraudulent exploits which are practifed, by the tacit confent, as it
were, of the parties, may dazzle and furprize a fuperficial obferver; but a ferious honeft mind will
generally condemn them, as inconfiftent with the
obligations of religion and virtue, and, except under

* Lord Kaims's Hiftory of Man, vol. iv. p. 158.
† Ductor Dubitant. p. 498.

very particular circumſtances, injurious to the contending powers themſelves. For as integrity is the
beſt policy in the conduct of individuals towards each
other, it will appear to be equally ſo in the tranſac-
tions between ſtates and communities, if an extenſive
view be taken of their great and permanent intereſts.
Cicero, in one of his dialogues, introduces Scipio as
maintaining the following excellent maxim: *non modo*
FALSUM effe illud, SINE INJURIA non poffe, fed hoc
veriffimum, fine SUMMA JUSTITIA rempublicam regi
non poff. "It is ſo far from being true, that go-
"vernment cannot be carried on without injury to
"others, that nothing is more certain than that it
"cannot be well adminiſtered without an inviolable
"adherence to the ſtricteſt juſtice." And the propriety of this obſervation ſeems to be acknowledged
in ſome of the regulations of war, now univerſally
adopted in civilized countries.

But a diſtinction ſhould be made between art or
ſtratagem, and perfidy or falſehood.* The wiſeſt
and beſt moraliſts admit, that we may deceive our
enemies, when we have a juſt cauſe of war, by any
ſuch ſigns as import no profeſſion of communicating
our ſentiments to them. Thus I have heard that the
Duke of Marlborough, when he commanded the
allied army in Germany, called a council of war on
a particular occaſion, to determine whether he ſhould
attack the enemy on the ſucceeding day. His general
officers were unanimous in recommending the mea-

* See Appendix, ſect. vi.

fure; but the Duke expreffed his objections to it in
the ftrongeft terms, and the council fubmitted to his
fuperior judgment. When he retired into his tent,
Prince Eugene followed him, and lamented the dis-
grace in which fuch a decifion would involve them.
" My refolution," faid the Duke, " is fixed to give
" battle to-morrow; and I fhall inftantly iffue the
" neceffary orders. But I oppofed this plan in
" council, becaufe I had received fecret information,
" that our enemies had concerted the means of be-
" coming acquainted with the refult of our delibera-
" tions. And you will agree with me in the neceffity
" of deceiving them."

But men of true courage and honour muft hold
in deteftation all treachery and falfehood. The Earl
of Peterborough, in conjunction with the Prince of
Darmftadt, carried on the fiege of Barcelona, about
the beginning of the prefent century. The governor
offered to capitulate, and came to a parley with Lord
Peterborough at the gates of the city. The articles
were not yet figned; when fuddenly loud fhouts and
huzzas were heard in the town. " You have perfi-
" dioufly betrayed us!" faid the governor to the
Earl; " whilft we are capitulating with unfufpecting
" honour and fincerity, your Englifh foldiers have
" entered the city by the ramparts, and are now
" committing rapine, murder, and every kind of vio-
" lence." " You do injuftice to the Englifh," replied the General; " this treachery is chargeable
" only on the troops of Darmftadt. But permit me

" to enter into the town with my foldiers, and I will
" inftantly reprefs the outrage, and return to the gate
" to finifh the capitulation."

The offer was made with an air of truth and fincerity; and accepted with a generous confidence.
Peterborough haftened into the ftreets, where he
found the Germans and Catalans pillaging the houfes
of the principal inhabitants. He drove them away; and
obliged them to leave the booty which they were carrying off: and after having quieted all difturbances, he
rejoined the governor, and completed the capitulation,
without demanding any new or more advantageous
terms. The Spaniards were aftonifhed at the magnanimity of the Englifh, whom they had generally
regarded before as faithlefs barbarians.*

Sophron remarked, that the glory on this occafion
appeared to belong chiefly to Lord Peterborough, as
an individual. But I recollect, continued he, a trans-
action in the Grecian hiftory, which feems to evince
an equal fenfe of honour, and deteftation of perfidy,
in the whole body of the Athenians. Thefe people
were inflamed with the ambition of governing Greece;
and Themiftocles, a favourite general, exerted all his
talents to accomplifh the defign. One day he affembled the citizens of Athens, and informed them,
he had a moft important plan to propofe; but that
he could not communicate it to them, becaufe the
fuccefs of it depended upon fecrecy. He therefore requefted them to appoint a confidential perfon, to

* See Voltaire's Siecle de Louis XIV.

whom he might explain his views, and whofe approbation of them might have the force of public authority. Ariftides was unanimoufly chofen; and
Themiftocles laid open to him the project, which he
had conceived, of burning the whole fleet of the
Grecian ftates, then lying unguarded in a neighbouring port; the deftruction of which, he faid, could not
fail to fecure the dominion of Athens. Ariftides
returned to the affembly, and declared, that the project of Themiftocles promifed the greateft benefit to
the commonwealth; but that it was perfidious and
unjuft. The people inftantly, and with one voice,
rejected the propofal. But the Athenians were foon
afterwards corrupted by profperity: and Thucy-
dides informs us, it became with them a maxim of
ftate, " that nothing is difhonourable, which is
" advantageous."*

Here I could not forbear to mention a noble and
long-continued exertion of public faith and commercial honour, though it was a flight digreffion from
the topic of difcourfe. The Spanifh galeons, deftined
to fupply Terra Firma, and the kingdoms of Peru
and Chili, with almoft every article of neceffary confumption, touch firft at Carthagena, and then at
Porto-Bello. In the latter place a fair is opened;
the wealth of America is exchanged for the manufactures of Europe; and during its prefcribed term
of forty days, the richeft traffic on the face of the
earth is begun and finifhed, with unbounded confi-

* Thucydid. lib. vi.

dence, and the utmoſt ſimplicity of tranſaction. No
bale of goods is ever opened, no cheſt of treaſure is
examined. Both are received on the credit of the
perſons to whom they belong; and only one inſtance
of fraud is recorded, during the long period in which
trade was carried on with this liberal confidence.
All the coined ſilver which was brought from Peru
to Porto-Bello, in the year 1654, was found to be
adulterated, and to be mingled with a fifth part of
baſe metal. The Spaniſh merchants, with their uſual
integrity, ſuſtained the whole loſs, and indemnified
the foreigners by whom they were employed. The
fraud was detected; and the treaſurer of the revenue
in Peru, the author of it, was publicly burnt.*

Are we not every day guilty of lying, purſued
Philocles, in the common forms of civility; and in
various modes of ſpeech, which cuſtom has introduced?

Surely not, replied Sophron; for if theſe be well
underſtood, no one is deceived by them.

I do not entirely accord with you, Sophron, ſaid
I; and I believe it will not be eaſy to juſtify, upon
the principles either of wiſdom or ſtrict morality,
many complimental expreſſions uſed in converſation.
You remember the letter of the ambaſſador from
Bantam, which is inſerted in one of the volumes of
the Spectator. This honeſt ſtranger informs his
maſter, that the people of England call him and his
ſubjects barbarians, becauſe they ſpeak 'the truth;'
and account themſelves polite and civilized, becauſe

* Robertſon's Hiſt. of America, vol. ii. note 93, b. viii.

they fay one thing, and mean another. " On my
" firft landing," fays he, " one told me that he
" fhould be glad to do me any fervice in his power.
" I defired him, therefore, to carry my portmanteau;
" but inftead of ferving me according to his promife,
" he laughed, and ordered another to do it. I
" lodged the firft week at the houfe of a perfon, who
" intreated me to think myfelf at home, and to con-
" fider his houfe as my own. Accordingly, the next
" morning I began to knock down one of the walls,
" in order to let in the frefh air; and packed up
" fome of the houfhold goods, of which I intended
" to make thee a prefent. But the falfe varlet foon
" fent me word, that he would have no fuch doings
" in his houfe." Perhaps, however, I may incur
the charge of falfehood, by quoting the letter of an
ambaffador who never exifted.

Such fictions, Philocles remarked, partake not of
the nature of lies. They are intended to convey
amufement or inftruction, not to ferve the purpofes
of deceit.

Nor is the cafe effentially different, with refpect
to the common forms of civility. Their import is
known to all who ufe them; and, as they are expreffive of urbanity and benevolence, they tend,
under proper reftrictions, to foften the afperities, and
heighten the pleafures, of focial intercourfe. Genuine
courtefy has, indeed, its feat in the heart; and implies the defire of gratifying others, in the fubordinate
offices of life, by the facrifice of our own eafe or in-

tereſt. It is eſſential, therefore, to every amiable character; and can only diſplay itſelf in ſuch appropriated modes as cuſtom has eſtabliſhed in different countries, or amongſt different ranks of men. But, when the *ſubſtance* is wanting, ſome benefit is derived to the world even from its *forms:* and to the ruſtic, who claims the privilege of ſpeaking improper truths, or of acting with rude and malicious ſincerity, we may juſtly addreſs the words of Shakeſpeare:

> . . . . " This is ſome fellow,
> " Who, having been praiſed for bluntneſs, doth affect
> " A ſaucy roughneſs, and conſtrains the garb
> " Quite from his nature. He can't flatter, he,
> " An honeſt mind, and plain; he muſt ſpeak truth,
> " And they will take it ſo; if not, 'tis plain."

On this account, I cannot but condemn the affected ſeverity of Paulinus biſhop of Nola, who reproves his correſpondent Sulpicius Severus for having ſubſcribed himſelf his ſervant. " Beware," ſays this primitive writer, " thou ſubſcribe not thyſelf HIS " SERVANT, who is thy BROTHER; for flattery is " ſinful; and it is not a teſtimony of humility to " give thoſe honours to men, which are only due to " the One Lord, Maſter, and GOD."* We find the patriarch Abraham actuated by no ſuch ſcruples, though he lived in the period of paſtoral ſimplicity, and was highly diſtinguiſhed for his virtue and integrity. *And he lift up his eyes and looked; and lo, three men ſtood by him. And when he ſaw them, he an to meet them from the tent door, and bowed him-*

* See Barclay's Apology, p. 525.

*self toward the ground; and said, My lord, if now I
have found favour in thy sight, pass not away, I pray
thee, from thy servant.**

Lot, alfo, is reprefented, in the book of Genefis, as
accofting, in fimilar terms, two ftrangers, with whofe
dignity he was then unacquainted. *And he faid,
Behold now, my lords, turn in, I pray you, into your
fervant's houfe, and tarry all night, and wafh your
feet; and ye fhall rife up early, and go on your ways.*†

The conduct and expreffions of thefe venerable
patriarchs might, I obferved, be perfectly confiftent
with the nicest adherence to truth and fincerity. For
though they ftyled themfelves the *fervants* of the
ftrangers, whom they addreffed, they could not mean
to extend the term beyond fuch *fervices* as the laws
of hofpitality required.

Similar laws, anfwered Philocles, which general
confent has eftablifhed, bind every man, in the common intercourfe of life, to reftrain his angry paffions,
to filence his fevere judgments, to fupprefs his pride
and arrogance, and not only to correct whatever is
offenfive in his manners, but to fhew that urbanity
of fpirit, which, by its benevolent attentions, contri-
butes to alleviate mifery, and to increafe the fum of
public happinefs and order. Miftake me not, however, by fuppofing that I would recommend forward
profeffions, a fawning demeanour, or unlimited com-
plaifance. Integrity of heart and fteadinefs of principle forbid all finful conformity with the world:

* Gen. xviii. 2, 3. † Gen. xix. 2.

and I would neither flatter folly, countenance vice, nor yield up one important duty to artificial politenefs. But the facrifice of my own pride, refentment, caprice, or ill-nature, to focial eafe and enjoyment, may often be required: and he, who, like Diogenes, neither poffeffes the fubftance nor the form of courtefy, fhould be banifhed from the world. This cynic, you remember, when he paid a vifit to Plato, who united a tafte for elegance with the love of philofophy, exulted in the rudenefs of reproof, and bedaubing with his dirty feet the fine carpet which covered the floor, cried out, " Thus I trample on the pride of Plato." " But with far greater pride," retorted Plato, with a farcaftic feverity, which the occafion fully juftified. Lord Bacon mentions two noblemen of his acquaintance, one of whom kept a very magnificent table, but treated his guefts with illiberal freedom: the other, when he entertained the fame guefts, probably with humbler cheer, but more politenefs, ufed to afk them, " Tell truly, was there never a flout, or " dry blow, given at my lord's table?" To which the guefts anfwered, " Such and fuch a thing paffed." " I thought," faid this nobleman, " he would mar " a good dinner."*

Urbanity has been admirably chara&terized, by a celebrated writer, under the appellation of GENTLE-NESS. " This virtue," he obferves, " is founded " on a fenfe of what we owe to Him who made us, " and to the common nature of which we all fhare.

---

* Bacon's Effays, xxxii.

" It arifes from reflection on our own failures and
" wants, and from juft views of the condition and
" the duty of man. It is native feeling, heightened
" and improved by principle. It is the heart which
" eafily relents, which feels for every thing that is
" human, and is backward and flow to inflict the
" leaft wound. It is affable in its addrefs, and mild
" in its demeanour; ever ready to oblige, and will-
" ing to be obliged by others; breathing habitual
" kindnefs towards friends, courtefy to ftrangers,
" long-fuffering to enemies. It exercifes authority
" with moderation, adminifters reproof with tender-
" nefs, confers favours with eafe and modefty. It
" is unaffuming in opinion, and temperate in zeal.
" It contends not eagerly about trifles; is flow to
" contradict, and ftill flower to blame; but prompt
" to allay diffention, and to reftore peace. It nei-
" ther intermeddles unneceffarily with the affairs, nor
" pries inquifitively into the fecrets, of others. It
" delights above all things to alleviate diftrefs, and,
" if it cannot dry up the falling tear, to footh at leaft
" the grieving heart. Where it has not the power
" of being ufeful, it is never burdenfome. It feeks
" to pleafe, rather than to fhine and dazzle; and
" conceals with care that fuperiority, either of talents
" or of rank, which is oppreffive to thofe who are
" beneath it. In a word, it is that fpirit, and that
" tenour of manners, which the Gofpel of CHRIST
" enjoins, when it commands us *to bear one another's*

" *burdens; to rejoice with thofe who rejoice, and to*
" *weep with thofe who weep; to pleafe every one his*
" *neighbour for his good; to be kind and tender-*
" *hearted; to be pitiful and courteous; to fupport the*
" *weak, and to be patient towards all men.*"*

Sophron appeared to be much imprefled with this animated and ftriking picture of courtefy; but he fuggefted to Philocles, that amongft the inferior offices of focial life, he had not noticed the duties of Counsel and Reproof. Thefe, faid he, I fear, cannot be adminiftered by a mind under the influence of gentlenefs, without the concealment, and fometimes even the violation, of truth.

The former part of your allegation, replied Philocles, may perhaps be granted; but the latter I cannot admit. Advice and reprehenfion require, indeed, the utmoft delicacy; and painful truths fhould be delivered in the fofteft terms, and expreffed no farther than is neceffary to produce their due effect. A courteous man will alfo mix what is conciliating with what is offenfive; praife with cenfure; deference and refpect with the authority of admonition; fo far as thefe can be done in confiftency with probity and honour. For the mind revolts againft all cenforian power, which difplays pride or pleafure in finding fault; and is wounded by the bare fufpicion of fuch difgraceful tyranny. But advice, divefted of the harfhnefs, and yet retaining the honeft warmth of

* Blair's Sermons, vol. i. p. 150.

truth, " is like honey put round the brim of a veffel
" full of wormwood."* Even this vehicle, however, is fometime infufficient to conceal the draught
of bitternefs; of which we are furnifhed with an
admirable and diverting inftance in the hiftory of Gil
Blas. This young man became the favourite of the
Archbifhop of Grenada, in whofe family he enjoyed
a lucrative and agreeable office, and future profpects
of much higher preferment. The archbifhop regarded him as a perfon of tafte and fentiment; and
one day entered into the following converfation with
him. " Liften with attention to what I am going
" to deliver. My chief pleafure confifts in preaching;
" the Lord gives a bleffing to my homilies; they
" touch the hearts of finners, make them ferioufly
" reflect on their conduct, and have recourfe to in-
" ftant repentance. This fuccefs fhould alone be a
" fufficient incitement to my ftudies: neverthelefs, I
" will confefs to thee my weaknefs, and acknow-
" ledge that I propofe to myfelf another reward, a
" reward with which the delicacy of my nature re-
" proaches me in vain. The honour of being reck-
" oned a perfect orator has charmed my imagination:
" my performances are thought equally nervous and
" refined; but I am anxious to avoid the misfortune
" of thofe who write too long; and I wifh to retire
" without forfeiting one tittle of my reputation.
" Wherefore, my dear Gil Blas, what I exact of thy
" zeal is, that whenever thou fhalt perceive a fa lure

* Memoirs of Brandenburgh, by the King of Pruffia.

" in my genius, or the leaſt mark of the imbecility
" of old age in my compoſitions, that thou wilt im-
" mediately advertiſe me of it. I dare not truſt to
" my own judgment, which may be ſeduced by ſelf-
" love; but make choice of thine, becauſe I know it
" to be good, and am reſolved to ſtand by thy deciſion." Some time after this diſcourſe, the prelate was
ſeized with a fit of apoplexy. He was however ſoon
relieved; and ſuch ſalutary medicines were administered, that his health ſeemed to be re-eſtabliſhed.
But his underſtanding ſuffered a ſevere ſhock, which
was plainly perceptible in the firſt homily that he
compoſed. The ſucceeding one proved perfectly
deciſive; as it abounded in repetitions, vain arguments, and falſe pathos. " Now," ſaid Gil Blas to
himſelf, " maſter homily-critic, prepare to exerciſe
" the office which you have undertaken. You ſee
" that the faculties of his grace begin to fail. It is
" your duty to give him notice of it, not only as the
" depoſitory of his thoughts, but likewiſe left you
" ſhould be anticipated by ſome other of his friends."
But the embaraſſment was, how to convey the mortifying intimation to his patron. Fortunately the
archbiſhop extricated him from the difficulty, by enquiring what people ſaid of him, and if they were
ſatisfied with his laſt diſcourſe. Gil Blas anſwered,
that the homily had not ſucceeded ſo well as the
others, in affecting the audience. ' How?' replied
the prelate with aſtoniſhment; ' has it met with any
' Ariſtarchus?' " No, Sir," ſaid Gil Blas, " by

" no means: but fince you have laid your injunctions
" upon me to be open and fincere, I will take the
" liberty of telling you, that your late difcourfe, in
" my judgment, has not altogether the energy of
" your prior performances." The archbifhop grew
pale at thefe words; and faid, with a forced fmile,
' So then, Mr. Gil Blas, this piece is not to your
' tafte? You think my underftanding enfeebled,
' don't you?' " I fhould not have fpoken fo
" freely," anfwered Gil Blas, " if your grace had
" not commanded me. I do no more, therefore,
" than obey you; and I moft humbly beg that you
" will not be offended at my freedom." ' GOD
' forbid,' cried the prelate, with precipitation;
' GOD forbid that I fhould find fault with it. This
' would be extremely unjuft. I am not angry that
' you fpeak your fentiments: it is the fentiment only
' that I condemn. Know that I never compofed a
' better homily than that of which you difapprove;
' for my genius, thank heaven, hath yet loft nothing
' of its vigour. Henceforth, however, I will choofe
' an abler confidant than you are. Go,' added he;
pufhing Gil Blas out of his clofet by the fhoulders,
' go, tell my treafurer to give you a hundred ducats.
' I wifh you all manner of profperity, with a little
' more tafte.'*

But we have enlarged fufficiently on this part of
our fubject. Permit me, therefore, Sophron, to pro-

---

* Gil Blas, vol. iii

ceed, by enquiring, whether SECRECY, in certain cafes, be not a branch of faithfulnefs or veracity?

It is a very important one, anfwered Sophron. To betray the confidence that is repofed in us, whether we have tacitly or by a promife bound ourfelves to fidelity, evinces a weak underftanding or a bad heart. Levity, an eagernefs to communicate, or the defire of feeming to be important, are the moft frequent caufes of the breach of fecrecy; but it is to be feared, that it fometimes originates from bafenefs and malevolence.

This offence was deemed infamous by the ancient Perfians. For it was their opinion, fays Quintus Curtius, that however deficient a man might be in the talents requifite to the attainment of excellency, the negative virtues were, at leaft, in his power; and that he might be filent, although he could not be eloquent.

Here Philocles judicioufly remarked, that the laws of fecrecy are not, in all cafes, to be regarded as inviolable; for we are under antecedent obligations, of a nature ftill more forcible and binding. If any atrocious defign, either againft an individual or the ftate, be communicated in confidence to us, it is our duty to diffuade the party, if poffible, from the execution of it. But fhould our endeavours appear to be unavailing, the concealment of what we know might involve us in the guilt of the offence; and we fhould be juftly punifhable, as acceffaries to the crime. At Florence, and in other ftares of Italy, a a man apprifed of a plot againft the government is put to death for not revealing it.* In England, *mifprifion* of *treafon* is punifhed by forfeiture of rents and of goods, and by imprifonment during life: and *mifprifion* of *felony*, by imprifonment for a difcretionary term, and by fine and ranfom, at the pleafure of the king's judges.†

If fuch *mifprifions* be really culpable, how comes it to pafs, I afked, that informers are almoft univerfally held in contempt and deteftation?

Becaufe few villains, faid Philocles, will communicate their wicked defigns to any but thofe, whom they believe inclined to participate in the commiffion of them. Hence there is generally a prefumption of previous guilt in the informer: and to this guilt we fuperadd that of bafenefs and perfidy, as we are not willing to fuppofe that he is influenced to perform this public act either by motives of private virtue or of patriotifm. However, we fhould be careful not to carry our prepoffeffion againft informers, even of this clafs, too far. They do effential fervice to the community; and may, perhaps, think this fervice the beft atonement for their paft guilt, and the fulleft proof of their prefent repentance.

There is another branch of faithfulnefs, which it is alfo difhonourable to violate, and which lays us under an obligation to avoid TATTLING, TALE-BEARING, and CENSORIOUSNESS. In the unguarded hours of focial intercourfe, and ftill more in the commerce of

---

* Guiccardini's Hift. † Blackftone's Commentaries.

domeftic life, the wifeft and the beft of men fpeak their thoughts without referve; and cafting off all reftraint, may fometimes deviate, both in their words and actions, from the rules of ftrict propriety. To relate fuch inadvertencies, is meannefs; to ridicule them, is ill-nature; and to exaggerate them, is calumny.*

Sophron now turned our attention to a moft important branch of moral truth, by inquiring whether INSINCERITY in RELIGION may not be deemed a highly criminal fpecies of lying?

Certainly it may, returned Philocles. GOD is a being of fpotlefs purity, who fearches the heart, and commands us to worfhip Him " *in fpirit and in truth.*" " *Lying lips,*" whether employed in falfe profeffions of faith or of piety, " *are an abomination to the* " *LORD.*" And he who can habitually practife infincerity and hypocrify, in thofe ferious and important tranfactions with his Creator, Benefactor, and Judge, which have eternity for their object, is not likely to pay any fteady regard to temporary interefts, refulting from the laws of fociety, or the ordinary obligations of morality. When one of the kings of France folicited M. Bogier, who was a Proteftant, to conform to the Roman Catholic religion, pro nifing him

---

*   " Abfentem qui rodit amicum,
   " Qui non defendit, alio culpante; folutos
   " Qui captat rifus hominum, famamque dicacis;
   " Fingere qui non vifa poteft; commiffa tacere
   " Qui nequit; hic niger eft; hunc tu, Romane, caveto."
                 HOR, lib. i. fat. iv.

in return a commiffion or a government; "Sire,"
replied he, " if I could be perfuaded to betray my
" GOD for a marfhal's ftaff, I might be induced to
" betray my king for a bribe of much lefs value." .

It was a noble reply! cried Sophron, with ingenuous warmth; and the recital of it brings to my
memory a ftory which the Duke of Sully has recorded
of Ambrofe Parè, a zealous Huguenot, and furgeon
to Charles the Ninth of France. He was with the
king during the time of the maffacre of Paris, when
fo many thoufand innocent and virtuous perfons were
inhumanly butchered in cold blood; and was perhaps
a witnefs of the monarch's firing with a carbine upon
the wretched Calvinifts, who fled from their mur-
derers by the windows of the palace. The courtiers,
as they came into the royal prefence, vied with each
other in boafting of the barbarities which they had
committed; and Charles faid to Parè, whofe religious
opinions he well knew, "The time is now come,
" when I fhall have none but Catholics in my domi-
" nions." ' Sire,' anfwered he, without embarraffment or perturbation, ' can you forget your pro-
' mife to me, that I fhould never be obliged to go to
' mafs!' The Duke of Sully feems to be of opinion,
that the edict which Charles iffued the fucceeding
day, to prohibit the continuance of the maffacre, was
partly owing to the intrepidity and influence of Pare.

The conduct of Parè, faid Philocles, on fo trying
an occafion, affords a ftriking proof of firmnefs and
fincerity in the profeffion of religious faith. But ex-

amples of much higher degrees of fimilar fidelity are
to be found in the earlier annals of the Chriftian
church.   Nor are inftances wanting, even in the
heathen world, of a zealous and fearlefs attachment
to thofe rites which ignorance deemed facred, and
which individuals or bodies of men bound themfelves
by folemn engagements to perform.   When the
Gauls were become mafters of Rome, they befieged
the capitol, and clofely guarded every avenue, to
prevent the efcape of a fingle Roman citizen.   Under
thefe circumftances of danger, Caius Fabius Dorfo, a
young man of an illuftrious family, defcended from
the capitol, bearing certain holy utenfils in his hands;
and paffed through the midft of the enemy, regardlefs
of their menaces, to offer a facrifice to the gods on
the hill Quirinalis.   This facrifice it was the cuftom
of his anceftors to perform yearly, on a ftated day;
and when he had finifhed the folemnity, the Gauls,
though a fierce and barbarous people, fuffered him
to return unmolefted, admiring his piety, and aftonifhed at his intrepidity.*   Facts like thefe fhould
make us blufh at indifference, and abhor diffimulation,
in religion.   But whilft we allow fuch impreffions to
produce their full influence on our hearts, let us
beware of paffing judgment upon others with rafhnefs or unchriftian feverity.   Intemperate zeal is apt
to beget a malignancy of fpirit, no lefs incompatible
with the love of God, than with benevolence to man.
The conviction of the mind in matters of faith often

* Vide Liv. Hift.

depends more upon education and authority than on the exertions of reafon: and if we fee men profeffing to believe what is unintelligible or abfurd, we fhould be well affured that they have not deceived themfelves, before we accufe them of mocking their Creator, and impofing on the world.

We may pity ignorance, and lament credulity; but hypocrify, urged Sophron, merits from us no indulgence: and this fpecies of falfehood is fo characteriftically marked, that it cannot be miftaken. Who, that obferves a man fanctified in his behaviour, and affiduous in his public devotions, whilft he is at the fame time felfifh, malevolent, bigoted, and oppreffive, will hefitate to charge him with the groffeft and moft infamous diffimulation?

If there be fufficient proof that this is really his temper of mind, I acknowledge, faid Philocles, that you may and ought to brand him with the name of hypocrite. But no man fhould be charged with a crime univerfally odious, on flight or equivocal evidence. There is a fpecies of devotion, which having its feat chiefly in the imagination and the paffior, bears no exact proportion to the virtue of the character in which it is found: and charity, together with an humble fenfe of our own infirmities, will always lead us to put the moft favourable conftruction on the conduct of our fellow-creatures. We fhould remember alfo, that enthufiafm and fuperftition have often appeared with the external marks of diffimulation. The famous Lord Herbert, of Cherbury, had

written an elaborate work againſt Chriſtianity, which
he entitled, *De Veritate, prout diſtinguitur à Revelatione.* But knowing that it would meet with much
oppoſition, he remained ſome time in anxious ſuſpenſe
about the publication of it. Providence, however,
as he informs us, kindly interpoſed, and determined
his wavering reſolutions. Hear the marvellous tale
which he relates!

   " Being thus doubtful in my chamber, one fair day
" in the ſummer, my caſement being opened towards
" the ſouth, the ſun ſhining clear, and no wind ſtir-
" ring, I took my book *De Veritate* in my hand, and
" kneeling on my knees, devoutly ſaid, *O thou eternal*
" *God, I am not ſatisfied enough whether I ſhall pub-*
" *liſh this book. If it be for thy glory, I beſeech Thee*
" *give me ſome ſign from heaven; if not, I ſhall ſup-*
" *preſs it.* I had no ſooner ſpoken theſe words, but
" a loud, though yet gentle, noiſe came from the
" heavens, which did ſo comfort and cheer me, that
" I took my petition as granted, and that I had the
" ſign I demanded; whereupon alſo I reſolved to
" print my book."*

It muſt appear ſtrange that a man who had ſpent a
conſiderable part of his life in courts and camps,
ſhould poſſeſs ſuch a deluded imagination. And this
deluſion will be ſtill more ſuſpicious, when you are
told that Lord Herbert's chief argument againſt
Chriſtianity is, the improbability that Heaven ſhould
reveal its laws only to a portion of the earth. For

* See the Life of Lord Herbert, written by himſelf.

how could he, who doubted of a *partial*, believe an *individual* revelation? Or is it poffible, that he could have the vanity to think his book of fuch importance as to extort a declaration of the Divine will, when the intereft and happinefs of a fourth part of mankind were deemed by him objeƈts inadequate to the like difplay of goodnefs?* Do thefe arguments convince you of Lord Herbert's hypocrify? Your conclufion is hafty and unjuft. Read his life, and you will be fatisfied that the warmth of his temper might expofe him to felf-deception; but that he was incapable of obtruding on the world what he knew to be a falfehood.

Sophron modeftly acknowledged, that the figns of religious diffimulation might be lefs decifive than he had fuppofed. But allow me, faid he, to contraƈt your inftance of Lord Herbert with two faƈts concerning Oliver Cromwell; to fhew that the charge of hypocrify may be juftly grounded on fingle aƈtions, without taking into our view the whole tenour of a man's life. Suppofe a ftranger, ignorant of the craftinefs and ambition of Cromwell, to have been prefent in the long parliament, when the ordinance for the trial of Charles I. was read and affented to; would he have hefitated to think him a hypocrite, after hearing him deliver the following words? " Should any one have voluntarily propofed to bring " the king to punifhment, I fhould have regarded " him as the greateft traitor; but fince Providence

* See Walpole's Catalogue of Royal and Noble Authors.

" and neceffity have caft us upon it, I will pray to
" GOD for a bleffing on your counfels; though I am
" not prepared to give you my advice on this im-
" portant occafion. Even I myfelf, when I was lately
" offering up a petition for his Majefty's reftoration,
" felt my tongue cleave to the roof of my mouth;
" and confidered this fupernatural movement as the
" anfwer which Heaven, having rejected the king,
" had fent to my fupplications."*

Let us farther fuppofe that this ftranger attended
the high court of juftice, and faw Cromwell, when he
took the pen in his hand to fign the warrant for the
king's execution, jocularly bedaub the face of his
neighbour with the ink; could he forbear to exprefs
his difguft at the levity which he then obferved, and
his abhorrence of the grofs diffimulation to which he
had been before a witnefs?

You have drawn your example, replied Philocles,
from that diftracted period of our hiftory when truth
appears to have been banifhed from public life. The
defpotic views of a monarch who was under the influence of a Popifh queen, a bigoted prelate, and a
corrupt ftatefman, led him to the practice of deceit
and falfehood;† and the parties who united in op-
pofing his encroachments on the civil and religious
rights of the people, foon deviated from their original
principles; and availing themfelves of the gloomy
enthufiafm of the times, concealed their perfidy and
ambition under the mafk of pious zeal and divine

---

* Whitlock.　　　　† See Appendix, fect. v.

illuminations. That Cromwell was guilty of hypocrify, may with too much probability be inferred
from numerous and undoubted facts. But I know
not whether the two which you have related would
have authorized a ftranger to charge him publicly
with this reproachful offence. Cromwell poffeffed a
vigorous, active, and enlarged underftanding; and
could affume, whenever he pleafed, that dignity of
manners which befitted his high ftation. But when he
relaxed himfelf from the toils of war, or the cares of
government, his amufements frequently confifted in
the loweft buffoonery. Yet in thefe apparently unguarded moments he was upon the watch to remark
the characters, defigns, and weakneffes of men; and
to penetrate into the inmoft receffes of their hearts.
Before the trial of Charles, a meeting was held between the chiefs of the republican party and the
general officers, to concert the model of the intended
new government. After the debates on this moft
interefting and important fubject, Ludlow informs us,
that Cromwell, by way of frolic, threw a cufhion
at his head; and when Ludlow took up another
cufhion to return the joke, the general ran down
ftairs, and was in danger of breaking his bones in
the hurry.* It is evident, therefore, that this extraordinary man might really be ferious, under the
appearance of levity. But this topic has engroffed
too much of our attention; and I will only add, that

* Hume's Hiftory.

the more we cultivate moral or religious fincerity in ourfelves, the lefs difpofed we fhall be to fufpect the want of it in others.

There is a character, faid Sophron, of genuine dignity and importance, not ufurped like that of Cromwell, the luftre of which has been tarnifhed by the charge of religious diffimulation. This charge, you know, is laid in the ftrongeft terms againft the apoftle Peter, by St. Paul himfelf, who writes thus to the Galatians: *But when Peter came to Antioch, I withftood him to the face, becaufe he was to be blamed. For before that certain came from James, he did eat with the Gentiles; but when they were come, he withdrew, and feparated himfelf, fearing them which were of the circumcifion. And the other Jews diffembled likewife with him, infomuch that Barnabas was carried away with their diffimulation. But when I faw that they walked not uprightly, according to the Gofpel, I faid unto Peter before them all, If thou, being a Jew, liveft after the manner of Gentiles, and not as do the Jews, why compelleft thou the Gentiles to live as do the Jews?*

The conduct of Peter on this occafion is the more extraordinary, as he appears to have had the fulleft conviction of the abolition of the Jewifh ceremonies, by the promulgation of the Gofpel of CHRIST:* a conviction founded on an immediate revelation from heaven; in confequence of which he baptized the centurion Cornelius and his family. *And he faid*

---

* Acts v. 7, 8.

*unto them, Ye know how that it is an unlawful thing
for a man that is a Jew to keep company with or come
unto one of another nation: but* GOD *hath shewed me,
that I should not call any man common or unclean. For
of a truth I perceive that* GOD *is no respecter of persons;
but in every nation, he that feareth Him, and worketh
righteousness, is accepted with Him.**

The enemies of Chriftianity, anfwered Philocles,
have indecently and unjuftly triumphed in this difpute
between the apoftles; and its friends, with a zeal no
lefs heated and erroneous, have anxioufly fought to
difavow or to evade it. Two primitive fathers† of
the church have even reprefented it as a ftratagem
or deceit, concerted privately for the benefit of the
Jewifh converts; but Auftin rejects this defence with
proper indignation, as difhonourable to the character
of Paul, and inadequate to the juftification of Peter,
whofe conduct he confeffes to have been worthy of
reprehenfion. The truth, indeed, feems to be, that
this great Apoftle fuffered himfelf to be governed on
the unfortunate occafion now alluded to, as on feve
others of his life, by the warmth and impetuofity of
his paffions. But diffimulation is not the concomitant
of fuch a temper of mind: and as the hiftory of Peter
fufficiently evinces that this vice was foreign to his
nature, it could originate only in the prefent inftance
from the fudden impreffion of fear on one, not yet
completely difciplined in the fchool of fortitude. Let
us learn therefore, Sophron, from the feverity of St

---

* Acts x.   † Chryfoftom and Jerom.

Paul's rebuke, to avoid all mean prevarications or time-ferving compliances, inconfiftent with our religious principles; and *to walk uprightly, according to the truth of the Gofpel, holding faft the liberty with which* CHRIST *has made us free.*

May we remember alfo, in the judgments which we form concerning the faith and practices of others, that our great Mafter and Lawgiver has invefted them with the fame freedom which we ourfelves enjoy; and that if an apoftle was not authorized to impofe a yoke on others, we can have no claim to prefide over confcience, however erroneous it may be, or to affume any power in fpiritual matters, but what arifes from the perfuafive influence of fuperior reafon: and even in the exercife of this faculty, our language and treatment fhould be fuch, as to manifeft the benignity and gentlenefs of Chriftian toleration.

I could not hear the term *toleration* from the mouth of Philocles, without expreffing fome objections to it, although it has been adopted by Mr. Locke, and other writers of the firft diftinction. For words, I obferved, have a confiderable influence on opinions; and the prefent term appears to be injurious to that religious liberty which it is defigned to import. It implies a *right* to impofe articles of faith and modes of worfhip; that non-conformity is a crime; and that the *fufferance* of it is a matter of favour or lenity. But the non-conformift in every country, whether he be a Chriftian at Conftantinople, a Proteftant at Rome, an Epifcopalian in Scotland, or a Prefbyterian in Eng-

land, if his rational principles be confonant to his practice, will regard this claim of *right* as ufurpation, and
will urge, that it has neither been conferred by JESUS
CHRIST, nor delegated by the people. Our Saviour
exprefsly declares, *My kingdom is not of this world:*
and his religion was perfecuted and oppreffed, during
the period of its greateft purity and perfeftion, and
when the minifters of it had gifts and powers which
are now unknown. The people could not delegate
fuch a right to any man, or body of men: for the
human mind is fo mutable, that no individual can
fix a ftandard of his own faith, much lefs can he
commiffion another to eftablifh one for him and his
pofterity. And this power would in no hands be
fo dangerous, as in thofe of the ftatefman or prieft,
who has the folly and prefumption to think himfelf
qualified to exercife it.

Philocles, by his filence, feemed to acquiefce in
what I had advanced: and when I apologized afterwards for the interruption which I had more than
once occafioned to the methodical difcuffion of the
fubject in debate, he very politely replied, that the
freedom of converfation admits not of a rigid adherence to the precife rules of fyftem. But were it
otherwife, faid he, the mind is relieved from weari-
nefs, and animated to more attention by feafonable
digreffions, if not too long, or too often repeated.
That I am not averfe to enter into them myfelf, you
may already have obferved, and will now find, by my
recalling to Sophron's memory the difpute between

the Apoftles Paul and Peter; and deducing from it an argument in favour of the truth of Chriftianity. It is obvious, I think, from this incident, that there was no combination to deceive mankind amongft the firft preachers of the Gofpel; and that if, on ordinary occafions, they were actuated by the common weakneffes and prejudices of human nature, they neither attempted to conceal nor to extenuate them. With the fimplicity of truth they related facts as they occurred, whether advantageous or otherwife to their characters. And every unprejudiced judge will difcover, in the records of the Gofpel, fuch internal marks of fidelity, as no other hiftory, either of ancient or modern periods, can difplay. Juftly, therefore, may we apply to the writings of the Evangelifts that maxim of Cicero, *Quis nefcit primam effe hiftoriæ legem, ne quid falfi dicere audeat; deinde, ne quid veri non audeat?*

—— A paufe enfued, and the converfation feemed to be concluded. But Sophron taking up Locke's Effay on the Human Underftanding, which happened to lie on the table before him, read the diftinction which that author makes between moral and metaphyfical truth. This fuggefted frefh matter of difcuffion, and gave rife to a variety of obfervations on the danger of error, and on the conduct of reafon in our intellectual purfuits. Philocles particularly enlarged on the pernicious confequences of fupporting FALSE OPINIONS, for the fake of argument, in public or private difputations; and reprefented this practice

Cicero de Oratore, lib. ii.

as one great fource of fcepticifm and infidelity amongft
literary men.* The imagination, faid he, is ftruck
with novelty; it appears honourable to fhake off the
fetters of vulgar prejudice; and pride is doubly gratified by the humiliation of an opponent, and the
triumph over authority. Thus the paffions become
engaged on the fide which the fceptic efpoufes;
fophiftry is miftaken for found logic; he becomes ena-
moured of difcoveries, made by his fuperior penetration; and the fingularity of his notions or principles,
which would create doubt and hefitation in a wife
man, tends only to ftrengthen his conviction of their
certainty. Milton, defcribing the character of Belial,
one of the fallen angels, fays, in emphatic language,

- - - - - - - - - - - - " His tongue
" Dropp'd manna, and could make the worfe appear
" The better reafon, to perplex and dafh
" Matureft counfels."†

Does not the philofopher's maxim, faid Sophron,
Nullius jurare in verba magiftri, feem to recommend
a ftrict fcrutiny into every fubject? And what more
judicious method can be devifed, of correcting our
prejudices, in favour of an eftablifhed opinion, than
by fetting ourfelves boldly in oppofition to it?

Would you free yourfelf, Sophron, from a trifling
malady, by incurring a fevere and dangerous one?
Then, urged Philocles, you may correct a flight prejudice by adopting another that is greater. In our

---

* See Appendix, fect. vi.
† Paradife Loft, book ii. l. 912.

inquiries into truth, we ought to diveſt ourſelves, as
much as poſſible, of every prepoſſeſſion. But it is
ſurely a reaſonable deference to the judgment of the
public, concerning any doctrine or opinion, that we
ſhould firſt examine with attention the arguments in
its favour, before we admit the objections which may
be raiſed againſt it. And by this method the mind
will be leaſt unfairly biaſſed in her deciſions, and will
reſt on them with a degree of confidence and ſatisfaction, which can never reſult from partial or prejudiced inveſtigation. Young men of lively parts
and acute underſtandings, when they enter upon the
field of controverſy, are ſometimes ſo proud of their
polemic ſkill, as to engage indiſcriminately on any
ſide of the queſtion in debate. This is a dangerous
practice, and cenſured even by Socrates himſelf; whoſe
labours were devoted to the diſcuſſion of truth, and
the detection of error. " If thou continueſt to take
" delight in idle argumentation," ſaid he to Euclides,
" thou mayeſt be qualified to combat with the ſo-
" phiſts, but wilt never know how to live with men."
And Lord Bacon, the great luminary of ſcience, appears to have entertained ſimilar ideas; for, ſpeaking
of the logic of Ariſtotle, he terms it, " a philoſophy
" for contention only, but barren in the production
" of works for the benefit of life."* Many lamentable proofs have I ſeen of the tendency of this habit
of altercation to create indifference, not only to intellectual, but alſo to moral and religious truth. Cato

* Biog. Brit. vol. i. ſecond edit. p. 449.

the cenfor, prophefied the ruin of the Roman conftitution, whenever this fort of learning fhould become
the fafhionable ftudy of his countrymen. He conceived his diflike to it on the following occafion. "In
" the year of Rome 599, the Athenians fent three
" of their principal philofophers on an embaffy to
" the republic. At the head of thefe was Carneades,
" a very celebrated leader of the academic fect. While
" he was waiting for an anfwer from the fenate, he
" employed himfelf in difplaying his talents in the
" art of difputation: and the Roman youth flocked
" round him in great numbers. In one of thefe
" public difcourfes he attempted to prove, that *juftice*
" *and injuftice depend altogether on the inftitutions of*
" *civil fociety, and have no foundation in nature.* The
" next day, agreeably to the manner of that fect, and
" in order to fet the arguments on each fide of the
" queftion in full view, he fupported with equal
" eloquence the reverfe of his former propofition.
" Cato was prefent at both thefe difputations; and
" and being apprehenfive that the moral principles
" of the Roman youth might be fhaken, if they fhould
" become converts to this mode of philofophizing,
" he was anxious to prevent its reception; and did
" not reft till he had prevailed with the fenate to dis-
" mifs the ambaffadors with their final anfwer."*

Perhaps the verfatile opinions and principles of the
Jefuits may be afcribed to this caufe; for I have been
informed by feveral of them with whom I have con-

* Plut. in Vit. Caton. Melmoth's Cato, p. 190.

verfed, that their academical exercifes are chiefly directed to make them fubtle difputants. How far the
fame obfervation may be applicable to the members
of a learned profeffion, highly refpected in this country, I will not prefume to determine. But there is
too much reafon to apprehend, that the cuftom of
pleading for any client, without difcrimination of
right or wrong, muft leffen the regard due to thofe
important diftinctions, and deaden the moral fenfibility of the heart.*

I have been too ftrongly impreffed with the love of
truth, replied Sophron, to debate with indifference
about it; and therefore, to guard againft deception,
from " what the nurfe and what the prieft have
" taught," I would examine my moft ferious opinions, and try whether I cannot, by direct oppofition,
or by the teft of ridicule, invalidate their authority.

I have already given you my reafons againft this
practice, anfwered Philocles; and I could enforce
them by many examples of the pernicious confequences
of it, which have fallen under my obfervation. But
private hiftory is invidious; and I fhall therefore confine myfelf to a few cafes of public notoriety. The
academy of Dijon many years ago propofed the following whimfical prize-queftion, viz. " Whether the
" fciences may not be deemed more hurtful than be-
" neficial to fociety?" M. Rouffeau became a candidate for the laurel, and affumed the affirmative fide
of the queftion; probably becaufe it furnifhed him

* See Appendix, fect. vii.

with a better opportunity of difplaying his genius and powers of perfuafion.* His difcourfe was received with the higheft applaufe; he became the dupe of his own rhetoric, and adopted as a philofopher the maxims which he had delivered as an orator. From this period commenced his fame, his paradoxes, and his misfortunes.† He combated the common fenfe of mankind with all the zeal of a reformer; and his writings proved like the bubble which glitters, expands, and burfts in the fun-fhine: they were dazzling, empty, and foon forgotten. I am inclined to fufpect that Machiavel's Prince, the Fable of the Bees, and other productions of this nature, originated from caufes fomewhat fimilar to thofe which gave rife to the chimeras of Rouffeau. And it is faid that a celebrated adverfary of Chriftianity, by yielding up his judgment and imagination to a particular fet of arguments, became fucceffively a Proteftant, a Papift, and an Infidel.‡

But permit me, Sophron, to fuggeft to you a caution of ftill higher importance, which regards fuch of your intellectual purfuits as relate to the Deity. Religion may be confidered both as a fpeculative fcience, and as a practical principle. In the former view, it conftitutes the fublimeft object of the underftanding, and the moft interefting topic of rational inveftigation:

---

* " Major eft ille qui judicium abftulit, quam qui meruit."—Cic.
" Nefcio quomodo, dum lego affentior, cum pofui librum, affenfio
" omnis illa elabitur."—Idem.   † Helvetius.

‡ See an account of Mr. Tindal, in the Britifh Biography, vol. ix. p. 314.

In the latter, it is a fpring of motion, and excites all
the devout affections of veneration, gratitude, and
love.   When you contemplate as a philofopher the
character of the Divine Being, you muft be ftruck
with reverence at the proofs which offer themfelves
of his boundlefs power, univerfal prefence, and infinite duration: and thefe attributes, reflecting dignity
and luftre on the more amiable perfections of his
nature, will heighten the impreffion made by the relation which He ftands in to you, as your Creator,
Benefactor, and Friend.   Thus the principle of piety
will fubfift in your mind in its full force, fupported
by the authority of reafon, and harmonizing with all
the feelings of your heart.   But if you defcend from
thefe general and exalted views of the Divine Being
into minute difquifitions concerning his effence, the
freedom of his agency, and other fubtilties beyond the
human ken, you will foon damp the ardour of devotion in your breaft; and fhould you make thefe inquiries the common matter of academical difputation,
or of familiar debate, the facred flame will be extinguifhed altogether.*   The poet lately quoted has
defcribed fome of the fallen angels, who had been
driven from heaven for impiety and rebellion, as
" fitting on a hill retired, and reafoning high"

> " Of Providence, foreknowledge, will, and fate;
> " Fix'd fate, free-will, foreknowledge abfolute;
> " And found no end, in wand'ring mazes loft."†

* See Dr. Gregory's Comparative View, and Mrs. Barbauld on
Devotional Tafte.

† Milton's Paradife Loft, book ii, l. 559.

I mean not, however, to condemn indifcriminately all metaphyfical refearches of this kind. It is natural for men of a fpeculative turn to extend their views of theology beyond the clear limits either of reafon or of revelation: and if their inquiries be conducted with that humility and reverence which fuch fubjects fhould infpire, they may tend to invigorate the underftand-ing without depraving the heart. The example of Locke, Newton, Clarke, Hartley, and other diftin-guifhed philofophers, affords fufficient confirmation of this truth; and at the fame time evinces a ftill more pleafing and important one, that religion numbers, amongft her votaries, men who have dignified and adorned human nature by their genius, virtue, and learning. I would particularly recommend to your notice, Sophron, I need not fay to your imitation, the conduct of Mr. Boyle, who had fo profound a vene-ration for the Deity, that the name of GOD was never mentioned by him without a paufe in his difcourfe.* This great philofopher alfo had fuch delicate notions of veracity, and was fo fenfible of the imperfection of human knowledge, even when derived from expe-riment, that in the preface to his Effays he makes an apology for the frequent ufe of the words *perhaps, it feems, 'tis not improbable,* as implying a diffidence of the juftnefs of his opinions: and this diffidence arofe, as he informs us, from repeated obfervation, that what pleafed him for a while, was afterwards difgraced by fome further or more recent difcovery.

* Britifh Biography, vol. vi. p. 248.

Here Philocles was interrupted by the arrival of a ſtranger, whoſe preſence put an end to the converſation.

ON THE

INFLUENCE

OF

HABIT and ASSOCIATION.

———⟨◇⟩———

- - - - - - - " VIRESQUE ACQUIRIT EUNDO."
VIRGIL.

- - - - - - - - - - - - " ANGIT,
" IRRITAT, MULCET, FALSIS TERRORIBUS IMPLET."
HOR. Ep. I. lib. ii.

MISCELLANEOUS

OBSERVATIONS

ON THE INFLUENCE OF

HABIT AND ASSOCIATION.

SECTION I.

THE laws of HABIT and ASSOCIATION form a moſt important branch both of phyſiology and of ethics. And as *the proper ſtudy of mankind is man,* every faČt muſt be deemed intereſting, which tends to elucidate either the animal, intelleČtual, or moral œconomy of his nature. The following obſervations have a reference to one or other of theſe objeČts. But no particular regard has been paid to ſyſtem in the arrangement of them: and I have attempted only, as Lord Verulam expreſſes it, " to write certain brief " notes, ſet down rather ſignificantly than curiouſly."

I. MUSCULAR ACTIONS, perfeČtly ſpontaneous, may be excited without apparent volition, ſo as to become completely automatical, by the recurrence of thoſe impreſſions with which they have been long aſſociated. I ſhall give a ſtriking example of the truth of this propoſition.

Several years ago the. Countefs of **** fell into
an apoplexy, about feven o'clock in the morning.
Amongft other ftimulating applications, I directed a
feather dipped in hartfhorn to be frequently introduced into her noftrils. Her Ladyfhip, when in
health, was much addicted to the taking of fnuff; and
the prefent .irritation of the olfactory nerves produced
a junction of the fore-finger and thumb of the right
hand, the elevation of them to the nofe, and the
action of fnuffing in the noftrils. When the fnuffing
ceafed, the hand and arm dropped down in a torpid
ftate. A frefh application of the ftimulus renewed
thefe fucceffive efforts; and I was a witnefs to their
repetition till the hartfhorn loft its power of irritation,
probably by deftroying the fenfibility of the olfactory
nerves. The Countefs recovered from the fit about
fix o'clock in the evening; but though it was neither long nor fevere, her memory never afterwards
furnifhed the leaft trace of *confcioufnefs* during its
continuance.

Does not this inftance of a complex feries of actions, ordinarily. fpontaneous, in circumftances which
feem to preclude both volition and confcioufnefs,
reflect fome light on the obfcure queftion concerning
the fleep of the foul, fo much agitated in the time of
Mr. Locke? Is not the opinion of this celebrated
philofopher confirmed by it, that the perception or
contemplation of ideas is to the mind what motion is
to the body, not its effence but one of its operations:
and that an unceafing energy of the underftanding

and the will is the fole prerogative of that infinitely-perfect Being, who, according to the language of the Pfalmift, *never flumbers or fleeps.*

II. Slight PARALYTIC AFFECTIONS of the organs of fpeech fometimes occur without any correfpondent diforder in other parts of the body. In fuch cafes the tongue appears to the patient too large for his mouth, the faliva flows more copioufly than ufual, and the vibratory power of the *glottis* is fomewhat impaired. Hence the effort to fpeak fucceeds the volition of the mind flowly and imperfectly, and the words are uttered with faltering and hefitation. Thefe are facts of common notoriety: but I have never feen it remarked, that in this local palfy the pronunciation of PROPER NAMES is attended with peculiar difficulty; and that the recollection of them becomes either very obfcure, or entirely obliterated; whilft that of perfons, places, things, and even of abftract ideas, remains unchanged. Such a partial defect of memory, of which experience has furnifhed me with feveral examples, confirms the theory of affociation, and at the fame time admits of an eafy folution by it. For as words are arbitrary marks, and owe their connection with what they import to eftablifhed ufage, the ftrength of this connection will be exactly proportioned to the frequency of their re-currence; and this recurrence muft be much more frequent with generic than with fpecific terms. Now proper names are of the latter clafs; and the idea of a perfon or place may remain vivid in the mind, with-

out the leaſt ſignature of the appellative which diſtin-
guiſhes each of them.   It is certain alſo that we often
think in words; and there is probably at ſuch times
ſome ſlight impulſe on the organs of ſpeech, analogous to what is perceived when a muſical note or
tune is called to mind.   But a leſion of the power of
utterance may break a link in the chain of aſſociation,
and thus add to the partial defeĉt of memory now
under conſideration.

The following very curious fâĉt I have received
from unqueſtionable authority.   Mr. S———, a
Welchman by birth, and miniſter of a congregation
at W——, had a paralytic ſtroke in 1783, at the
age of ſixty, which deprived him entirely of the power
of ſpeaking Engliſh, after he had preached in that
language thirty or forty years.   He could ſtill con-
verſe in the Welſh tongue with facility, and continued
to underſtand thoſe who ſpoke to him in Engliſh, though
he was unable to make any reply in the ſame language.

III. Dr. Willis relates the ſtory of an IDEOT, who,
reſiding within the ſound of a clock, regularly amuſed
himſelf with counting aloud the hour of the day,
whenever the hammer of that inſtrument ſtruck: but
being afterwards removed to a ſituation where there
was no clock, he retained the former impreſſions ſo
ſtrongly, that he continued to diſtinguiſh the ordinary diviſion of time, repeating at the end of every
hour the preciſe number of ſtrokes which the clock
would have ſtruck at that period.*   Mr. Addiſon

* Willis *De Anima Brutor.* pars i. cap. xvi. p. 85.

has quoted this fact in one of the Spectators, not from the original, but from Dr. Plott's History of Staffordſhire; and has deduced from it many important moral reflections. Whatever may be thought of the authenticity of this narrative, an inſtance has lately occurred within the circle of my own obſervation ſomewhat ſimilar, and which no leſs clearly evinces the power of habit to renew former mechanical impreſſions, independently of any external cauſe.

Mr. W—— had been long confined to his chamber, by a palſy and other ailments. Every evening about ſix o'clock he played at cards with ſome of the family. He was ſeized in June, 1780, at three o'clock in the afternoon, with a fit, which terminated in deſipiency. At the ſtated hour of card-playing, he fancied himſelf to be engaged in his uſual game; talked of the cards as if they were in his hand; and was very angry at his daughter when ſhe endeavoured to rectify his miſtaken imagination. His fatuity was of ſhort continuance; but when recovered from it, he expreſſed no recollection of what had paſſed.

IV. A celebrated French writer* has remarked, that " the greater degree of ſagacity any one is maſter of, " the more ORIGINALS will he diſcover in the cha- " racters of mankind." This *originality* may doubtleſs depend on the primary conſtitution of the mind; but I am perſuaded alſo, that it is often the reſult of particular aſſociations. When theſe are unnatural or inordinate, they produce partial alienations of the

* Paſchal.

underſtanding: and to this ſource we may trace the
viſions of enthuſiaſm, the perſecuting zeal of bigotry,
the ſanguinary honour of duelling, the ſordid purſuits
of avarice, and the toilſome ſolicitudes of ill-directed
ambition. Theſe and numberleſs other quixotiſms
of the mind give the phantoms of imagination an
aſcendancy over reaſon, and produce a temporary in-
ſanity, varying according to its object, degree, and
duration. If the predominant train of ideas be foreign to the offices of life, there will be little chance
of breaking the magic combination; and the habitual
indulgence of this tyranny of paſſion, or fancy, will
at laſt render it fixed and uncontrollable.

According to Shakeſpeare, " the lunatic, the lover,
"·and the poet, are of imagination all compact."
But as our great dramatiſt obſerves, on another occaſion, " 'twere to conſider too curiouſly to conſider
" ſo.*" At leaſt, we ſhould reſtrict our concluſions,
that they may not involve ſo large a portion of mankind, as to injure the honour even of human nature
itſelf. Beſides, paſſion is the ſpring of the mind,
which gives vigour and energy to all its movements:
and, if not extravagantly diſproportionate to the value
of its object, it may be indulged, not only with innocence, but ſometimes even with ſingular advantage.
For, the ardour inſpired by it is the ſource of all that
is excellent in genius, and ſublime in conduct: and
without the ſalutary aid of this ſpecies of enthuſiaſm
we ſhould ſink into a ſtate of torpid apathy.

* Hamlet.

But though it be difficult to define the precife boundaries of rationality, it can neither be denied, nor concealed, that partial infanity may fubfift with general intelligence. A few years fince, a gentleman came from Buxton to Manchefter to confult me. He had been fent by his phyfician to ufe the bath, and to drink the waters of that place: but fome gouty fymptoms fupervening, he was unwilling to proceed in the courfe enjoined him, without further advice. I received from him a well-connected, minute, and rational account of his complaint; and after giving fuch directions as the cafe feemed to require, I arofe to take my leave of him. He defired me to fit down again, and told me he had lately read the MORAL TALES, which I had publifhed; and from a little experiment related in one of them, hoped that I had made the nature of found a particular object of my ftudy. I have a friend, continued he, who is conftantly tortured, whenever he travels, with the moft diftracting noife in his ears; a noife produced by an inftrument in the poffeffion of his implacable enemy. On expreffing my difbelief of the poffibility of fuch a fact, he averred the truth of it with much emotion; informed me that he was himfelf the fufferer; defcribed, in the moft lively manner, the acute pains which he felt in his ear; and charged the bifhop of ———, in confequence of a family quarrel, with being the author of them. I was now fully aware of my patient's mental infirmity, and inftead of attempting to reafon with him about the delufion of his imagi-

nation, I tried to footh him with the hope that the
bifhop of ——, whom I had the honour of perfonally knowing, might be prevailed with to difcon-
tinue the exercife of fo extraordinary a power of
torture. But finding it impoffible to give him comfort by infpiring expectations, which he rejected as
groundlefs and abfurd, I had the good fortune to
fuggeft a mode of relief that perfectly coincided with
his own ideas. The painful impreffion, faid I, produced by the bifhop on your ear, muft confiderably
depend upon the ftate of that organ; and if you can
diminifh its fenfibility, and deaden the vibrations of
the tympanum, you may again be reftored to fome
degree of eafe and enjoyment. A little olive oil
poured twice or thrice every day into your ears will,
in all probability, completely anfwer thefe purpofes
if it do not, a fmall quantity of opium may be combined with it. He liftened to me with eager attention; joy fparkled in his eyes at the fuggeftion of a
remedy, which excited his hope and confidence; and
I left him under the moft happy conviction, that he
might now fet his ideal enemy at defiance.

This cafe recalls to my memory the very fingular
and affecting one of Mr. Simon Browne, of which it
may not be unfeafonable to give a fhort recital.
He was a diffenting clergyman of exemplary life,
and eminent intellectual abilities; but having been
feized with melancholy, he defifted from the duties of
his function, and could not be perfuaded to join in
any act, either of public or of private worfhip. The

reafon which, after much importunity, he affigned for this change in his conduct, was, "that he "had fallen under the difpleafure of GOD, who "had caufed his rational foul gradually to perifh, "and left him only an animal life, in common with "brutes: that it was therefore profane in him to "pray, and improper to be prefent at the prayers of "others." In this opinion he remained inflexible, at the time when all the powers of his mind feemed to fubfift in full vigour; when his judgment was clear, and his reafoning ftrong and conclufive. For at this period he publifhed a defence of the *Religion of Nature*, and of the *Chriftian Revelation*, in anfwer to *Tindal's Chriftianity as old as the Creation:* and the work is univerfally allowed to be the beft which that celebrated controverfy produced. But in a dedication of it to Queen Caroline, which fome of his friends found means to fupprefs, he difplays the very extraordinary phrenfy under which he laboured. Speaking of himfelf, he informs her Majefty, "that "by the immediate hand of an avenging GOD, his "very thinking fubftance has, for more than feven "years, been continually wafting away, till it is "wholly perifhed out of him, if it be not utterly "come to nothing."

This remarkable and humiliating example of vigour and imbecility, rectitude and perverfion of the fame underftanding, I have related on the authority of Dr. Hawkefworth,* who has preferved the entire

* See the Adventurer,

copy of the dedication, from which only a brief extract is here made. Our ignorance of the hiftory of
Mr. Browne renders it impoffible to trace to its fource
this mental malady. But there is reafon to prefume,
that it originated from fome ftrong impreffion, and
fubfequent invincible affociation, connected with, or
perhaps producing, a change in the organization of
the brain. Perhaps, having acquired an early predilection for the writings of Plato, he might afterwards, in fome feafon of hypochondriacal dejection,
fall into the gloomy myfticifm of the later followers
of that amiable philofopher: for Plotinus, who flourifhed in the third century after the Chriftian æra,
taught that the moft perfect worfhip of the Deity
confifts, not in acts of veneration and of gratitude,
but in a certain felf-annihilation, or total extinction of
the intellectual faculties.*

I am inclined to believe, that the celebrated M.
Pafchal laboured under a fpecies of infanity, towards
the conclufion of his life, fimilar to that of Mr. Simon
Browne: and having hazarded fuch a furmife, it is
incumbent on me to fhew on what it is founded.
This very extraordinary man difcovered the moft
aftonifhing marks of genius in his childhood; and
his progrefs in fcience was fo rapid, that at the age
of fixteen he wrote an excellent treatife of Conic
Sections. He poffeffed fuch a capacious and reten-
tive memory, that he is faid " never to have for-

* See Collier's Hift. Dict. Alfo, Maclaurin's Account of Sir
Ifaac Newton's Difcoveries, p. 397.

" gotten any thing which he had learned." And it was his practice to digest and arrange in his mind a whole series of reflections before he committed them to writing. This power was at once so accurate and extensive, that he has been heard to deliver the entire plan of a work, of which he had taken no notes, in a continued narration, that occupied several hours. But it is related by the editor of his *Thoughts on Religion and other subjects*,* " that it pleased GOD so to " touch his heart, as to let him perfectly understand, " that the Christian religion obligeth us to live for " GOD only, and to propose to ourselves no other ob-" ject." In consequence of this persuasion, he renounced all the pursuits of knowledge, and practised the most severe and rigorous mortifications ; living in the greatest penury, and refusing every indulgence which was not absolutely necessary for the support of life. It appears from some of his pious meditations, that this resolution of mind proceeded from the visitation of sickness. And the following solemn addresses to the Deity clearly indicate an imagination perverted by the most erroneous associations:—

" O LORD, Thou gavest me health to be spent in " serving Thee, and I applied it to an use altogether " profane. Now Thou hast sent sickness for my " correction.—I know, O LORD, that at the instant " of my death, I shall find myself entirely separated " from the world, stripped naked of all things, stand-" ing alone before Thee, to answer to thy justice

* See the Preface to that Work.

" concerning all the motions of my thoughts and
" fpirits. Grant that I may look on myfelf as dead
" already, feparated from the world, ftripped of all
" the objects of my paffion, and placed alone in thy
" prefence. I praife Thee, O GOD, that Thou haft
" been pleafed to anticipate the dreadful day, by
" already deftroying all things to my tafte and
" thoughts, under this weaknefs, which I fuffer from
" thy providence. I praife Thee, that Thou haft
" given me this divorce from the pleafures of the
" world." Was it confonant with foundnefs of underftanding, for a man to take a fudden difguft at
all the liberal ftudies, and innocent enjoyments, which
had before engaged and gratified his mind? And
was it not as much the fiction of a diftempered fancy,
that GOD enjoined poverty, abftinence, and ignorance,
to one poffeffing rank, fortune, and the nobleft endowments of the mind; as the belief of Simon Browne,
that he was divefted of that rationality, which at the
fame time he fo eminently difplayed? Whenever
falfe ideas, of a practical kind, are fo firmly united as
to be conftantly and invariably miftaken for truths, we
very juftly denominate this unnatural alliance INSA-
NITY. And if it give rife to a train of fubordinate
wrong affociations, producing incongruity of behaviour, incapacity for the common duties of life, or
unconfcious deviations from morality and religion,
MADNESS has then its commencement.

In the foregoing examples, the force of habit and
affociation is clearly manifeft: and man, whilft under

the influence of their authority, however defpotic or
perverted, ftill retains a capacity for action and enjoyment, though he ceafes to be a rational or moral
agent.   But the fufpenfion of their operation ftops
at once all the movements of the mind, and feems to
annihilate every energy of the underftanding, the
affections, and the will.   On the 25th of October,
1778, a fea-faring perfon, about forty years of age,
was recommended as a patient to the Lunatic Afylum
in York.*   During his abode in the hofpital, he was
never obferved to exprefs any defire for fuftenance, or
to fhew any preference of it to his medicines.   The
firft fix weeks after his admiffion, he was fed in the
manner of an infant; a fervant undreffed him at
night, and dreffed him in the morning; after which
he was conducted to his feat in the common parlour,
where he remained all day, with his body bent, and
his eyes fixed upon the ground.   Every thing was
indifferent to him; and he was regarded by all about
him as endued with little more than vegetable life.
In this ftate of infenfibility he remained five years
and fix months.   But, the 14th of May, 1782, on
his entrance into the parlour, he faluted the convalefcents with the words, *Good-morrow to you all.*
He then thanked the fervants of the houfe in the
moft affectionate manner for their tendernefs to him, of
which he had begun to be fenfible fome weeks before,

---

* This cafe was lately tranfmitted to me, by my friend Dr. Hunter, of York, to be communicated to the Literary and Philofophical
Society of Manchefter. I have given only an abridgment of it.

but till then had not refolution to exprefs his gratitude. A few days after this unexpected recovery,
he was permitted to write a letter to his wife, in which
he expreffed himfelf with becoming propriety. At
this time he feemed to take peculiar pleafure in the
enjoyment of the open air, and in his walks converfed
with freedom and ferenity. On making inquiry
concerning what he felt during the fufpenfion of his
intellectual and fenfitive powers, he replied, that his
mind had been *totally loft*; but that about two months
before his full reftoration to himfelf. he began to have
thoughts and fenfations, which at firft ferved only to
excite in him fears and apprehenfions, efpecially in
the night-time. On the 28th of May, 1782, he returned to his family, and has now the command of a
fhip employed in the Baltic trade.

SECTION II.

I. IT is highly inftructive, as well as curious, to
contemplate the progreffive influence of particular
affociations on the affections and the judgment, as
they gradually acquire the force of habit by time,
and vividnefs by frequent renewal. Dr. Swift, in a
letter to Lord Bolingbroke, dated 1729, expreffes
himfelf in the following terms: " I remember, when
" I was a little boy, I felt a great fifh at the end of
" my line, which I drew up almoft on the ground,
" but it dropt in, and the difappointment vexes me
" to this very day, and I believe it was the type of
" all my future difappointments." This little incident, perhaps, gave the firft wrong bias to a mind
predifpofed to fuch impreffions; and by operating
with fo much ftrength and permanency, it might
poffibly lay the foundation of the Dean's fubfequent
peevifhnefs, paffion, mifanthropy, and final infanity.
The quicknefs of his fenfibility furnifhed a fting to
the flighteft difappointment; and pride feftered thofe
wounds which felf-government would inftantly have
healed. As children couple hobgoblins with darknefs, every contradiction of his humour, every obftacle
to his preferment, was by him affociated with ideas
of malignity and evil. By degrees, he acquired a

contempt of human nature, and a hatred of mankind, which, at laſt, terminated in the total abolition of his rational faculties.

This is no exaggerated picture, and we have the Dean's own authority for its accuracy. "The chief "end," ſays he, in a letter to Mr. Pope, "I propoſe "to myſelf in all my labours, is to vex the world, "rather than divert it; and if I could compaſs that "deſign, without hurting my own perſon or fortune, "I would be the moſt indefatigable writer you have "ever ſeen. I have ever hated all nations, profeſ- "ſions, and communities; and all my love is towards "individuals. For inſtance; I hate the tribe of "lawyers, but I love Counſellor ſuch a one, and "Judge ſuch a one. 'Tis ſo with phyſicians, (I will "not ſpeak of my own trade,) ſoldiers, Engliſh, "Scotch, French, and the reſt. But principally I "hate and deteſt that animal called man, although "I heartily love John, Peter, Thomas, and ſo forth. "This is the ſyſtem upon which I have governed "myſelf many years, (but do not tell,) and ſo I ſhall "go on till I have done with them."*

This letter is not written in a ſtrain which will ſuffer the moſt indulgent critic to aſcribe it to jocularity. And in the epitaph which the Dean compoſed for himſelf long afterwards, and which is inſcribed on his monument in the cathedral of St. Patrick's, he has left a ſolemn and deciſive memorial of his miſanthropy.

* Pope's Works, vol. ix. lett. 2.

HIC DEPOSITUM EST CORPUS
JONATHAN SWIFT, S. T. P.
UBI SÆVA INDIGNATIO
ULTERIUS COR LACERARE NEQUIT,
&c.

The ftrongeft tint in the complexion of the human character may be fometimes formed by a circumftance or event apparently cafual; which, by forcibly impreffing the mind, produces a lafting affociation, that gives an uniform direction to the efforts of the underftanding, and the feelings of the heart.

Dr. Conyers Middleton, one of the moft learned, various, and elegant writers of the prefent age, is faid to have been much more addicted, in the early part of his life, to mufic than to fcience. But he was roufed from his favourite amufement, and ftimulated to the clofeft application to ftudy, by a farcafm of his rival and enemy, the celebrated Dr. Bentley, who ftigmatized him with the name of fidler.* And indignation made him eager to convince the Doctor and the world that he could *write* as well as *fiddle*; a conviction, of which his opponent had afterwards the moft painful experience.†

The author of the *Night Thoughts,* a poem which contains the tendereft touches of nature and paffion, and the fublimeft truths of morality and religion, intermixed with frivolous conceits, turgid obfcurities, and gloomy views of human life, wrote that work under the recent preffure of forrow for the lofs of his

* Gent. Mag. 1773, page 387.   † Britifh Biog. vol. ix.

wife, and of a fon and daughter-in-law, whom he
loved with paternal tendernefs. Thefe feveral events
happened within the fhort period of three months, as
appears from the following apoftrophe to death:

" Infatiate archer! could not *one* fuffice?
" Thy fhaft flew *thrice*; and *thrice* my peace was flain;
" And *thrice*, ere *thrice* yon moon had fill'd her horns."*

But though time alleviated this diftrefs, his mind,
probably, acquired from it a tincture of melancholy,
which continued through life, and caft a fable hue
even on his very amufements. The like difpofition
alfo difcovered itfelf in his rural improvements. He
had an alcove in his garden, fo painted as to feem at
a diftance furnifhed with a bench or feat, which
invited to repofe; and when, upon a nearer approach,
the deception was perceived, this motto at the fame
time prefented itfelf to the eye—

Invifibilia non decipiunt.
The things unfeen do not deceive us.†

The following witty allufion bears the marks of a
fimilar turn of thought. The Doctor paid a vifit to
Archbifhop Potter's fon, then rector of Chiddinftone,
near Tunbridge. This gentleman lived in a country,
where the roads were deep and miry; and when Dr.
Young, after fome danger and difficulty, arrived at
his houfe, he inquired, " Whofe field is that which I
" have croffed?" ' It is mine,' anfwered his friend.

* Night Thoughts.
† Britifh Biography, vol. ix.

"True," faid the Poet, "*Potter's field, to bury*
"*ſtrangers in.*"*

II. It is a very important office of education to
guard the underſtanding againſt the union of ideas
which have no natural or proper connection. Yet
this object is lefs attended to than any other; and we
often find men diftinguiſhed for genius, erudition,
and even ſtrength of mind, warped by the falfe conceptions, and governed by the prejudices of puerility.
Creduloufnefs is the concomitant of the firſt ſtages of
life; and is indeed the principle on which all inſtruction muſt be founded. But it lays the mind open to
impreſſions of error, as well as of truth: and when
fuffered to combine itfelf with that paſſion for the
marvellous which all children difcover, it fofters the
rankeſt weeds of chimera and fuperſtition; rooting
firmly in the mind *all that the nurfe, and all the prieſt
have taught.* Hence the awful folemnity of *darknefs
viſible*, and of what the poet has denominated *a dim
religious light:* together with the terrors of evil
omens, of haunted places, and of ghaſtly fpectres:

  " Of calling ſhapes, and beckoning ſhadows dire;
  " And airy tongues, that fyllable men's names
  " On fands, and ſhores, and defert wilderneſſes."†

Hiſtory prefents us with few characters fuperior to
thofe of Henry the Fourth of France, and his prime
miniſter the Duke of Sully. But notwithanding the
wifdom, knowledge, and difcernment of thefe great

* Gent. Mag. July 1781, p. 319.   † Milton's Comus.

men, they appear on feveral occafions to have been actuated by their juvenile affociations in favour of aftrology. What can be more foreign to the events of human life, what lefs adapted to excite fear or hope in the mind of an intelligent man, than the afpect of a diftant ftar, or the variegated lines of his hand? Yet Sully confeffes, that an early prepoffeffion had made him weak enough to give credit to predictions derived from this fanciful origin: and though he informs us that the king, his mafter, was of opinion religion ought to infpire a contempt of fuch prophecies, the converfation which he relates at the fame time, evidently betrays Henry's confidence in them. This matter is put beyond difpute by an incident which occurred foon after the birth of the Dauphin; the particulars of which I fhall recite from the memoirs of this excellent writer.

" La Riviere was the king's firft phyfician,* a man " who had little more religion than thofe generally " poffefs who blend it with judicial aftrology. Henry " already felt a tendernefs for his fon, which filled him

---

* It fhould feem that aftrology was confidered formerly as an effential part of the learning of a phyfician; for Chaucer, in the prologue to the Canterbury Tales, has thus characterized him:

" With us there was a doctor of phyfik,
" In al the worlde was ther non hym lyk,
" To fpeke of phyfik and of furgerye;
" For he was groundit in aftronomy.
" He kept his pacient a ful gret del
" In hourys by his magyk naturel;
" Wel couth he fortunen the afcendent
" Of his ymagys for his pacient."

" with an eager anxiety to know his fate; and having
" heard that La Riviere succeeded wonderfully in
" his predictions, he commanded him to calculate
" the Dauphin's nativity with all the ceremonials of
" art. To aid this business, he had carefully sought
" for the most accurate watch which could be pro-
" cured; that the precise moment of the prince's
" birth might be exactly ascertained. About a fort-
" night afterwards, the king and Sully being alone
" together, their conversation turned upon the pre-
" diction of the astrologer La Brosse, concerning his
" majesty. This renewed Henry's solicitude with
" respect to his son; and he ordered La Riviere to
" be called. ' Monsieur La Riviere,' said the king,
" what have you discovered relative to the Dauphin's
" destiny?' " I had begun my calculations," replied
" Riviere, " but I left them unfinished, not caring
" to amuse myself any longer with a science which I
" have always believed to be in some degree cri-
" minal." The king, dissatisfied with this answer,
" commanded his physician to speak freely, and with-
" out concealment, on pain of his displeasure. La
" Riviere suffered himself to be pressed still longer;
" but at last, with an air of apparent discontent, he
" delivered himself in the following terms: ' Sire,
" your son will complete the common period of
" human life, and will reign longer than you shall do;
" but his turn of mind will be widely different from
" yours. He will be obstinate in opinion, often
" governed by his own whims, and sometimes by

" thofe of others.   Under his adminiftration it will
" be fafer to think than to fpeak.   Impending ruin
" threatens your former fociety.   He will perform
" great exploits, be fortunate in his defigns, and make
" a diftinguifhed figure in Europe.   There will be a
" viciffitude of peace and war in his time.   He will
" have children, and after his death affairs will grow
" worfe and worfe.   This is all you can know from
" me,' concluded La Riviere, ' and more than I had
" I refolved to tell you.'   His Majefty and the Duke
" of Sully remained a long time together, making re-
" flections on the words of the aftrologer, which left
" a ftrong impreffion on the mind of the king."

III. Ludicrous Associations, not founded in
truth or nature, are peculiarly unfavourable to the
principles and practice of virtue and religion.   Reafon,
efpecially during the period of youth, affords but a
feeble barrier againft the attacks of ridicule; and the
mind that is enflaved by its influence, may be fo far
deluded or depraved, as to lofe the fufceptibility of
good impreffions, or to contemplate the moft amiable
moral affections with derifion, fhame, and even difguft,

-------------- " Here fubdued
" By frontlefs laughter, and the hardy fcorn
" Of old unfeeling vice, the abject foul
" With blufhes half refigns the candid praife
" Of temperance and honour ; half difowns
" A free man's hatred of tyrannic pride;
" And hears with fickly fmiles the venal mouth
" With fouleft licence mock the patriot's name."*

* Akenfide's Pleafures of Imagination, book iii.

The celebrated Dr. Pitcairn was no lefs diftinguifhed for wit than learning. It is recorded, that
as he paffed one day along the ftreets, he beheld the
affecting fpectacle of a mafon killed by the fall, and
buried in the ruins, of a chimney, which he had juft
completed. " Bleffed are the dead who die in the
" Lord," faid he, " for they reft from their la-
" bours, and their works follow them." Such a
humorous conjunction of refembling yet incongruous
ideas probably ftifled in his breaft the fentiments of
compaffion: and I have been informed by a very
humane friend, that on the relation of a melancholy
event, fimilar in its circumftances, the recollection of
this ludicrous remark fubftituted in his mind emotions
of laughter for thofe of commiferation.

The natural propenfity of Dean Swift led him to
the indulgence of this fpecies of drollery, very much
to the prejudice of every finer feeling of the heart.
In one of his letters he laments the mortal illnefs of
his amiable friend Arbuthnot; but mixes with his
expreffions of forrow certain whimfical reflections,
which convert his mourning into grimace. " There
" is a paffage in Bede," fays he to Mr. Pope,
" highly commending the piety and learning of the
" Irifh in that age; where, after abundance of
" praifes, he overthrows them all, by lamenting, that
" alas! they kept Eafter at a wrong time of the
" year. So our Doctor has every quality and virtue
" that can make a man amiable or ufeful; but *alas!*
" he hath *a fort of flouch in his walk.* I pray God

" protect him, for he is an excellent Christian, though
" not a Catholic."*

When the mind has been long habituated to the
assemblage of ludicrous ideas, they recur on very
improper occasions, not only spontaneously, but even
in despite of every effort of the judgment and the will.
In this state, elevation of thought and dignity of
character are unattainable; and seriousness, when
assumed, is always marked with some glaring and
risible inconsistency. Swift, in his last testament,
bequeaths three old hats, and other still more trifling
and absurd legacies, with farcical solemnity: and the
celebrated Hogarth could not help displaying traits of
humour in his gravest historical paintings. I have
heard it remarked by one who was sometimes the
companion of his walks, that he would interrupt the
most interesting conversation to laugh at any oddity
which presented itself, and that his eyes were con-
stantly cast about in search of objects singular and
diverting. When a man of this turn applies himself
to books, it is not instruction or rational criticism, but
hilarity, that is his pursuit: and he finds food for his
prevailing appetite, equally palatable, both in the
beauties and the blemishes of his author. For Tully
has well observed, that the *verbum ardens*, the glowing boldness of expression which sublimity of senti-
ment inspires, may be easily rendered ludicrous by
an illiberal paraphrase. Even entire productions of
some of the best writers have been thus misrepresented

* Pope's Works, vol. ix. lett. 11.

and deformed, for the purpofe of merriment, under
the title of Travefties: and the bulk of mankind are
readily deceived into the belief that what gives rife
to laughter is in itfelf ridiculous. For this reafon, a·
reader of fenfibility, who has the intereft of virtue
and religion at heart, will perufe with pain and difguft
the *Meditations on a Broomftick, written according to
the ftyle and manner of the Honourable Robert Boyle.**
" To what a height," fays Lord Orrery, " muft·
" the fpirit of farcafm arife in an author, who could
" prevail upon himfelf to ridicule fuch a man as Mr.
" Boyle! But the fword of wit, like the fcythe of
" time, cuts down friend and foe, and attacks every
" thing that accidentally lies in its way." It muft be
confeffed, however, that this great and good philofopher has indulged in his theological writings certain
conceits, which will draw a fmile from his warmeft
admirers, A zeal to promote the habit of pious and
moral reflections has fometimes tempted him to force
ideas into the moft unnatural alliance; and to deduce
very important analogies from objects or circumftances not only incongruous, but low and con-
temptible. Thus, from the ftumbling of a horfe in a
good road, he infers the danger of profperity; from
being let blood in a fever, he juftifies the wifdom of
the Deity, in depriving his creatures of fpiritual
fuperfluities; and from a diftafte of the fyrups prefcribed by his phyfician, he concludes that the good
things of life are not objects of envy, becaufe

* Swift's Works, vol. v. p. 372.

not always relifhed as enjoyments. But I feel a
reluctance to point out fuch trivial exuberances in the
works of Mr. Boyle. It is ungenerous to injure the
well-earned wreath of laurel which he wears, by
faftidioufly culling a few folitary leaves that are
withered. We fhould remember alfo, that dignity
and meannefs, grace and vulgarity, have, in many
inftances, no fixed ftandard; and are dependent on
certain acceffary affociations, which vary in different
countries, at different periods of time, and with different perfons even of the fame age and place. Jacob
is reprefented in the holy fcriptures, as calling his fons
together before his death, to deliver to each of them
his benediction; and in the language of metaphor
and prophecy, he fays, *Iffachar is a ftrong afs,*
couching down between two burdens : from which it
appears, that this animal was not then regarded as a
fymbol of ftupidity and infignificance. Ajax, retreat-
ing between two armies, is compared by Homer to
the lion for undaunted courage, and to the afs for
fullen and unyielding flownefs.* But Mr. Pope, in
his tranflation, has omitted the latter allufion, to ac-
commodate his word to the ftate of modern opinion.
The fame fublime poet exhibits the awful uncertainty
of victory, in the engagement between the Greeks
and Trojans, by the image of a poor woman weighing
wool in a pair of fcales; and Euftathius fays it was a
tradition, that Homer derived this fimile from the
occupation of his mother, who maintained herfelf by

* Iliad, lib. xi.

fuch manual labour.* But a ftill more remarkable comparifon occurs in the writings of this ancient bard: for Ulyffes, toffing about through the whole night, with reftlefs anxiety, is likened to a fat pudding frying on the fire.† Even Virgil, whofe elegance and correctnefs are univerfally acknowledged, has drawn the fimilitude of a queen (Amata, the wife of king Latinus) under the violence of paffion, from a company of boys whipping a top.‡

I do not recollect one coarfe allufion or low image in the whole poem of *Paradife Loft*; though feveral contained in it are fantaftical, being derived from the fictions of heathen mythology. But it is more than probable that Milton, when tranflated by foreigners, will not appear to deferve the character of undeviating dignity. For the correfpondent terms, in other languages, may have fecondary ideas of meannefs affixed to them, from which in the original they are exempt. The fame remark is applicable to other works; and it is particularly to be wifhed that the books of the Old and New Teftament, in the common verfion, were always perufed with a candid attention to it.

I have been told of a picture, which exhibits a burlefque view of the tablature, reprefenting the judgment of Hercules. The young hero is painted as a tall grenadier, Virtue as a methodift preacher, and Pleafure as a drunken ftrumpet. The parody, if this term can be applied to painting, may anfwer

---

* See the Notes of Dacier, Pope, and other commentators.

† Od. lib. xxi. ‡ Æn. lib. vii.

the purpofe of exciting laughter, but will counteract in the fpectator's mind all the beneficial effects of the moft inftructive and philofophical apologue of antiquity.

" Difcit enim citius, meminitque libentius illud,
" Quod quis deridet, quam quod probat et veneratur."

HOR.

PARODY is a favourite flower both of ancient and of modern literature.* It is a fpecies of ludicrous compofition, which derives its wit from affociation; and never fails to produce admiration and delight, when it unites tafte in felection with felicity of application. Even licentious fpecimens of it move to laughter; for we are always inclined to be diverted with mimickry, or ridiculous imitation, whether the original be an object of refpect, of indifference, or of contempt. A polifhed Athenian audience heard, with burfts of mirthful applaufe, the difcourfes of the venerable Socrates burlefqued upon the ftage; and no Englifhman can read the Rehearfal, without fmiling at the medley of borrowed abfurdities which it exhibits. Mr. Pope's *Dunciad*, and *Rape of the Lock*, abound with the moft admirable parodies; but fome of them may appear, to a religious mind, chargeable with levity and profanenefs. I fhall quote an example, both of the excellent and exceptionable; as the beauty of the one, and the fault of the other, equally relate to the fubject of the prefent effay.

---

* See Diog. Laertius, Lucian. Dialog, Boileau, Cervantes, Butler, Swift, &c. &c.

When the fatal rape was committed by the baron on Belinda's Lock, she is reprefented as attempting to revenge herfelf by her bodkin:—

> " Now meet thy fate, incens'd Belinda cry'd,
> " And drew a deadly bodkin from her fide.
> " The fame, his ancient perfonage to deck,
> " Her great great grandfire wore about his neck,
> " In three feal rings; which after, melted down,
> " Form'd a vaft buckle for his widow's gown:
> " Her infant grandame's whiftle next it grew,
> " 'The bells fhe jingled, and the whiftle blew;
> " Then in a bodkin graced her mother's hairs,
> " Which long fhe wore, and now Belinda wears."*

The unlearned reader will be ftruck with this fplendid genealogical defcription of an infignificant bodkin: but he who is verfed in the writings of Homer, will perufe it with additional delight, from the recollection of the analogy which it bears to the progrefs of Agamemnon's fceptre. In the third canto of the incomparable poem above referred to, a game of ombre is defcribed with all the *pathos* and folemnity which the heroic mufe can call forth; and the cards in Belinda's hand being pompoufly enumerated, viz.

> . . . . . " Four kings, in majefty rever'd,
> " With hoary whifkers, and a forky beard:
> " And four fair queens, whofe hands fuftain a flow'r,
> " Th' expreffive emblem of their fofter power."

The two following lines fucceed—

> " The fkilful nymph reviews her force with care,
> " *Let fpades be trumps! fhe faid; and trumps they were.*"

* Canto v. l. 87.

This parody of one of the moſt ſublime paſſages
in the Old Teſtament, *And God ſaid, Let there be
light, and there was light*, may, I think, be juſtly
deemed reprehenſible; as it tends to connect a ludicrous idea with that Being who ought never to be
thought of but with reverence.* But ſhould this
remark appear to be an overſtrained refinement, it
will be acknowledged that, in leſs dignified caſes,
very ſlight aſſociations of the burleſque kind have an
aſtoniſhing effect on the ſentiments and taſte of thoſe
who form them. When Thomſon's tragedy of Sophoniſba was firſt repreſented on the ſtage, the higheſt
expectations were formed of its theatrical merit. But
a waggiſh parody on the following line,

　　" O! Sophoniſba! Sophoniſba! O!"

---

* Pope ſeems to have been peculiarly fond of alluſions to this
paſſage of the Old Teſtament; but has been a little unfortunate in
the application of them. The truth is, that the ſentiment is too
ſublime either for burleſque or for compliment: and the extravagance of theſe lines, in his epitaph on Sir Iſaac Newton, offends
almoſt equally with the parody quoted above:—

　　" Nature, and Nature's laws, lay hid in night;
　　" God ſaid, *Let Newton be!* and all was light!"

This hyperbolical encomium is ſuch a profanation of ſacred writ
to monumental flattery, that it was juſtly ſatirized in the following
epigram, written by a young man, who has diſcloſed only the
initials of his name:—

　　" If Newton's exiſtence enlighten'd the whole,
　　" What part of expanſion inhabits the fool?
　　" If light had been total, as Pope hath averr'd,
　　" I. T. had been right, for he could not have err'd;
　　" But Pope has his faults, ſo excuſe a young ſpark;
　　" Bright Newton's deceas'd, and we're all in the dark."

damned the reputation of the play, and for a while
the town echoed with

O! Jemmy Thomſon! Jemmy Thomſon, O!*

It happened not long ſince, that a perſon of mean
rank was elected provoſt, or chief magiſtrate, of Aber-
deen. In the firſt moments of elevation, and whilſt
receiving the congratulations of his friends, he laid
his hands upon his breaſt, and very emphatically declared, that *after all he was but a mortal man.*

Is it poſſible for any one, under the impreſſion of
this ludicrous ſtory, to read without ſmiling the fact
related by Ælian, and quoted with great applauſe by
many other hiſtorians, viz. that Philip king of Macedon kept a perſon in his ſervice, whoſe office it
was to deliver to him daily the following admonition,
Remember, Philip, that thou art mortal! Perhaps if
ſuch an incident had occurred in Greece, during the
reign of that monarch, it might have turned into
ridicule the admiration in which his inſtitution was
held, by expoſing at once the abſurdity, pride, and
affected humility, on which it was founded.

The people improperly, becauſe opprobriouſly,
called Quakers, certainly merit a very high degree of
eſteem from their fellow-citizens, on account of their
induſtry, temperance, peaceableneſs, and catholic
ſpirit of charity. For notwithſtanding the enthuſi-
aſtic pretenſions of their founders to ſuperior ſanctity
and Divine inſpiration, they diſclaimed all dominion

* Johnſon's Lives of the Poets; Article—Thomſon.

over faith and confcience: and Barclay, their learned
apologift, wrote ably in defence of. religious liberty;
whilft Penn, as a law-giver and civil magiftrate, eftablifhed it, on the broadeft foundation, in his new
government of Pennfylvania.*   At a period, when
bigotry and perfecution were predominant through
the Chriftian world, fuch rational fentiments and
liberal conduct reflect the higheft honour on this fect.
But the fingularity of their apparel, manners, and
forms of worfhip, has expofed them to the keeneft
fhafts of ridicule.   And however illiberally and un-
juftifiably fuch offenfive weapons may have been
employed, they would in all probability have prevailed, if the converts and youth of this fect had not
been fortified againft them by the moft unremitting
ftrictnefs of their inftitutions.   Thefe are admirably
calculated to correct, or to prevent, all ludicrous
affociations; and to fupprefs, if poffible, the very
principle of laughter, as inconfiftent with the *ferious*

* This venerable man was fufpected of being a papift in difguife;
owing to the favour fhewn him by King James II.   To obviate fo
unjuft an opinion, feveral letters were written by him to Dr. Tillotfon, then dean of Canterbury, who, amongft others, had adopted
it; and in one of them he thus expreffes himfelf.   " I know not a
" jefuit or a prieft in the world : and yet I am catholic, though not a
" Roman.   I have bowels for mankind, and dare not deny others,
" what I crave for myfelf, I mean, liberty for the exercife of my
" religion; thinking faith, piety, and providence, a better fecurity
" than force; and that, when truth cannot prevail with her own
" weapons, all others will fail her.   I am no Roman Catholic, but
" a Chriftian, whofe creed is the Scripture, of the truth of which I
" hold a nobler evidence than the beft Church authority in the
" world."—Brit. Biog. vol. vii.

*nefs, gravity, and godly fear of the Gofpel.** It is
aftonifhing to obferve, in a large body of people, the
efficacy of a fet of practical maxims, utterly repugnant to nature: and the influence of them is early
vifible, even in their children, who difplay an invariable fteadinefs of countenance and deportment,
under circumftances which cover others of the fame
age, but differently educated, with the blufhes of
bafhful confufion. But there is now an increafing
relaxation of difcipline amongft the members of this
refpectable community; and their diftinguifhing modes
will gradually ceafe, as they become more and more
combined with the painful ideas of obloquy and
derifion in the minds of thofe who adopt them.

Piety to GOD, whether it refpects the inward fentiments and affections of the foul, or the outward
expreflions of them in homage and prayer, ought to
elevate us far above the reach of raillery, or the influence of low and ludicrous affociations. But unhappily, both the principle and practice of devotion
are too often debafed by fuperftition, deformed by
enthufiafm, and counterfeited by hypocrify: and as
thefe conftitute legitimate objects of ridicule and contempt, the fterling value of piety itfelf becomes de-
preciated by the union of a bafe and foreign alloy.
Such numbers *draw near to the Deity with their lips,
whilft their hearts are far from Him,* that a noble
writer has farcaftically obferved, " If we are told a
" man is religious, we ftill afk, what are his morals?

* Barclay's Apology for the Quakers, p. 136.

" But if we hear at firſt that he has honeſt morals,
" and is a man of natural juſtice and good temper,
" we ſeldom think of the other queſtion, whether he
" be religious and devout."* Theſe are conſiderations, which operate powerfully on the mind: and
if they be ſtrengthened by the ideas of ungraceful
geſtures, diſſonant tones of voice, or other extravagancies in devotion, ſuch a degree of timidity and
falſe delicacy may be created, as entirely to depreſs
the fervour which theſe exerciſes are adapted to excite. Prayer may then be performed as a duty, but
will not be felt as a privilege; and the creature will
even bluſh at the higheſt honour he can enjoy, that
of holding communion with his Creator. Many an
ingenuous youth has been deſpoiled of this glorious
diſtinction of humanity by the ſneers and jeſts of his
companions: and of the military profeſſion it is ſaid,
that an officer would rather face the mouth of a
cannon, than be found privately in the poſture of
ſupplication. Dr. Swift ſeems to have been governed, in his religious obſervances, by ſome ſuch
ill-grounded aſſociation. His conſtant preſence at
church, whilſt he reſided at the deanery of St. Patrick's, he knew would be expected; but he was
ſeduloufly careful to conceal whatever had the appearance of voluntary devotion. When he was in London, therefore, he never attended divine ſervice but
at a very early hour in the morning: and though
he practiſed family prayer in his houſe, his ſervants

* Lord Shafteſbury's Claracteriſtics.

affembled, as it were, by ftealth ; fo that Dr. Delany
lived fix months with him before he difcovered it.*

I hope it will not be underftood from what has
been advanced on the topic of ludicrous affociations,
that I am averfe to laughter, or an enemy to wit and
pleafantry. Human life, without their exhilarating
influence, would be a fcene of anxious care or phlegmatic dulnefs. Nor is the harfher controul of ridicule to be wholly condemned or rejected. It is
neceffary to reftrain the irregular fallies of folly ; and,
as thefe often proceed from a lively imagination, the
fenfe of it is happily acuteft, where its correction is
moft required.

IV. There are few people who have not, at particular feafons, experienced the effect of certain accidental affociations which obtrude one impertinent
idea, or fet of ideas, on the mind, to the exclufion of
every other. Mr. Locke has noticed this weaknefs,
and he humoroufly defcribes it, " as a childifhnefs of
" the underftanding, wherein, during the fit, it plays
" with and dandles fome infignificant puppet, without
" any end in view."† Thus a tune, a proverb, a

* Brit. Biog. vol. viii. Johnfon's Lives of the Poets; article Swift.
—Dr. Swift furnifhes an excellent fubject for the moral anatomift.
His life was eventful; his paffions were various and ftrong; and his
fenfibilities acute in the extreme. Self-indulgence gave every fpring
to action, within him, its full power; and pride prevented the concealment of its operation. Hence the motives, which directed his
conduct, were feldom either extraneous or complex; and they are
generally eafy to be traced to their fource.

† Lock's Conduct of the Underftanding.

H 2

scrap of poetry, or some other trivial object, will
steal into the thoughts, and continue to possess them
long after it ceases to be amusing. Persuasives to
dismiss a guest that proves so troublesome can hardly
be necessary; and bodily exertion is generally the
best remedy for this mental infirmity. But there is
another state of mind dependent on the laws of
association, which is more dangerous, because it invites to indulgence. It consists in reveries, gay visions
of fancy, the creation of air-built castles, and cobweb
hypotheses. Men of genius alone are incident to these
flattering delusions; and they too often implicitly give
way to them. But in proportion as they prevail,
reason and judgment are impaired, study becomes
formal dullness, activity toilsome, and the necessary
offices of life are neglected. Thomson has thus beau-
tifully pictured such a character:—

" There was a man of special grave remark;
" A certain tender gloom o'erspread his face,
" Pensive, not sad, in thought involv'd, not dark;
" As sweet this wight could sing as morning lark,
" And teach the noblest morals of the heart:
" But these his talents were y' buried stark.
" To noon-tide shades incontinent he ran,
" Where purls the brook with sleep-inviting sound,
" There would he linger till the latest ray
" Of light sat trembling on the welkin's bound.
" Oft has he travers'd the cœrulean field,
" And mark'd the clouds, that drove before the wind;
" Ten thousand glorious systems would he build,
" Ten thousand great ideas fill'd his mind;
" But with the clouds they fell, and left no trace behind."

CASTLE OF INDOLENCE, Canto I.

V. It has been remarked, that gameſters, ſailors, and others who are under the influence of what is vulgarly, but very improperly, termed *chance*, that is, of cauſes not within the reach of human power to direct, nor of human ſagacity to diſcern, are extremely prone to ſuperſtition. Their hopes and fears, their confidence and deſpair, are founded on circumſtances which bear only a fanciful relation to the events that are to come. Imagination connects the ideas of magnitude and importance with the ſlighteſt cauſes, which are viewed in obſcurity, as objects appear largeſt to our ſenſes during twilight. A gameſter lays great ſtreſs on the luck of a ſeat, or the ſhake of a die: and I remember in croſſing a ferry, whilſt it was very calm, the boatman whiſtled more than three hours a particular ſet of notes, to forward the motion of his veſſel, crying out at ſhort intervals, *Blow, good wind, blow; blow a briſk gale!* and if a gentle gale ſprung up, he redoubled his efforts in the fulleſt aſſurance of ſucceſs. The abſolute truſt, repoſed in empirical medicines, ariſes from a ſimilar deception; and the miraculous operation often aſcribed to them even by perſons of judgment and education, is a proof of the aſtoniſhing power of wrong aſſociations. The wiſe Emperor Marcus Aurelius was ſo firmly perſuaded of the efficacy of a certain antidote, called *theriaca*, to reſiſt every ſpecies of poiſon, that he made uſe of it daily, to the great injury of his health; for his head became affected to ſuch a degree that he dozed in the midſt of buſineſs;

and when opium was left out of the compofition, an
obftinate watchfulnefs enfued.*

The fame principle of affociations explains the
dogmatifm of the critic and the antiquarian, whofe
pofitivenefs refpecting the conftruction of a fentence,
or the letters of a worn-out infcription, is often in
exact proportion to their uncertainty. When any
one foars with great ardour into the regions of conjecture, the airy phantoms which he meets with will
be contemplated by him as fubftantial realities; and
he will purfue truth, not with a temperate and rational zeal, but with the blind enthufiam of love; dig-
nifying, like a paffionate *inamorato*, every conceit of
his mind, and admiring difcoveries which exift no
where but in his own brain. Thefe reflections have
been in part fuggefted by the perufal of the memoirs
of Mr. Whifton; a man whofe genius, learning, and
integrity, might have placed him high in the fcale of
excellence, had he not fuffered a perverted imagination to ufurp the juft authority of judgment. " The
" warmth of his temper difpofed him to receive any
" fudden thoughts, any thing that ftruck his fancy,
" when favourable to his preconceived fcheme of
" things, or to any new fchemes of things, which
" ferved, in his opinion, a religious purpofe."†
With fuch propenfities he wrote *An Effay on the Revelation of St. John:* and being appointed the following year (1707) to preach Mr. Boyle's lectures,

* Galen de Antidotis, lib. i. cap. 1.
† Mr. Collins.

he chofe for his fubject, the *accomplifhment of Scripture prophecies.* In 1712, when Prince Eugene of Savoy was in England, he dedicated a work to him in which *he interpreted the end of the hour, and day, and month, and year, for the Ottoman devaftations,* (Apoc. ix. 15,) *to have been put by his glorious victory over the Turks, September 1ft,* 1697, *(O. S.) or the fucceeding peace of Carlowitz,* 1698.* His favourite conceptions were now fo ftrongly riveted in his mind, that he difcerned clearly all the revolutions of paft and future ages in the writings of the Prophets, or the Revelations of St. John. Such indeed was the afcendancy of thefe abfurd affociations over his underftanding, that he gave entire credit to the impudent impofture of Mary Tofts, a woman of Godalmin, who pretended to be delivered of rabbits, becaufe her monftrous births were deemed by him to be the exact completion of an old prediction in Efdras.†

In almoft every cafe of wrong affociations, the underftanding either voluntarily fufpends its controuling and directing power, or is deluded into a conformity with fancy; and the mind ftill retains a confcioufnefs of freedom, and of moral agency. But there are certain habits which ufurp, by *force,* the dominion of reafon, and compel the will to gratify inordinate defires, by the choice of known evil in pre-

* Prince Eugene feems to have been pleafed with the honour of the difcovery, that he was the object of fo ancient a prediction; for he prefented Mr. Whifton, on this occafion, with a purfe of gold.—See Brit. Biog. vol. viii. p. 247.

† Gent. Mag. July, 1781, p. 321.

ference to acknowledged good. The lamentation of
the poet, *video meliora proboque, deteriora sequor*, seems
also to have been felt by St. Paul, who says, Rom.
vii. 11, *That which I do, I allow not; for what I
would, that I do not; but what I hate, that I do. If
then I do that which I would not, I consent unto the
law, that it is good. Now then it is no more I that
do, but sin that dwelleth in me.* If an enlightened
Apostle speak in such abasing terms of himself, with
how much more truth and propriety might the same
language have been adopted by a late advocate for
the divine dispensation of the Gospel. For charity
inclines me to hope, that the learned author of the
Christian Hero *wrote* in consistency with, whilst he
acted in opposition to, his most serious conviction.
This work, Sir Richard Steele informs us,* was composed by him principally with a view to contrast im-
pressions of piety and virtue with the strong propensity
which he experienced to licentious pleasures. For he
says, even when rioting in scenes of debauchery, he
was deeply conscious of the impropriety of his conduct, and condemned those unlawful gratifications
which he had not resolution to renounce. His
Christian Hero, however, whilst the treatise remained
privately in his own hands, afforded but a weak and
ineffectual check to his vicious pursuits. He therefore determined to publish it, that by thus placing
himself in a new light before his acquaintance, he
might be restrained from guilt by an explicit and

---

* See his Apology for himself and his writings.

avowed teftimony in favour of goodnefs. But it
does not appear that this fingular experiment proved
fuccefsful. Steele forfook not his debaucheries; and
by having affected the faint, he aggravated, in the
opinion of his friends, his condemnation as a finner.
Yet Mr. Pope, who knew him well, juftified him
from the imputation of hypocrify; and always regarded him as a real lover of virtue in *theory*, though
a flave to vice in *practice.**

Many other examples might be adduced of the
force of evil habits, and the pernicious influence of
falfe affociations, whether intellectual or moral;
but to dwell long on the fhades of the human character is apt to abate our benevolence to mankind,
and to impair the principle of veneration towards
the great Author of our nature. More pleafing would
be the tafk, and I will add, more eafy to vindicate the wifdom of the Divine laws, by fhewing, that
the power of habit, and the propenfity to combine
ideas together, are effential to the juft conftitution of
the mind; and that without their well-regulated aid,
knowledge would be unattainable, virtue a tranfient
emotion or defultory act, and life itfelf a fcene of indifference and infipidity.

* Ruffhead's Life of Pope, p. 493. Brit. Biog. vol. viii.

ON

INCONSISTENCY OF EXPECTATION

IN

LITERARY PURSUITS.

——⫸⟨◇⟩⫷——

" RETINUIT, QUOD EST DIFFICILLIMUM, EX SAPIENTIA
" MODUM." TACIT. VIT. AGRICOL.

INCONSISTENCY OF EXPECTATION

IN

LITERARY PURSUITS.

———

" He, who hath treafures of his own,
" May leave a cottage, or a throne;
" May quit the world to dwell alone,
" Within his fpacious mind."

———

WHERE, amongft the men of fcience, is the archetype to be found of a picture fo flattering to human pride? The original, from which it appears to have been drawn, was indeed an exalted character; but at the fame time, alas! a feeble valetudinarian, who muft have experienced thofe mortifying impediments to mental exertion, which arife from a conftitution naturally delicate, and broken by laborious refearches into truth. Under fuch circumftances, could it be affirmed, that

" Locke had a foul,
" Wide as the fea,
" Calm as the night,
" Bright as the day;
" There might his vaft ideas play,
" Nor feel a thought confin'd."

The amiable poet,* who has thus pourtrayed, with the glowing colours of admiration and refpect, one of the moft diftinguifhed ornaments of the human fpecies, paffed himfelf a life of lingering ficknefs: and though his genius was fertile, and his induftry wonderfully and varioufly productive, yet fuch was his fenfibility of the obftructions he had to furmount, that he made a painful and humiliating calculation of the days, months, and years, which he had loft even by his flighteft malady, the tooth-ach. The celebrated Mr. Pafchal languifhed four years under a diftemper, which, without manifefting itfelf by many outward figns, or occafioning confinement, debarred him of the pleafures and improvements of ftudy; and it was the anxious office of his friends to guard him from writing or fpeaking on any topics which might exercife much thought or attention.† Mr. Pope's vital functions were fo difordered, that his life is emphatically faid to have been a *long difeafe*. The head-ach was his moft frequent affailant; and he ufed to relieve it by inhaling the fteams of coffee, which he often required during thofe hours that fhould have afforded the refrefhment of fleep. Such was his earneftnefs and folicitude in the pro- fecution of his literary undertakings, that Swift complains he was never at leifure for converfation : and one of Lord Oxford's domeftics related, that in the fevere winter of 1740, fhe was called from her bed four times in one night to fupply him with

* Dr. Watts.   † Preface to Pafcal's Thoughts.

paper, that he might not lofe a thought.* The learned biographer who farcaftically records this fact, acknowledges in the preface to the moft laborious of his works, that he himfelf *triumphed* in the acquifitions which he fhould difplay to mankind, and indulged all the dreams of a poet, doomed at laft to wake a lexicographer. For he found that " one " inquiry only gave occafion to another; that book " referred to book; that to fearch was not always " to find; and to find was not always to be in- " formed; and that thus to purfue perfection was, " like the firft inhabitants of Arcadia, to chace the " fun, which, when they had reached the hill where " he feemed to reft, was ftill beheld at the fame " diftance from them." There is a paffage in Thomfon's *Caftle of Indolence* fo applicable to this kind of folly, that I am tempted to tranfcribe it:

" This globe pourtray'd the race of learned men,
" Still at their books, and turning o'er the page
" Backwards and forwards: oft they fnatch the pen,
" As if infpir'd, and in a Thefpian rage,
" Then write and blot, as would your ruth engage.
" Why, authors! all this fcrawl and fcribbling fore?
" To lofe the prefent, gain the future age,
" Praifed to be, when you can hear no more:
" And much enrich'd with fame, when ufelefs worldly ftore?"†

The examples which I have recited are of men occupied chiefly, if not folely, in the walks of literature: but the tafte for knowledge may be cultivated fuccefsfully in the bufy fcenes of active life. And

* Johnfon's Lives of the Poets.
† Thomfon's Caftle of Indolence, Canto I.

under thefe circumftances aftonifhing proficiency has been made by the combined powers of genius and induftry. The works of Tully, Pliny the elder, Bacon, Temple, and Bolingbroke, not to mention various other names of ancient and modern times, are fufficient evidences of this fact. But neither the efforts of genius nor of induftry can ward off ficknefs, obviate folicitude, or ftop thofe unacountable ebbings of the mind, which even a lowering fky will fometimes produce. Cicero, notwithftanding all his exultation on the foothing influence of philofophy, found himfelf under the neceffity of retiring at certain feafons to one of his country villas, fituated near Aftura; and in this folitary refidence, which was covered with a thick wood cut into fhady walks, he ufed to pafs his hours of fpleen and melancholy.*

But could we fuppofe health to be enjoyed without interruption, the fpirits to be always lively and active, and all the intellectual faculties in a ftate of uniform compofure and energy; yet ftill the progrefs in knowledge would be retarded by error, and obftructed by the want of thofe materials for which we muft depend on the accuracy, induftry, and attainments of others. The temple of fcience requires for its elevation the united labours of myriads of different artifts; and the conftruction of it will be perpetually incident to delays, by the indolence, unfkilfulnefs, and miftakes of thofe who are employed in the undertaking. In fuch circumftances, to unite ardour with ferenity, an en-

* Middleton's Life of Cicero, vol. iii. page 296.

thufiafm for fcience with patience under all the obftructions of purfuit, from outward accident or inward
infirmity, is a happinefs of which few can boaft.*
And the page of biography is filled with narratives
of the queruloufnefs, impaired health, and mental
imbecility of thofe, who, by their writings, have informed, enlightened, and charmed mankind. Juft
views of the defigns of Providence in the government
of the world, and particularly in the ftructure of the
human mind with refpect to the progreffive evolution
of its faculties, would tend to obviate thefe evils, by
reftraining the inordinate afpirations of literary ambition, and by correcting the inconfiftency of expectation from which they proceed.

Man is evidently conftituted for two great ends;
the attainment of virtue, and of knowledge. All his
mental endowments have a reference to one or other
of thefe final caufes: on them, therefore, muft depend
the *perfection* and *felicity* of his nature. But his
moral powers feem more circumfcribed in their operation, and confequently to admit of lefs extenfive
culture, than thofe of his underftanding. For they
are confined within the limits of rational, or at moft
of fenfitive being, and with fuch they can hold only a
partial and contracted correfpondence; whilft the intellectual faculties have for their object the whole
fyftem of nature, the infinitude of which is, perhaps,

* Sir Ifaac Newton affords a fingular example of temperate ardour, unremitting energy, and almoft invariable equanimity.

not lefs apparent in its minutenefs than immenfity
From thefe confiderations I am inclined to believe,
that our ftation in the prefent world is intended for
near approaches towards the *maturity* of *virtue*;
but for the *infancy* only of *knowledge*. And the
wifdom of this ordinance of the Deity is fufficiently
difcernible: for as *knowledge* is *power*, the antecedent
poffeffion of goodnefs, to direct it, muft be effentially
neceffary to beatitude: The paffions and affections
are of fpeedy growth, and often manifeft great vigour
in that feafon of life which is marked by the feeble-
nefs of reafon. Increafing years modify, direct, and
meliorate them; but the difcipline of experience
ferves rather to balance and reftrain, than to augment,
their native ftrength and energy. On the contrary,
the mind proceeds by flow and regular gradations,
in the attainment of fcience: and our acquifitions
confift not folely in the difcovery of new objects or
phœnomena; but in the comparifon of thefe with
what we already know,* and in afcertaining their reciprocal dependencies, relations, or contrarieties. Thus
knowledge is multiplied beyond the fum of its feparate and component parts; and every acceffion to it
increafes the ftock in a 'ratio, that, we may devoutly
truft, will become greater and greater through all
eternity.

But the bulk of mankind, in this ftage of exiftence,
are in circumftances which preclude any confiderable

---

* Maclaurin's View of Sir Ifaac Newton's Philofophy.

advancement in learning: and we may obferve, that the difpenfation of the Gofpel gives no *direct* encouragement to it,† but applies all its precepts and exhortations to the cultivation of the heart. For the principles and practice of virtue are accommodated to every period and condition of life; and are exercifed, refined, and exalted, even by poverty, infirmity, ficknefs, and old age; all which check the exertions and deprefs the vigour of human genius. Rectitude of difpofition and of conduct bears a precife and permanent relation to all times, perfons, and occurrences. And if we afcend from particular to general excellence, by contemplating the duty of man in the aggregate, we may form a diftinct and adequate idea of *moral perfection.* But what mind can expand itfelf to the conception of *complete intelligence!* Every ftep of our afcent on the hill of fcience prefents to the view a widening horizon; and the boundary of darknefs increafes, in proportion to the amplitude of thofe enlightened regions which it encircles.

It is this endlefs progreffion of knowledge which is apt to give the *love* of it an inordinate afcendancy over every other principle, fo as to render it the *ruling paffion* of the mind. And as this paffion does not,

† Many paffages in the New Teftament, according to a literal interpretation, feem *directly levelled againft* human learning; which is defcribed as vain, deceitful, traditionary, confifting of endlefs genealogies, idle bablings, and profane fables. But the beft commentators are of opinion that thefe cenfures have a reference only to the abfurd philofophy of the Gnoftics or Sophifts, which was derived from the Egyptians.

like the love of virtue, temper its particular exertions,
by preferving a due fubordination in the powers which
it calls forth into action, the wildeft extravagancies of
emotion and of conduct have been difplayed by thofe
who fubmit to its uncontrouled dominion.   A great
philofopher has rufhed naked from the bath into the
ftreets of a populous city, frantic with joy on the
folution of an interefting problem.   Tacitus informs
us, that his excellent father-in-law, Agricola, " was
" inclined to have engaged more deeply in the ftudies
" of philofophy and law than was fuitable to a
" Roman and a fenator, if the difcretion of his mother
" had not reftrained the warmth and vehemence of
" his difpofition : for his high fpirit, inflamed by the
" charms of glory and exalted reputation, led him to
" the purfuit with more eagernefs than judgment.
" Reafon, and ripcr years, mitigated his ardour;
" and what is a *moft difficult tafk*, *he preferved mo-*
" *deration in fcience itfelf.*"*   The emperor Marcus
Antoninus, in one of his Meditations, expreffes
fervent gratitude to the gods, that by their favour he
had made no further advances in rhetoric, poetry,
and other amufing ftudies; that he had not beftowed
too much time on voluminous reading, logical difputations, or refearches into phyfics; becaufe thefe
might have engroffed his mind, or diverted his attention from the peculiar duties of his elevated

---

* Tacitus in vit. Agric. See alfo Mr. Aikin's elegant tranflation
of this admirable piece of biography page 65.

ſtation.† Juſt and weighty, therefore, is the maxim of another ancient moraliſt, with which I ſhall conclude theſe reflections, that *we ſhould not reſt ſatisfied with the* WORDS *of wiſdom, without the* WORKS; *nor turn philoſophy into an idle pleaſure, which was given us for a ſalutary remedy.**

† Marcus Antoninus, lib. i.   * Seneca.

ON THE

ADVANTAGES OF A TASTE

FOR THE GENERAL

BEAUTIES OF NATURE,

AND OF ART.

————

" ME VERO PRIMUM DULCES ANTE OMNIA MUSÆ
" ACCIPIANT!" - - - - - - -   VIRG.

" QUID MINUAT CURAS, QUID TE TIBI REDDAT AMICUM."
                                              HOR.

SECTION I.

ON THE

BEAUTIES OF NATURE.

THAT fenfibility to beauty, which, when cultivated and improved, we term Tafte, is univerfally diffufed through the human fpecies: and it is
moft uniform with refpect to thofe objects, which,
being out of our power, are not liable to variation,
from accident, caprice, or fafhion. The verdant lawn,
the fhady grove, the variegated landfcape, the boundlefs ocean, and the ftarry firmament, are contemplated
with pleafure by every attentive beholder. But the
emotions of different fpectators, though fimilar in
kind, differ widely in degree: and to relifh with full
delight the enchanting fcenes of nature, the mind muft
be uncorrupted by avarice, fenfuality, or ambition;
quick in her fenfibilities, elevated in her fentiments,
and devout in her affections. He who poffeffes fuch
exalted powers of perception and enjoyment, may almoft fay with the poet,

    " I care not, Fortune! what you me deny;
    " You cannot rob me of free Nature's grace;
    " You cannot fhut the windows of the fky,

" Through which Aurora fhews her bright'ning face;
" You cannot bar my conftant feet to trace
" The woods and lawns, by living ftream, at eve:
" Let health my nerves and finer fibres brace,
" And I their toys to the great children leave:
" Of fancy, reafon, virtue, nought can me bereave."*

Perhaps fuch ardent enthufiafm may not be compatible with the neceffary toils, and active offices,
which Providence has affigned to the generality of
men.   But there are none to whom fome portion of·
it may not prove advantageous; and, if it were che-
rifhed by each individual, in that degree which is
confiftent with the indifpenfable duties of his ftation,
the felicity of human life would be confiderably augmented.   From this fource the refined and vivid pleafures of the imagination are almoft entirely derived:
and the elegant arts owe their choiceft beauties to a
tafte for the contemplation of nature.   Painting and
fculpture are exprefs imitations of vifible objects. and
where would be the charms of poetry, if divefted of
the imagery and embellifhments which fhe borrows
from rural fcenes?   Painters, ftatuaries, and poets,
therefore, are always ambitious to acknowledge themfelves the pupils of nature; and, as their fkill increafes,
they grow more and more delighted with every view
of the animal and vegetable world.   But the pleafure
refulting from admiration is tranfient; and to cultivate tafte, without regard to its influence on the paffions and affections, " is to rear a tree for its bloffoms,
" which is capable of yielding the richeft and moft

* Thomfon's Caftle of. Indolence.

" valuable fruit."* Phyſical and moral beauty bear
ſo intimate a relation to each other, that they may
be conſidered as different gradations in the ſcale of
excellence; and the knowledge and reliſh of the former ſhould be deemed only a ſtep to the nobler and
more permanent enjoyments of the latter.

Whoever has viſited the Leaſowes, in Warwick-
ſhire, muſt have felt the force and propriety of an
inſcription, which meets the eye at the entrance into
thoſe delightful grounds.

> " Would you then taſte the tranquil ſcene?
> " Be ſure your boſoms be ſerene;
> " Devoid of haſte, devoid of ſtrife,
> " Devoid of all that poiſons life:
> " And much it 'vails you, in their place
> " To graft the love of human race."†

Now ſuch ſcenes contribute powerfully to inſpire
that ſerenity, which is neceſſary to enjoy and to
heighten their beauties. By a ſecret ſympathy, the
ſoul catches the harmony which ſhe contemplates,
and the frame within aſſimilates itſelf to that which
is without. For,

> " Who can forbear to ſmile with Nature? Can
> " The ſtormy paſſions in the boſom roll,
> " While every gale is peace, and every grove
> " Is melody?"‡

* Shenſtone.   † Id.   ‡ Thomſon's Seaſons, firſt edit.

Horace, when he breaks forth into the animated exclamation,

> " O rus! quando ego te aſpiciam? quandoque licebit
> " Nunc veterum libris, nunc ſomno et inertibus horis
> " Ducere ſolicitæ jucunda oblivia vitæ?"

ſeems to regret the want of that heart-felt complacency, which the
buſtle, pomp, and pleaſures of imperial Rome could not afford.

In this ftate of fweet compofure, we become fuſ
ceptible of virtuous impreſſions from almoſt every
furrounding objeſt. The patient ox is viewed with
generous complacency; the guilelefs ſheep with pity;
and the playful lamb raiſes emotions of tendernefs
and love. We rejoice with the horſe in his liberty
and exemption from toil, whilſt he ranges at large
through enamelled paſtures; and the frolics.of the
colt would afford unmixed delight, did we not recol-
leſt the bondage which he is foon to undergo. We
are charmed with the ſongs of birds, foothed with the
buzz of infeſts, and pleaſed with the fportive motions
of fiſhes, becauſe theſe are expreſſions of enjoyment;
and we exult in the felicity of the whole animated
creation. Thus an equal and extenſive benevolence
is called forth into exertion; and having *felt* a common intereſt in the gratifications of inferior beings,
we ſhall be no longer indifferent to their fufferings,
or become wantonly inſtrumental in producing them.

It feems to be the intention of Providence, that
the lower orders of animals ſhould be fubfervient to
the comfort, convenience, and fuſtenance of man.
But his right of dominion extends no farther; and, if
this right be exerciſed with mildnefs, humanity, and
juſtice, the fubjeſts of his power will be no leſs be-
nefited than himfelf. For various fpecies of living
creatures are annually multiplied by human art, improved in their perceptive powers by human culture,
and plentifully fed by human induſtry. The relation,
therefore, is reciprocal between ſuch animals and man;

and he may fupply his own wants by the ufe of their
labour, the produce of their bodies, and even the facrifice of their lives; whilft he co-operates with all-
gracious Heaven in promoting HAPPINESS, the great
end of exiftence.

But though it be true that *partial evil*, with refpect
to different orders of fenfitive beings, may be *univerfal
good;* and that it is a wife and benevolent inftitution
of nature to make deftruction itfelf, within certain
limitations, the caufe of an increafe of life and enjoyment; yet a generous perfon will extend his compaf-
fionate regards to every individual that fuffers for
his fake: and whilft he fighs

> " E'en for the kid, or lamb, that pours its life
> " Beneath the bloody knife;"*

he will naturally be folicitous to mitigate pain, both
in duration and degree, by the gentleft modes of inflicting it.

I am inclined to believe, however, that this fenfe
of humanity would foon be obliterated, and that the
heart would grow callous to every foft impreffion,
were it not for the benignant influence of the fmiling
face of nature. The Count de Lauzun, when im-
prifoned by Louis XIV. in the caftle of Pignerol,
amufed himfelf, during a long period of time, with
catching flies, and delivering them to be devoured
by a rapacious fpider. Such an entertainment was
equally fingular and cruel, and inconfiftent, I believe,
with his former character, and fubfequent turn of

* Lord Lyttelton.

mind. But his cell had no window, and received
only a glimmering light from an aperture in the roof.
In lefs unfavourable circumftances, may we not prefume, that, inftead of fporting with mifery he would
have releafed the agonizing flies, and bidden them
enjoy that freedom of which he himfelf was bereaved?

But the tafte for natural beauty is fubfervient to
higher purpofes than thofe which have been enumerated: and the cultivation of it, not only refines and
humanizes, but dignifies and exalts the affections.   It
elevates them to the admiration and love of that Being,
who is the Author of all that is fair, fublime, and
good in the creation.   Scepticifm and irreligion are
hardly compatible with the fenfibility of heart,*
which arifes from a juft and lively relifh of the wisdom, harmony, and order, fubfifting in the world
around us: and emotions of piety muft fpring up
fpontaneoufly in the bofom that is in unifon with all
animated nature.   Actuated by this divine infpiration,
man finds a fane in every grove: and glowing with
devout fervour, he joins his fong to the univerfal cho-
rus, or mufes the praife of the ALMIGHTY in more
expreffive filence.   Thus they

" Whom Nature's works can charm, with GOD himfelf
" Hold converfe; grow familiar, day by day,
" With his conceptions; act upon his plan;
" And form to his the relifh of their fouls."†

* See Gregory' Comparative View.   † Akenfide.

SECTION II.

ON

A GENERAL TASTE FOR THE

FINE ARTS.

THE analogy of phyſical to moral beauty, and the connection ſubſiſting between a good heart and a juſt reliſh for the general works of nature, have, I truſt, been fully eſtabliſhed. But though all mankind are endued with the principle or faculty of taſte, it often lies almoſt entirely dormant for want of cultivation. The ſavage Indian, wholly occupied in providing for the neceſſities of life, traverſes the deſert, and the flowery lawn, with equal indifference. Eager in the chace, he ſcarcely turns his eye, as he paſſes along, to contemplate the golden beams of the ſetting ſun, reflected from the lake of Erie. Or if he quit his native wilds in the ſummer ſeaſon, to fiſh in the river Ohio, he ſits in his canoe, inattentive to the awful cataract, and views the moſt ſplendid ſcene in

the creation with flight and tranfient emotions. Nor
are the generality of men, even in civilized fociety, or
in the higher walks of life, fully qualified to comprehend or to admire the *affemblage* of beauties, which
the vifible creation prefents to the view of an enlightened imagination. Single objects, or detached
parts, attract the notice and engrofs the attention:
and the mind, by an eafy tranfition, paffes to the recognition and relifh of thofe operations of human
fkill, which are their fymbols or reprefentations. For
the elegant arts are all imitative in their effence and
origin. Thus mufic, by the variation of its movements and tones, calls up into the mind ideas, both
of the natural, animal, and rational world. The
murmuring brook, and boifterous ocean; the ftormy
wind, and gentle zephyr; the wild roar of the lion,
the bleating of the lamb, and the plaintive melody of
the nightingale; are all within the compafs of its
mimetic enchantments. Thefe are extended even to
the paffions and emotions of the human heart, fo as
to typify anger pity, remorfe, delight, and forrow.
Painting occupies a ftill wider field of fimilitude and
affociation, difplaying all thofe objects which are
known to us in nature, by diverfity of figure, or the
various fhades of colour. Even motions and founds
may be expreffed by this wonderful art. For, as they
are accompanied, in many inftances, with a certain
configuration or pofition of parts, the fign is readily
adopted for the thing fignified: and we fee or hear
upon the canvas, the horfe *ftarting* aghaft at the

fudden view of the lion; the foldier *running* towards his dying general with the news of victory; the cock *crowing* at the denial of Peter; and the water-fall *dafhing* againft the rocks below.*

Poetry, under which term I mean to comprehend all numerous and rhetorical compofition, derives moft of its charms from allufions, fimilies, metaphors, or defcriptions; and thefe are obvioufly imitative. In this way its powers are fo tranfcendent, that even a fingle epithet will fometimes produce a reprefentation more picturefque than the pencil of Pouffin, or Salvator Rofa, ever exhibited. The firft line in the following ftanza of Gray's elegy will afford an example and a proof of what is here advanced:

" Now fades the *glimmering* landfcape on the fight,
" And all the air a folemn ftillnefs holds,
" Save where the beetle wheels his droning flight,
" And drowfy tinklings lull the diftant folds."†

The accuracy and force of the word *glimmering* muft be felt by any one who has viewed with attention an extenfive profpect, about an hour after fun-fet.

The mimetic arts have fome advantages over nature herfelf; for the imitations with which they prefent us are generally agreeable, even though their archetypes be in themfelves indifferent or difgufting. The mind delights in comparifon; and this pleafure is heightened by the recognition of refemblance, and by the contemplation of ingenious defign or mafterly

* Mr. Stubbs's Picture. The death of General Wolfe; &c.
† Gray's Elegy;

execution. Who can read Mr. Gay's defcription of
a poor benighted traveller, without being charmed
at the verifimilitude of the narration, which is at
once fo clear, fo difcriminative, and circumftantial,
that we become, as it were, fpectators of a fcene,
which, either in its parts, or in the whole, is exactly
correfpondent to our recollection and experience.

It is evident, therefore, that the fine arts have for
their object the gratification of the fame faculty which
perceives and relifhes the charms of nature. And
by analogy we may infer, that the exercife which
they give to the tafte is favourable to the virtuous
affections of the heart. This truth has been fo long
acknowledged, that the obfervation of the poet is
now received as an eftablifhed maxim in ethics;

" Ingenuas didiciſſe fideliter artes
" Emollit mores, nec finit eſſe feros."*

But the validity of this canon is not to be admitted
without fome reftriction. The energies of mufic,
painting, and poetry, are fo powerful and multifarious,
that they have at command all the emotions and paffions of the foul,

- - - - - " Pectus inaniter angunt,
" Irritant, mulcent, falfis terroribus implent."†

They may excite or reftrain, kindle or extinguifh paffion; and thus, according to their application, become
the inftruments either of vi e or of virtue. They are
incident, likewife, to numberlefs adventitious affocia-

* Ovid.   † Hor. Epift. I. lib. ii.

tions, which, counteracting or diverfifying their natural and original tendency, may make them adminifter
to vanity, oftentation, pride, envy, and jealoufy. Such
difpofitions are fometimes found in the profeffors of
thefe arts; and the difplay of them, in men of diftinguifhed genius and merit, raifes in our minds a painful ftruggle of difcordant emotions.*

Whoever, therefore, yields himfelf implicitly to the
magic delufions of the fine arts, is in danger of having
his judgment impaired, his heart corrupted, and his
capacity deftroyed for the ordinary duties and enjoyments of life. To this fource may be traced all the
follies and extravagance of what is termed VERTU.
Admiration ftimulates the defire of poffeffion, however immoderate the price; poffeffion turns the admiration of the object to ourfelves; and this is fucceeded
by a fond and abfurd impatience to difplay a fuperiority over others, both in tafte and property.

" What brought Sir Vifto's ill-got wealth to wafte?
" Some dæmon whifper'd, ' Vifto, have a tafte.'
" Heav'n vifits with a tafte the wealthy fool;
" And needs no rod, but Ripley with a rule.†

But it is further to be obferved, that as an acute
relifh for beauty, and a quick difcernment of deformity,
are, in a certain proportion, neceffarily connected to-

* " Who would not laugh, if fuch a one there be?
" Who would not weep, if Atticus were he?" POPE.

No reflection is meant, by the quotation of thefe lines, on the
very refpectable character to whom they allude. They were dictated
by refentment, and reprobated by fome of the Poet's beft friends.

† Pope's Moral Effays.

gether; the latter may become predominant through pride, affectation, or too frequent indulgence. Whenever this happens, taste will prove the instrument of pain, and not of pleasure: and the fastidious feelings of disgust, so often excited, will be transferred from the works of human skill to human life, rendering the temper petulant, morose, and selfish. But a perversion of the powers of the imagination is no argument against their proper culture and well-regulated application. For reason itself is liable to abuse; and philosophy and religion have been rendered subservient to scepticism and superstition.

MISCELLANEOUS

OBSERVATIONS

ON THE ALLIANCE OF

NATURAL HISTORY, and PHILOSOPHY,
WITH POETRY.

—◆◆◆◆—

. . . . NIL SCRIBENS IPSE DOCEBO,

UNDE PARENTUR OPES; QUID ALAT FORMETQUE POETAM.

. . . . VATIBUS ADDERE CALCAR.

HOR.

MISCELLANEOUS

OBSERVATIONS

ON THE ALLIANCE OF

NATURAL HISTORY, and PHILOSOPHY,

WITH POETRY.*

———◄◄◊►►———

THE maxim of Lord Verulam, that " knowledge is power," is no lefs applicable to poefy
than to philofophy.   For whether we engage in this
delightful purfuit as an art, or as a fcience, it is evident that the ability to convey and the capacity to
relifh its peculiar pleafures, muft be exactly proportioned to our acquaintance with the means either of
communicating or enjoying them.   The works of
creation are the great ftorehoufe where thefe means
are to be fought; and an inquifitive attention to
every furrounding object is effential to the poet, and
highly ufeful to the lover of poetry.   He who ex-

* In this Effay, the author has confined his views chiefly to the
application of natural knowledge to that branch of the poetic art
which relates to DESCRIPTION; referving for fome future occafion
the alliance of phyfics with POETICAL IMAGERY and MORAL
ANALOGY.

tends his refearches beyond the furface of things, will find that the treafures of nature are inexhauftible. For it is literally no lefs than metaphorically true, that

- - - - " Many a gem, of pureft ray ferene,
" The dark unfathom'd caves of ocean bear;
" Full many a flower is born to blufh unfeen,
" And wafte its fweetnefs on the defert air."*

Yet few have been the labourers in this rich harveft of fcience, fince the days of Theocritus; and the paftoral defcriptions and images of that ancient Sicilian bard, have been ufed like hereditary property by all fucceeding poets. In the ruder ages of the world, the modes of life were peculiarly favourable to the obfervation of nature. Rural fcenery was continually before the eyes; and the culture of land, or the care of fheep and cattle, conftituted the occupation of the greateft perfonages. This furnifhed a rich fupply of original materials, which muft for ever be withheld from thofe who immure themfelves in cities, and contemplate only the operations of art. Writers, therefore, of this clafs are humbly fatisfied to be mere copyifts of others; and adopt, without referve, the figures, allufions, and reprefentations, of their poetical predeceffors. But fcience, which is borrowed, is often mifunderftood: and it is not in the power, even of genius itfelf, to obviate the miftakes which are committed through ignorance. Who, for inftance, can notice the countenance of the ox, without perceiving that it difplays meeknefs, patience, and the moft

* Gray's Elegy.

inoffenfive difpofition;* and that the eyes of this animal are of no unufual dimenfion? Yet in many verfions of Homer, that divine poet, fo converfant with zoology, is made to ftyle the artful, proud, and paffionate queen of the gods, " Ox-eyed Juno." This miftake of the tranflators has evidently arifen, from the want of attention to nature: and M. Dacier has fhewn, that the particle Gᴈ is only an augmentative, fignifying *(valde)* large-eyed; and that it has no direct relation to the ox. The error which Dr. Young has fallen into, in his paraphrafe on Job, is more pardonable; becaufe an Englifh poet, who has never feen the CROCODILE, might be ignorant that his eyes are remarkably fmall. This animal is fuppofed to be the Leviathan, defcribed in the 41ft chapter of that book: and if the explanation be true, the following paffage muft have a reference to the brightnefs, and not to the magnitude, of his organs of fight, as my friend Mr. Aikin has judicioufly remarked.† *By his neezings a light doth fhine, and his eyes are like the eyelids of the morning.* Dr. Young, by a mifconception of the original, has rendered this ftrong figure ftill more hyperbolical—

> " Large is his front; and when his burnifh'd eyes
> " Lift their *broad* lids, the morning feems to rife."

* Thomfon thus defcribes the ox:
    - - - - " And the plain ox,
    " That honeft, harmlefs, guilelefs animal."

† See his elegant and ingenious Effay on the Application of Natural Hiftory to Poetry.

When the rebellious angels are defcribed by Milton, as converted into ferpents, he fays,

- - - - - - " Dreadful was the din
" Of hiffing through the hall,
" Scorpion and afp, and amphifbæna dire,
" Ceraftes horn'd, hydrus, and elops drear."*

A celebrated critic† afferts that it is a miftake to enumerate the fcorpion and the afp amongft the ferpents; and that the elops was a fifh, much admired by the ancients.   It has, been fhewn, however, that Milton, in this paffage, has the authority of Pliny, Lucan, and Nicander.

In a former effay I have remarked, concerning the mimetic powers of poetry, that a fingle word will fometimes produce a reprefentation more picturefque than the pencil of Pouffin, or of Salvator Rofa, ever exhibited.   And the obfervation was exemplified by this line of Mr. Gray;

" Now fades the glimmering landfcape on the fight,"

In which the accuracy and force of the epithet *glimmering* will be felt by any one, who has viewed with attention an extenfive profpect, about an hour after fun-fet.‡   But a gentleman of this county, who has

---

* Milton's Paradife Loft, book x.

† Dr. Bentley.—Dr. Johnfon, in the plan of his great Dictionary addreffed to Lord Chefterfield, when treating of the importance of the explanation of appellatives, fays that Milton, with fuch affiftance, would not have difpofed fo improperly of his *elops*, and his *fcorpion;* nor would Shakefpeare have made the *woodbine* entwine the *honeyfuckle.*

‡ Effay on the Advantages of a Tafte for Nature and the Fine Arts.

inferted the foregoing line in a very elegant little poem, by an unfortunate tranfpofition, has entirely deftroyed its beauty, truth, and energy.

" Now fades the landfcape on the *glimmering fight*."

Many original writers, of the moft diftinguifhed re-putation, have deviated widely from nature, by adopt-ing facts and opinions without examination, or on infufficient authority. Thus the poet Lucretius, who flourifhed about fifty years before the Chriftian æra, has fanctioned the vulgar error, that in the jaundice objects are painted on the retina of the fame colour with that which tinges the external coat of the eye; and has given a theory of it in conformity to the phi-lofophy of the Epicurean fchool :

" *Lurida præterea fiunt quæcunque tuentur*
" *Arquati, quia luroris de corpore eorum*
" *Semina multa fluunt, fimulacris obvia rerum;*
" *Multaque funt oculis in eorum denique mifta,*
" *Quæ contage fua palloribus omnia pingunt.*"*

" Befides, whatever jaundic'd eyes do view,
" Look pale, as well as thofe, and yellow too;
" For lurid parts fly off with nimble wings,
" And meet the diftant coming forms of things:
" And others lurk within the eyes, and feize,
" And ftain, with pale, the entering images."†

Mr. Pope has authorized the fame obfervation, in his Effay on Criticifm:

" All feems infected, that th' infected fpy;
" As all looks yellow to the jaundic'd eye."

* Lucretius, lib. iv. line 333.
† Creech's Tranfl. of Lucret. book iv. line 344.

And the like miftaken allufion is more than once repeated in an admirable poem, lately publifhed by
Mr. Hayley:

> " The bards of Britain, with unjaundic'd eyes,
> " Will glory to behold fuch rivals rife."*
>
> " On faireft names, from every blemifh free,
> " Save what the jaundic'd eyes of party fee."

I am inclined to believe there is no fufficient foundation for this opinion.   Galen indeed fpeaks of yellow
vifion, as common to ifteric patients; and Sextus
Empyricus has delivered the fame account; but their
relation is neither confirmed by experience, nor confonant to reafon.   In the worft cafes of the jaundice
now known, I believe this fymptom has no exiftence;
and I do not find it noticed in the records of Aretæus,
Celfus, or Hippocrates.

The fuppofition, that the fertilizing quality of
snow arifes from nitrous falts, which it is fuppofed
to acquire in the act of freezing, is void of foundation; becaufe the moft accurate experiments have
demonftrated, that it contains no nitre, and only a
fmall portion of calcareous earth.   Falfe philofophy,
fays an eminent chemift,† firft gave rife to this idea,
and poetry has contributed to diffufe the error,
Thus Mr. Philips:

> - - - - - - - - - " O may'ft thou often fee
> " Thy furrows whiten'd by the woolly rain,
> " Nutritious: fecret nitre lurks within
> " The porous wet, quickening the languid glebe."

----

* On Epic Poetry. Ep. iv.

† Dr. Watfon, now Bifhop of Landaff, in his Chemical Effays.

But the following lines of Mr. Thomfon do not appear to me to be liable to the fame objection: for the term *falts*, with the annexed epithet *little*, may be applied, without much poetical licence, to the cryftals of water, formed by freezing:

" What art thou, froft?
" Is not thy potent energy unfeen,
" Myriads of *little falts*, or hook'd, or fhap'd
" Like double wedges, and diffus'd immenfe
" Thro' water, earth, and ether ?"

The operation of froft is here afcribed to its me-chanical powers. For by binding the furface of the earth, it arrefts the exhalations as they afcend from the parts below, and thus retains a nutritious *pabu-lum*, to be applied at a proper feafon to the roots of plants. But it chiefly meliorates the foil, by pulve-rizing the particles which compofe it, and fitting them for the abforption of the vernal dews and rains.

Whenever PHILOSOPHY is introduced into poetry, truth, for the moft part, is effential to its power of giving pleafure: and our great epic writer feems to defcend fometimes from the majefty of his work, by mixing with modern difcoveries the groundlefs opi-nions of the ancients. Thus, when Raphael addreffes Adam, concerning the great fyftem of nature, he fays,

- - - - - - - - - - - - " Other funs, perhaps,
" With their attendant moons, thou wilt defcry,
" Communicating *male* and *female* light."*

The idea of *male* light being communicated by the *fun*, and *female* light by the *moon*, probably originated in the mind of Milton, from his intimate acquaintance

* Milton's Paradife Loft, book viii. line 148.

with the writings of Pliny; who mentions, as a tradition, " that the fun is a mafculine ftar, drying all " things; but that the moon is a foft and feminine " ftar, of diffolving power. And that thus the ba- " lance of nature is preferved ; fome of the ftars " binding the elements, and others loofening them."*

The HARMONY of the SPHERES, or mufical revolution of the heavenly bodies in their feveral orbits, was firft taught by the Pythagoreans ; who feem to have derived this fanciful doctrine from analogy. For it was obferved by thefe philofophers, that a mufical chord produces the fame note as one double in length, when the force is quadruple with which the latter is ftretched; hence they fuppofed that the gravity of a planet is quadruple the gravity of a planet at a double diftance. And as any mufical chord may become unifon to a leffer chord of the fame kind, if its tenfion be increafed in the fame proportion as the fquare of its length is greater ; fo the gravity of a planet may become equal to the gravity of another planet nearer to the fun, provided it be increafed in proportion as the fquare of its diftance from the fun is greater. If therefore mufical chords be extended from the fun to each planet, to bring them into unifon, it would be requifite to increafe or diminifh their tenfions, in the fame proportions as would be

---

* " Solis ardore ficcatur liquor; et hoc effe mafculum fidus acce-
" pimus, torrens cuncta forbensque. E contrario ferunt lunam femi-
" neum ac molle fidus, atque nocturnum folvere humorem. Ita pen-
" fari naturæ vices, femperque fufficere, aliis fiderum elementa
" cogentibus, aliis vere fundentibus."—Hift. Nat. lib. ii. cap. 100.
See alfo the notes to Newton's edition of Paradife Loft.

fufficient to render the gravity of the planets equal.* This notion of the Pythagoreans is fo pleafing to the imagination, that it is not furprizing the poets have adopted it: and Milton has given fuch a view of it, as wants nothing but philofophical truth to render it delightful:—

" Myftical dance, which yonder ftarry fphere
" Of planets, and of fix'd, in all her wheels
" Refembles neareft; mazes intricate,
" Eccentric, intervolv'd, yet regular,
" Then moft, when moft irregular they feem;
" And in their motions harmony divine
" So fmooths her charming tones, that GOD's own ear
" Liftens delighted."†

Mr. Pope has not only fuppofed the actual exiftence of this heavenly harmony, but that it is poffible the human ear might have been fo conftituted as to have been fenfible of it:—

" If Nature thunder'd in his opening ears,
" And ftunn'd him with the mufic of the fpheres;
" How would he wifh that Heav'n had left him ftill
" The whifp'ring zephyr, and the purling rill?"‡

Thofe who are in poffeffion of the firft or fecond edition of Thomfon's Seafons, will find a grofs geo-graphical miftake in the hymn which is annexed to them. Towards the clofe of this beautiful poem, the author expreffes his pious confidence in the uni-verfal wifdom and impartial benevolence of the Deity;

* Vid. Plin. lib. ii. cap. 22. Macrob. lib. ii. cap. 1. See alfo Maclaurin's Account of Sir Ifaac Newton's Philofophical Difcove-ries, page 34.

† Paradife Loft, book v. line 620.

‡ Effay on Man, epift. i. ver. 201.

and afferts, that the fame regular feafons, which he had defcribed with fuch fervour of delight in the preceding work, are equally experienced in every part of the globe.

> - - - - - - "God is ever prefent, ever felt,
> " In the void wafte, as in the city full;
> " Roll the *fame kindred feafons* round the world,
> " In all *apparent*, wife and good in all."

The two laft lines are omitted in the fubfequent editions of this poem.

The fyftem of PHILOSOPHY which is now received, independent of its fuperiority in point of truth, infinitely exceeds in extent, elevation, and grandeur, that of the ancients.   The poet, therefore, fhould be well verfed in the fcience of phyfics, not only becaufe he can feldom deviate from it,* without injury to his compofitions, but becaufe they may derive from it fublimity, embellifhment, or grace.   Aftronomy, in

---

* In the following lines, the thought becomes low, by being unphilofophical:

> - - - - - - - - - - - - - "O thievifh night,
> " Why fhould'ft thou, but for fome felonious end,
> " In thy *dark lanthorn* thus clofe up the ftars
> " That Nature hung in heaven, and filled their *lamps*
> " With everlafting *oil*."   MILTON's Comus.

The fentiment is more brilliant, in a fubfequent paffage of this poem, but not more folid: and it is rendered abfurd by the leaft reflection on the impoffibility of finking the vaft orbs of the fun and moon in the ocean; or as it is here improperly ftyled, the *flat fea* :—

> " Virtue could fee to do what virtue would,
> " By her own radiant light; though fun and moon
> " Were in the *flat fea* funk."

particular, furnishes such magnificent ideas and bound-
less views, that imagination can hardly grasp, much
less exalt or amplify them. "The objects which we
" commonly call great," says an eminent writer,
" vanish, when we contemplate the vast body of the
" earth; the terraqueous globe itself is soon lost in
" the solar system. In some parts it is seen as a distant
" star; in others it is unknown; or visible only at
" rare times, to vigilant observers. The sun itself
" dwindles into a star; Saturn's vast orbit, and the
" orbits of all the comets, crowd into a point, when
" viewed from numberless spaces between the earth
" and the nearest of the fixed stars. Other suns
" kindle light to illuminate other systems, where our
" sun's rays are unperceived; but they also are
" swallowed up in the vast expanse. Even all the
" systems of the stars that sparkle in the clearest sky,
" must possess a corner only of that space, through
" which such systems are dispersed: since more stars
" are discovered in one constellation by the telescope,
" than the naked eye perceives in the whole heavens.
" After we have risen so high, and left all definite
" measures far behind us, we find ourselves no nearer
" to a term or limit; for all this is nothing to what
" may be displayed in the infinite expanse, beyond
" the remotest stars that have hitherto been disco-
" vered."* This description, though delivered in
the chaste language of a mathematician, is in sen-

* Maclaurin's View of Sir Isaac Newton's Discoveries, p. 16.

timent fo truly fublime, that it wants nothing but numbers to conftitute it poetry; and in the following lines, it appears with all the charms of grace and harmony :

‑ ‑ ‑ ‑ ‑ ‑ ‑ ‑ ‑ ‑ ‑ " Seiz'd in thought,
" On Fancy's wild and roving wing I fail
" From the green borders of the peopled earth,
" And the pale moon, her duteous fair attendant;
" From folitary Mars; from the vaft orb
" Of Jupiter, whofe huge gigantic bulk
" Dances in ether, like the lighteft leaf;
" To the dim verge, the fuburbs of the fyftem,
" Where cheerlefs Saturn 'midft his wat'ry moons,
" Girt with a lucid zone, majeftic fits
" In gloomy grandeur, like an exil'd queen
" Amongft her weeping handmaids: fearlefs thence
" I launch into the tracklefs deeps of fpace,
" Where burning round ten thoufand funs appear,
" Of elder beam; which afk no leave to fhine
" Of our terreftrial ftar, nor borrow light
" From the proud regent of our fcanty day,
" Sons of the morning, firft-born of creation,
" And only lefs than Him who marks their track,
‑‑ And guides thrir fiery wheels.   Here muft I ftop
" Or is there aught beyond ?   What hand, unfeen,
" Impels me onward, through the glowing orbs
" Of habitable nature; far remote,
" To the dread confines of eternal night,
" To folitudes of vaft unpeopled fpace,
" The deferts of creation, wide and wild;
" Where embryo fyftems, and unkindled funs,
" Sleep in the womb of chaos!   Fancy droops,
" And thought, aftonifh'd, ftops her bold career."*

Homer, whofe knowledge of the magnitude and diftances of the heavenly bodies, muft have been very

Mrs. Barbauld's Evening Meditation.

confined, never difplays a more glowing imagination, than when he introduces them to our notice. And no one can view his animated picture of a moonlight and ftarry night, without feeling himfelf tranfported to the fcene which it exhibits.

> " As when the moon, refulgent lamp of night,
> " O'er heaven's clear azure fpreads her facred light;
> " When not a breath difturbs the deep ferene,
> " And not a cloud o'ercafts the folemn fcene;
> " Around her throne the vivid planets roll,
> " And ftars unnumber'd gild the glowing pole;
> " O'er the dark trees a yellower verdure fhed,
> " And tip with filver every mountain's head;
> " Then fhine the vales, the rocks in profpect rife,
> " A flood of glory burfts from all the fkies;
> " The confcious fwains, rejoicing in the fight,
> " Eye the blue vault, and blefs the ufeful light."*

Mr. Pope has tranflated this paffage with fingular felicity; and perhaps it may be the faftidioufnefs of criticifm to remark, that a *refulgent moon* is not compatible with *vivid* planets, and *glowing ftars*; becaufe thefe fainter lights are eclipfed by the fplendour of that luminary. But though Homer, probably, did not mean to introduce a full moon, as his commentator Euftathius has obferved, yet a judicious poet has chofen to leave this bright orb out of the evening fcenery which fhe has fo admirably pourtrayed.

> - - - - - - - - - " Nature's felf is hufh'd;
> " And but a fcatter'd leaf which ruftles thro'
> " The thick-wove foliage, not a found is heard
> " To break the midnight air."

---

* Pope's Homer's Iliad, book viii. line 687.

- - - - - - - - - - " 'Tis now the hour
" When contemplation, from her funlefs haunts,
" Moves forward; and with radiant finger points
" Where, one by one, the living eyes of heav'n
" Awake, quick kindling o'er the face of ether
" One boundlefs blaze; ten thoufand trembling fires
" And dancing luftres, where th' unfteady eye,
" Reftlefs and dazzled, wanders unconfin'd
" O'er all this field of glories."*

It may be amufing to contraft the foregoing defcriptions of the night with thofe recorded by Mr.
Macpherfon, in his tranflation of the poems of Offian.
Five bards, paffing the night in the houfe of a Cale-
donian chief, went out feverally to make their obfervations; and returned with an extempore defcription
of the night, which, as appears from the poem, was
in the month of October. I fhall here recite part of
the compofition of the fourth bard, as it is moft analogous to the paffages above quoted.

" Night is calm and fair; blue, ftarry, fettled is
" night. The winds, with the clouds, are gone.
" They fink behind the hill. The moon is upon the
" mountain. Trees glifter; ftreams fhine on the
" rock. Bright rolls the fettled lake; bright the
" ftream of the vale.

" The breezes drive the blue mift flowly over the
" narrow vale. It rifes on the hill, and joins its
" head to heaven. Night is fettled, calm, blue,
" ftarry, bright with the moon. Receive me not,
" my friends; for lovely is the night."†

* Mrs. Barbauld's Evening Meditation.
† Offian's Croma, p. 255, 4to edition.

In fouthern latitudes the HEAVENLY BODIES are far more refplendent, than when viewed through the thick atmofphere of Britain. It is faid, that in Jamaica, the *milky way* is tranfcendently bright; and that the planet Venus appears like a little moon, glittering with fo vivid a beam, as to render vifible the fhadows of trees, buildings, and other objects.* The fetting fun, in that ifland, exhibits a fpectacle peculiarly auguft. His apparent circumference being enlarged by his ftation in the horizon, and the re-fraction of the rays of light retaining in view his glorious orb, he feems to reft awhile from his career, on the fummit of the mountains. Then he fuddenly vanifhes, leaving a train of fplendour, that ftreaks the clouds with the moft lively and variegated tints which fancy can conceive.† In defcribing fuch a fpectacle as this, the majefty of the great luminary generally abforbs the whole attention of the poet; and he takes little notice of the effect of the fun's declination on terreftrial objects: yet it is certain, that a landfcape of fmall extent never appears more beautiful than at the clofe of a fummer's day. Several caufes then confpire to give a richnefs to the fcene, and no one fo powerfully as the heightened verdure of the her-bage, arifing probably from the combination of blue and yellow colours, reflected at the fame time, from the golden clouds and azure fky. Perhaps the in-creafed refraction and foftened luftre of the evening rays of light may alfo contribute to this effect. For

* Hift. of Jamaica, book ii. p. 371. † Ibid. 372.

the herbage at that time appears not only more green, but more copious too; infomuch that a pafture, which looks *bare* at noon, feems to abound in grafs at fun-fet. When thick black vapours hover about the weftern fun, and prefent only fmall illumined edges, I have obferved a circle of green furrounding his difk; an appearance which I know not how to account for, but from the union above defcribed of blue and yellow rays. This phœnomenon I faw in great perfection, as I was lately travelling over the mountains which divide the counties of Lancafter and York. The day was wet and ftormy; and the war of elements which I beheld gave me fome faint idea of what is experienced on the Alps and Andes; where the traveller views clouds at his feet, and cor-rufcations of lightning darting on all fides below him. Numberlefs meteors, which are unknown on the plain, prefent themfelves to his aftonifhed fight; fuch as circular rainbows, parhelia, the fhadow of the mountain projected on the air, and his own image adorned with a kind of glory round the head.* How tremendous is the account which Don Ulloa has given of his ftation on the top of Cotopaxi, a moun-tain in Peru, more than three geographical miles above the level of the fea. Here he was ftationed a confiderable length of time, for the purpofe of mea-furing a degree of the meridian; and the hardfhips which he fuffered from the intenfenefs of the cold,

* Ulloa, vol. i. Acad. Par. 1744. Prieftley on Light and Colours, page 599, &c.

and the ftorms to which he was expofed, almoft exceed
belief. "The fky," fays he, "was generally ob-
"fcured with thick fogs; but when thefe were dif-
"perfed, and the clouds moved by their gravity
"nearer the furface of the earth, they furrounded
"the mountain to a vaft diftance, reprefenting the
"fea, with our rock like an ifland in the centre of it.
"When this happened, we heard the horrid noifes
"of the tempefts which difcharged themfelves on
"Quito, and the neighbouring countries. We faw
"the lightnings iffue from the clouds, and heard the
"thunders roll far beneath us. And whilft the
"lower regions were involved in tempefts of thunder
"and rain, we enjoyed a delightful ferenity. The
"wind was hufhed, the fky clear, and the enlivening
"rays of the fun moderated the feverity of the cold."*
How would a fcene like this have been felt and defcribed by the poet, of whom it is faid,

- - - - - - - - - - - - "When lightning fires
"The arch of heaven, and thunders rock the ground;
"When furious whirlwinds rend the howling air,
"And ocean, groaning from his loweft bed,
"Heaves his tempeftuous billows to the fky:
"Amid the mighty uproar, while below
"The nations tremble, Shakefpeare looks abroad
"From fome high cliff, fuperior, and enjoys
"The elemental war."†

The awful and gloomy grandeur of the mountainous fcenery of Peru is, perhaps, lefs favourable to the

* Ulloa's Voyage, vol. i. p. 231.
† Akenfide's Pleafures of Imagination, book iii. line 599.

descriptive powers of the poet, than the prospects
which some of the Alpine countries of Europe afford.
In the cultivated districts of Switzerland particularly,
the views furnish the happiest combination of the
sublime and beautiful. And I shall give a short ab-
stract of the observations made by a late traveller on
the Mole, a mountain which rises near five thousand
feet above the lake of Geneva, and is situated about
eighteen miles eastward of that city. " In my ascent,"
says Sir George Shuckburgh, " I saw the sun rising
" behind one of the neighbouring Alps, with a most
" beautiful effect; and the shadow of the mountain
" we were then upon extended fifteen or twenty miles
" west. Before me, at some distance, was spread the
" plain, in which lay Geneva and the lake; behind
" me rose the Dole, and the long chain of Mont
" Jura. A little to the left, and much nearer, lay
" Mont Saleve, which, from this height, appeared an
" inconsiderable hill. To the right and left nothing
" but immense rocks and pointed mountains of every
" possible shape, forming tremendous precipices. In
" the vale beneath, several little hamlets, and the
" most beautiful pasturages, with the river Arve
" winding and softening the scene. From whence
" arose a thick evaporation, collecting itself into
" clouds, which on the lake, that was quite covered
" with them, had the appearance of a sea of cotton;
" the sun's beams playing on the upper surface of
" them with those tints which are seen in a fine
" evening. To the south west appeared the lake of

" Annecy; behind us lay the Glacieres, and amongſt
" them, towering above all the reſt, ſtood Mont
" Blanc. The circumference of the horizon might
" be about two hundred Engliſh miles; and though
" not one of the moſt extenſive, yet certainly one of
" the moſt varied in the world."*

It is with a reluctance, ſimilar perhaps to what
this philoſophical traveller experienced when he de-
ſcended from the Mole, that I quit the imaginary
viſion of this enchanting ſcene. But it is neceſſary
to remark, that however ſtriking ſuch complex and
ſublime repreſentations may be, they can only be
introduced occaſionally by the poet; whoſe talents
for deſcription ſhould be chiefly exerciſed in the judicious ſelection and picturesque diſplay of ſmall
groups, or individual objects. Like the magnet, he
muſt draw forth what is valuable, even from the
rudeſt materials; and nicely diſcriminate in every
ſurrounding object thoſe attributes which can be
rendered ſubſervient to his art. We are informed
that Thomſon was wont to wander whole days and
nights in the country: and in ſuch ſequeſtered walks
he acquired, by the moſt minute attention, a knowledge of all the myſteries of nature. Theſe he has
wrought into his Seaſons with the colouring of Titian,
the wildneſs of Salvator Roſa, and the energy of
Raphael.

Milton appears to have been no leſs familiar with
nature than Thomſon, and equally happy in his por-

* Philoſoph. Tranſ. 1777, p. 536.

traits of her moſt pleaſing forms. He catches every diſtinguiſhing feature; and gives to what he deſcribes ſuch glowing tints of life and reality, that we have it, as it were, in full view before our eyes. How per-fect is the image in the following lines!

> — — — — — — — — "The ſwan, with *arched neck*
> "Between her *white wings mantling, proudly rows*
> "Her ſtate, with *oary feet.*"*

Indeed the whole account of the creation, which the Archangel relates to Adam, is ſo engaging and pic-tureſque, that it would fully refute the criticiſm of a learned Italian, if the poem contained no other beau-ties of a ſimilar kind. " The poets beyond the Alps," ſays Abbé Winckelmann, " ſpeak *figuratively*, but " without *painting*. The ſtrange and ſometimes ter-" rifying figures, which conſtitute almoſt all the " grandeur of Milton, are by no means the *objects* of " a *pencil*, but rather ſeem beyond the reach of " *painting*."† Surely the deſcription of the ſwan, above recited, might be copied on the canvas, by any artiſt of tolerable genius. As Milton derived his knowledge of this beautiful bird from actual obſerva-tion, he has not fallen into the error of the ancient poets, who have almoſt univerſally aſcribed to it a muſical voice. Callimachus terms it, " Apollo's " tuneful ſongſter;" and Horace compliments Pindar

---

* Paradiſe Loſt, book vii. line 438.

† Hiſtoire des l'Arts chez les Anciens.

with the epithet "*Dircæan swan.*"* Such impro-
prieties clea ly evince the importance of natural
knowledge to the poet.

The polity of ROOKS is almoſt conſtituted with as
much order and wiſdom as that of ants, bees, and
beavers; and their attachment to places contiguous to
the dwellings of men not only affords us frequent opportunities of obſerving them, but intereſts us at the
ſame time in their well being and preſervation. Theſe
birds, therefore, furniſh the poet with various topics
for the diſplay of his art; and the following incident,
by a little colouring, might be wrought into a pathetic picture. A large colony of rooks had ſubſiſted
many years in a grove, on the banks of the river
Irwell, near Mancheſter. One ſerene evening, I
placed myſelf within the view of it, and marked with
attention the various labours, paſtimes, and evolu-
tions of this crowded ſociety. The idle members
amuſed themſelves with chacing each other, through
endleſs mazes; and in their flight they made the air
reſound with an infinitude of diſcordant noiſes. In
the midſt of theſe playful exertions, it unfortunately
happened that one rook, by a ſudden turn, ſtruck
his beak againſt the wing of another. The ſufferer
inſtantly fell into the river. A general cry of diſtreſs

* "*Multa Dircæum levat aura cycnum*
"*Tendit, Antoni, quoties in altos*
"*Nubium tractus.*" Ode II. lib. iv.
In the addreſs to Melpomene, he ſays,
"*O mutis quoque piſcibus*
"*Donatura cycni, ſi libeat, ſonum.*" Ode III.

enfued. The birds hovered, with every expreffion of anxiety, over their diftreffed companion. Animated by their fympathy, and perhaps by the language of counfel, known to themfelves, he fprung into the air, and by one ftrong effort, reached the point of a rock, which projected into the water. The exultation became loud and univerfal; but, alas! it was foon changed into notes of lamentation: for the poor wounded bird, in attempting to fly towards his neft, dropt again into the river, and was drowned amidft the moans of his whole fraternity.

The habitudes of the domeftick breed of POULTRY cannot poffibly efcape obfervation: and every one muft have noticed the fierce jealoufy of the cock,

" Whofe breaft with ardour flames, as on he walks,
" Graceful, and crows defiance."*

It fhould feem that this jealoufy is not confined to his rivals, but may fometimes extend to his beloved female: and that he is capable of being actuated by revenge, founded on fome degree of reafoning concerning her conjugal infidelity. An incident which lately happened at the feat of Mr. B******, near Berwick, juftifies this remark. "My mowers," fays he, " cut a partridge on her neft, and immediately " brought the eggs (fourteen) to the houfe. I " ordered them to be put under a very large beautiful " hen, and her own to be taken away. They were " hatched in two days, and the hen brought them

* Thomfon's Spring, line 772.

" up perfectly well till they were five or fix weeks
" old. During that time they were conftantly kept
" confined in an outhoufe, without having been feen
" by any of the other poultry. The door happened
" to be left open, and the cock got in. My houfe-
" keeper, hearing her hen in diftrefs, ran to her
" affiftance, but did not arrive in time to fave her life.
" The cock finding her with the brood of partridges,
" fell upon her with the utmoft fury, and put her to
" death. The houfekeeper found him tearing her
" both with his beak and fpurs, although fhe was
" then fluttering in the laft agony, and incapable of
" any refiftance. The hen had been formerly the
" cock's greateft favourite."

A writer of no inconfiderable merit,* has employed
his mufe on a fubject highly interefting to the Englifh
reader, in a didactic poem entitled the *Fleece*. In this
work, whatever relates to the management of fheep,
and the manufacture of wool, is largely difcuffed; and
the whole is adorned by the introduction of rural
imagery and amufing digreffions. But the performance might have been rendered much more enter-
taing, if it had comprehended a fuller account of the
natural hiftory of the fheep; and had difplayed a nicer
attention to the peculiar and pleafing character of
that innocent animal, and of her fportive offspring.
One fact fhould not have been omitted in fuch a
narrative; and I wonder it efcaped Mr. Dyer's obfervation. I am informed, that after the dam has

* Mr. Dyer.

been fhorn, and turned into the fold to her lambs, they become eftranged to her; and that a fcene of reciprocal diftrefs enfues, which a man of lively imagination and tender feelings might render highly interefting and pathetic. The poor fheep, when undergoing the operation of wafhing, and alfo when ftripped of her warm and graceful covering, is in both circumftances, a fpectacle of pity, and a proper object of poetical amplification. Had Mr. Sterne been the author of the Fleece, he would perhaps have introduced the following little epifode. "Dear Sen-"fibility; thou fometimes infpireft the rough peafant, "who traverfes the bleakeft mountains.—He finds "the lacerated lamb of another's flock. This mo-"ment I beheld him, leaning his head againft his "crook, with piteous inclination looking down upon "it.—Oh! had I come one moment fooner!—It "bleeds to death.—His gentle heart bleeds with it. "Peace to thee, generous fwain; I fee thou walkeft "off with anguifh; but thy joys fhall balance it. "For happy is thy cottage;—and happy is the fharer "of it;—and happy are the lambs which fport about "thee!"

SMOKE, iffuing from the chimney of a retired cottage fhaded with trees, is a pleafing object. The waving line of beauty, in which it gradually afcends, and the fucceffion of graceful forms which it affumes, before it is loft in the atmofphere, adapts it to poetical defcription or comparifon, as well as to the canvas of the painter. Mr. Dyer, in the poem above re-

ferred to, has thus reprefented its appearance, and
affociated with it ideas of comfort and plenty, which
tend to heighten the complacency of the beholder.

" Yet your mild homefteads, ever blooming, fmile
" Among embracing woods, and wait on high
" The breath of plenty, from the ruddy tops
" Of chimneys, curling o'er the gloomy trees,
" In airy azure ringlets, to the fky."*

The FLOATING MISTS, which are feen on the tops
and fides of hills, often put on a variety of agreeable
fhapes and colours. They conftitute an interefting
part of the fcenery of Offian's poems; and are introduced with peculiar propriety, as objects which, in
a mountainous country, were continually within the
view of his *dramatis perfonæ*. " The mift of Cromla
" curls upon the rock, and fhines to the beam of the
" weft. The foft mift pours over the filent vale.
" The green flowers are filled with dew. The fun
" returns in his ftrength; and the mift is gone."
Thefe beautiful forms fuggeft to a devout mind,
converfant with the writings of Milton, part of
Adam's morning invocation:

" Ye mifts and exhalations, that now rife
" From hill or fteaming lake, dufky or grey,
" Till the fun paint your fleecy fkirts with gold,
" In honour to the world's great Author rife;
" Whether to deck with clouds th' uncolour'd fky,
" Or wet the thirfty earth with falling fhowers,
" Rifing or falling, ftill advance his praife."†

The expreffion *fteaming lake*, in the fecond line, is
ufed with the ftricteft philofophical truth. Thomfon

* Dyer's Fleece, book i. line 509.   † Milton, book v.

has applied the fame epithet, with equal juftnefs, to that inteftine motion in the earth, by which Divine Providence

" Works in the fecret deep, fhoots *fteaming* thence
" The fair profufion, that o'erfpreads the fpring."

For it appears, from fome late experiments, that fixteen hundred gallons of water rife by evaporation, from an acre of ground, within the fpace of twelve hours, of a fummer's day.*

An inattentive obferver of nature would hardly remark the CURVILINEAR DIRECTION in the motion of animals. Yet certain it is, that neither birds, fifhes, infeɛts, quadrupeds, nor men, ever move long in a ftraight line. The final caufe of this feems to be, that eafe may be alternately given to the mufcles, on the right and on the left fide of the body. When the mufcles of the right fide are in a ftate of vigorous exertion, the direɛtion of the body will incline that way; and when they require relief, thofe of the left fide come into aɛtion, and produce an oppofite effeɛt. Whoever follows a draught horfe heavily laden will perceive the truth of this obfervation. And it is not more apparent on the beaten highway, than in the fheep-tracks on the heath, and in the paths, worn by the paffage of cattle to their watering-places. Hence it is a rule in the art of gardening, that walks and pleafure-grounds fhould be ferpentine: as that form is moft agreeable to nature,

* Watfon's Chemical Effays, vol. iii. p. 52.

and therefore moſt conſonant to an elegant and improved taſte.

Milton makes frequent mention of the FLAMING
SWORDS, borne by the angelic ſpirits, and particularly by the cherubim, who were ſtationed at the
gate of Paradiſe:

> " And on the eaſt ſide of the garden, place,
> " Where entrance up from Eden eaſieſt climbs,
> " Cherubic watch; and of a ſword, the flame
> " Wide waving, all approach far off to fright,
> " And guard all paſſage to the tree of life."
>
> PARADISE LOST, book xi. l. 120.

If the poet had been acquainted with the modern
diſcoveries in electricity, he might perhaps have ſeized
this occaſion of exerting his ſuperior talents for deſcription, by a more minute and pictorial diſplay of
the ſword of flame wide waving. The reader at leaſt
may aſſiſt his imagination to conceive a more lively
idea of it, by the following beautiful experiment.

Make a torricellian *vacuum,* in a glaſs tube, about
three feet long, and ſeal it hermetically. Let one end
of this tube be held in the hand, and the other applied to the electrical conductor; and immediately
the whole tube will be illuminated, and when taken
from the conductor, will continue luminous for a
conſiderable time. If it be then drawn through the
hand, the light will be uncommonly intenſe, from end
to end, without the leaſt interruption. After this
operation, which diſcharges it in a great meaſure, it
will ſtill flaſh at intervals, though held only at one
extremity, and quite ſtill. But if it be graſped by

the other hand at the fame time in a different place, ftrong flafhes of light will dart from one extremity to the other, and continue to do fo twenty-four hours, or perhaps longer, without frefh excitation.*

The foregoing experiment was made by Mr. Canton, to elucidate the nature of the Aurora Borealis, a phenomenon well fuited to exercife the fancy of the poet. But ftill more congenial to him are thofe illufive meteors, which fometimes occur in northern climates; and which literally give " to airy " nothing a local habitation and a name."—" I was " never more furprized," fays Crantz, in his Hiftory of Greenland, " than on a fine warm fummer's " day to perceive the iflands, that lie four leagues " weft of our fhore, putting on a form quite different " from what they are known to have. As I ftood " gazing upon them, they appeared at firft infinitely " greater than what they naturally are; and feemed as " if I viewed them through a large magnifying glafs. " They were thus not only made larger, but brought " nearer to me: I plainly defcried every ftone upon " the land, and all the furrows filled with ice. " When this deception had lafted for a while, the " profpect feemed to break up, and a new fcene of " wonder to prefent itfelf. The iflands feemed to " travel to the fhore, and reprefented a wood, or " a tall cut hedge. The fcene then fhifted, and " fhewed the appearance of all forts of curious " figures; as fhips with fails, ftreamers, and flags,

* See Dr. Prieftley's Hift. of Electricity, p. 540.

"antique elevated caſtles with decayed turrets; and "a thouſand forms, for which fancy found a reſem- "blance in nature. When the eye had been ſatis- "fied with gazing, the whole group ſeemed to riſe in "air, and at length vaniſh into nothing. At ſuch "times the air is quite ſerene and clear, but compreſt "with ſubtile vapours; and theſe, appearing between "the eye and the object, give it all that variety of "appearances, which glaſſes of different refrangibi- "lities would have done."*

Thomſon, in his Caſtle of Indolence, refers to appearances ſomewhat ſimilar, in the weſtern iſles of Scotland:—

"As when a ſhepherd of the Hebrid iſles,
"Plac'd far amid the melancholy main,
"(Whether it be lone fancy him beguiles,
"Or that aërial beings ſometimes deign
"To ſtand embody'd to our ſenſes plain,)
"Sees on the naked hill or valley low,
"The whilſt in ocean Phœbus dips his wain,
"A vaſt aſſembly moving to and fro,
"Then all at once in air diſſolves the wondrous ſhew."

However marvellous ſuch narratives may appear to a phlegmatic reader, they will not ſeem incredible to the poet; whoſe fancy can form a ſtill brighter and more gay creation, without the aid of aërial refractions cr reflections. And if theſe fictions deviate not too far from veriſimilitude, they agreeably agitate the mind with the mixed emotions of ſurprize and delight. But in delineations of nature, they have no legitimate place; and the judgment rejects with

* See Goldſmith's Hiſtory of the Earth, vol. i.

difguft whatever falfifies the truth of defcription by
its obvious incongruity. Myrtle groves, perennial
fprings, unfading flowers, and odoriferous gales, the
hackneyed Arcadian fcenery, accord not with an
Englifh landfcape. And equally unfuitable to our
climate, and to the views of this country, are the
fpicy beauties and pearly treafures of the Eaft. Yet
Milton, in his Comus, thus addreffes the goddefs
of the Severn:

  " May thy billows roll afhore
  " The beryl, and the golden ore!
  " May thy lofty head be crown'd
  " With many a tower, and terrace round;
  " And here and there, thy banks upon,
  " With groves of myrrh and cinnamon."

But the poet is not upon all occafions to be confined
within the precife boundaries of truth. What writer,
of lively fancy, in defcribing a morning walk on the
banks of Kefwick, would not embellifh the beauty of
the fcene by the MELODY OF BIRDS; and thus add
the charms of mufic to all the enchantments of vifion?
Yet, I believe, there is not a feathered fongfter to be
found in thofe delightful vales; probably, owing to
the terror infpired by the birds of prey, which abound
on the mountains that furround them. The fame
obfervation will perhaps juftify the author of the
DESERTED VILLAGE, when he attempts to magnify
the horrors of an American wildernefs, by introducing
the t·ger into the tremendous group; though this
animal has never yet been found in the Britifh trans-
atlantic fettlements:

" Thofe pois'nous fields, with rank luxuriance crown'd,
" Where the dark fcorpion gathers death around;
" Where, at each ftep, the ftranger fears to wake
" The rattling terrors of the vengeful fnake;
" Where *crouching tigers* wait their haplefs prey,
" And favage men, more murd'rous ftill than they;
" While oft in whirls the mad tornado flies,
" Mingling the ravag'd landfcape with the fkies."

I cannot clofe this Effay, without making an apology for the freedom of my ftrictures on poetical demerit: and I feel a peculiar diffidence with refpect to the animadverfions on a poet, who is juftly the boaft and glory of Britain. To pluck a leaf from the brow of Milton, may be deemed a facrilegious attempt to injure the laurels of our country. Should it not, however, be recollected, that error is moft dangerous, when dignified by high example; and that it is no difparagement to genius, however exalted, to afcribe to it fome portion of that imperfection, which is the common allotment of humanity?

ON THE

INTELLECTUAL AND MORAL CONDUCT

OF

EXPERIMENTAL PURSUITS.

————

HOMO, NATURÆ MINISTER ET INTERPRES, TANTUM FACIT ET
INTELLIGIT, QUANTUM DE NATURÆ ORDINE, RE VEL MENTE,
OBSERVAVERIT; NEC AMPLIUS SCIT, AUT POTEST.

BACON, NOV. ORGAN. APH. I.

INTELLECTUAL AND MORAL CONDUCT

OF

EXPERIMENTAL PURSUITS.*

———

THE very learned and ingenious author of Hermes†
has ſtigmatized the purſuits of modern philoſophy, by treating them as mere *experimental amuſe-
ments;* and charging thoſe who are engaged in ſuch
purſuits, with deeming nothing *demonſtration*, that is
not made *ocular*. Thus, inſtead of aſcending from
ſenſe to *intellect*, the natural progreſs of all true learning, he obſerves, that the philoſopher hurries into
the midſt of ſenſe, where he wanders at random, loſt
in a labyrinth of *infinite particulars*. It would be
eaſy to retaliate on this celebrated writer, by pointing
out the futility of the ſyllogiſtic mode of philoſophizing, inſtituted by his favourite Ariſtotle. I might

* Read before the Literary and Philoſophical Society of Mancheſter, and inferted in the ſecond volume of their Memoirs.

† See a philoſophical enquiry concerning Univerfal Grammar, by
James Harris, efq; p. 361.

alfo oppofe to his authority that of Lord Verulam, the brighteſt luminary of ſcience, who objeƈts in the ſtrongeſt terms againſt that reverence for ſpecula‑ tions purely intelleƈtual, "by means whereof," as he expreſſes himſelf, "men have withdrawn too "much from the contemplations of nature, and the "obſervations of experience, and have tumbled up "and down in their own reaſon and conceits. Upon "theſe intelleƈtualiſts, who are notwithſtanding com‑ "monly taken for the moſt ſublime and divine philo‑ "ſophers, Heraclitus gave a juſt cenſure, ſaying, *men* "*ſought truth in their own little worlds, and not in* "*the great and common world.**" **

But, without depreciating metaphyſics, a ſcience which I have always ſtudied with delight, and which invigorates the faculties of the mind, and gives pre‑ ciſion and accuracy to our rational inveſtigations, by inſtruƈting us in the nicer diſcriminations of truth and falſehood, no doubt ought to be entertained of the high importance and dignity of natural knowledge. To this we owe the neceſſaries, the conveniences, and all the gratifications of our being; and in the purſuit of it the underſtanding is exerciſed and improved, and the moral affeƈtions are elevated to ſuperior de‑ grees of piety towards our great and beneficent Cre‑ ator. Nor is modern philoſophy liable to the charges which have been thus contumeliouſly brought againſt it. For, I truſt, it has been conduƈted on the prin‑ ciples of genuine *logic*, by all its more diſtinguiſhed

* Bacon of the Advancement of Learning, book i. p. 20.

profeſſors, who have been ſedulouſly careful firſt to
eſtabliſh found premiſes, and then to deduce juſt
concluſions.

The immortal Newton, from an appearance which
we daily obſerve, the fall of bodies to the ground,
aſcended by patient inveſtigation, and by a regular
gradation of evidence, to the great law of gravity:
and having aſcertained this general principle, he extended it over the univerſe; explaining by it not only
the phænomena of our globe, but the revolutions of
the whole planetary ſyſtem. By the ſucceſſive adoption of the fame *analytic* and *ſynthetic* mode of rea-
ſoning, he demonſtrated his beautiful theory of light
and colours. Numberleſs other ſubſequent diſcoveries have been conducted on the ſame ſcientific plan,
as might be evinced by references to the writings of
our own and foreign philoſophers.

Even the chemiſts have long ſince deſerted their
jargon and myſterious conceits; and they now carry
on their reſearches in a perſpicuous and rational manner. That unknown principle, phlogiſton, to which
they referred ſo many operations of nature, explaining, as the logicians expreſs it, *ignotum per ignotius*,
has been lately ſhewn to be no creature of the imagination; and may be exhibited to the ſenſes, under
the form of inflammable air. Fire, ſubtle as it is in
its activity, and univerſal in its energy, has been
traced through all its modifications, meaſured by different ſtandards, and reduced to known, precife, and
permanent laws. It is therefore no juſt complaint,

that intelligent principles are neglected, and that em-
pyricifm in phyfics is honoured with exclufive encouragement. Yet, in the prevailing rage for experiments,
it cannot be unfeafonable to caution the young adventurer, not to deem the microfcope, the retort, or
the air-pump, unerring guides to truth; but to pro-
fecute his refearches into nature with a modeft conviction of the fallacy of his fenfes, and the limited
powers of his underftanding. " You will wonder,"
fays Mr. Boyle in the preface to his effays, " that I
" fhould ufe fo often *perhaps*, *it feems*, *'tis not im-*
" *probable;* words which argue a diffidence of the
" truth of the opinions I incline to. But I have
" hitherto not unfrequently found, that what pleafed
" me for a while, was foon after difgraced by fome
" further or new experiment."

Mr. Bewley, an eminent chemift, not long fince
informed me, that he concluded the prefence of the
vitriolic acid to be unneceffary to produce the fpontaneous accenfion of Homberg's pyrophorus; and
delivered this opinion to the public, on the evidence
of at leaft fifty different trials.* Yet, with minerals
taken from the fame bottle, the experiment afterwards
failed nearly as often, though the minuteft circumftances in the procefs were as much alike as attention
could render them. Contrarieties, equally humiliating, have often occurred in my own philofophical
purfuits. But the moft inftructive leffon of modefty

* See Prieftley on Air, vol. iii. Appendix, p. 395.

and referve, which I recollect in the courfe of my experience, is the one I fhall now briefly recite.

The favourable influence of fixed air on vegetation
I believed to have been afcertained by more than a
hundred experiments, which I made in the year
1775. Many of thefe experiments were repeated
afterwards by Mr. Henry, Mr. Bew, and others.
But Dr. Prieftley, whofe accuracy and fidelity are not
lefs diftinguifhed than his learning and ingenuity, has
fince drawn conclufions from the profecution of this
fubject, which militate totally with mine. - I refumed
the enquiry, and engaged feveral of my friends in it.
The refult of all our trials was uniformly the fame,
viz. that fixed air, in a due proportion, is fo favourable to vegetable growth, that it may juftly be deemed
a *pabulum* of plants. Dr. Prieftley's fubfequent experiments, however, were ftill contradictory to mine:
and in one of his friendly letters to me, he thus expreffes himfelf:—" In all thefe cafes you will fay, I
" choak the plants with too great a quantity of *whole-*
" *fome* nourifhment : and to all yours I fay, you do
" not give them enough of the *noxious matter* to kill
" them. Thus the amicable controverfy muft reft
" between us; and like all other combatants, we
" fhall both fing TE DEUM." But I felt little dis-
pofition to exultation on fuch an occafion, and dropt
the fubject; confcious that though nature be always the
fame, we often view her under fallacious appearances.
Time, however, and the refearches of foreign philofophers have thrown new lights on this difputed point.

And I am informed, by a letter from our common friend, Mr. Vaughan, that Dr. Priestley now admits the salubrity of fixed air to vegetable life. I shall copy the paragraph which contains the account.
" Dr. Priestley tells me of a very valuable book, writ-
" ten by a person of Geneva, on vegetation; parti_
" cularly as to the influence of light, which he main-
" tains to be a phlogisticating process, acting on the
" resinous parts of plants only.   He also affirms, to
" the satisfaction of Dr. Priestley, that not only phlo-
" giston is the grand pabulum of plants, but that its
" predominant form of reception is that of fixed air;
" which, in a proper degree and place of application,
" he shews to be salutary to all plants whatever."

Differences in the results of our inquiries, or in those of others, whilst they incite attention, and guard us against confidence and presumption, should neither diminish the veneration due to philosophy, nor re-press our temperate ardour in the pursuit of truth. We should recollect, that though the operations of nature are simple, uniform, and regular, they are only discovered to be such, when fully unfolded to our understandings: and that, when we endeavour to trace her laws by artificial arrangements, combinations, or decompositions, which is all that *experiment* can accomplish,* success may be sometimes frustrated by circumstances so minute, as to elude the most saga-

---

* Ad opera nil. aliud potest homo, quam ut corpora naturalia admoveat, et amoveat; reliqua natura ipsa intus transigit.—BACON, Nov. Organ.

cious obfervation. From the hiftory of electricity it appears, that the gentlemen firft engaged in the culture of that fcience afcribed oppofite effects to the ufe of boiling water in the Leyden phial. M. Jalabert, of Geneva, and others, invariably found that the electric powers of the bottle were increafed by the water; whereas Meffrs. Kinnerfly, Nollet, and Watfon, experienced the reverfe, in all their trials. It has fince been fhewn that the jarring decifions of thofe learned men were owing to the difference in the action of boiling water on the feveral kinds of glafs employed. Contradictory opinions are now held by two very celebrated chemifts concerning the nature of fteel; one afferting that its phlogifton is augmented, the other that it is diminifhed, in the procefs by which it is made. Both appeal to experiment in fupport of their opinions; and as the point in difpute is of importance to the arts, it merits a more complete and fatisfactory inveftigation.

To thefe examples I fhall add another, in which I have myfelf been particularly interefted. The Rev. Dr. Hales, whofe experimental inquiries were generally directed to the good of his fellow-creatures, difcovered a lithontriptic power in certain fermenting mixtures. But he acknowledges the impracticability of injecting fuch mixtures into the bladder, with fufficient frequency, to diffolve the ftone; and recites his experiments chiefly with a view to engage others in the fame laudable and important purfuit. The fubject however funk into oblivion, and no further

attempts of this kind were made, till the notice of the
public was again excited towards the properties and
ufes of factitious air, by the writings of various
learned and ingenious men.   At this time (1774) Dr.
Saunders, a phyfician in London, eminent for his
knowledge of chemiftry, renewed the experiments
which Dr. Hales had begun, and found that the fol-
vent power, afcribed to the fermenting mixtures,
refided only in the fixed air.   Hearing fome very imperfect accounts of this difcovery, curiofity and humanity engaged me in the purfuit of it.   I recollected
that Dr. Black and Mr. Cavendifh had proved the
folubility of various earthy bodies in water, either by
abftracting from or fuperadding to the fixed air which
they contain.   And as the human calculus is diffolved
in the former way, by lime-water and the cauftic alkali, it appeared to me highly probable, that the effect
would be produced in the fame fubftance by the latter
mode of operation.   Analogy feemed favourable to
the hypothefis, and a feries of experiments, which I
made with great care, in the fulleft manner confirmed
it.   Two years afterwards Dr. Falconer engaged in
the fame inquiry, and the refults of his trials exactly
coincide with thofe which I have related.   This united
evidence has been alfo ftrengthened by the fubfequent teftimony of Dr. Prieftley and Dr. Hulme.
Yet decifive as it appears to be, a friend of mine, who
is a very able and accurate experimenter, affures me,
that the *calculi*, which he has tried, uniformly refift
the action of mephitic water: and he further adds,

that not one of them has been found to contain a
single grain of abforbent earth; but that all of them
proved inflammable, like gall-ftones. Dr. Heberden
has alfo favoured me with fimilar information refpecting their analyfis. On the other hand, I have fhewn
that thefe fubftances vary in their ftructure and compofition; that calcination converts fome into quick-
lime; that others are confumed entirely in the fire;
and that a third fort yield, after burning, an infipid
refiduum, incapable of giving any impregnation to
water.* What then are we to infer from premifes,
apparently fo inconfiftent? Let us deduce from them
thefe falutary leffons; that dogmatifm is unbecoming
a philofopher; that fallacy may attend our cleareft
views; and that unperceived diverfities in the fubjects of our inveftigation may render truth compatible with contrariety of evidence.

An eagernefs to eftablifh fyftems, and a faftidious
difdain of perplexity, contradiction, or difappointment,
are difpofitions highly unfavourable to phyfical inveftigation. Lord Bacon has well obferved, " that one
" who begins with certainties, fhall end in doubts,
" but if he will be content to begin with doubts, he
" fhall end in certainties."† The progrefs of fcience
is ufually flow and gradual; and in all ordinary cafes
the *race is not to the fwift,* but to the fteady, the patient, and the perfevering. A man of lively parts and

* Philofoph. Medic. and Experim. Effays.

† Advancement of Learning, book i. p. 40.

fertile imagination generally engages in philofophical refearches with too much impetuofity; and if he be fortunate in the attainment of a few leading facts, he fupplies all remaining deficiencies by conjecture and hypothefis. But fhould his career be obftructed by contradictory phænomena, he quits the ftudy of nature with difguft, and concludes that all is uncertainty, becaufe he has had the mortification to find himfelf miftaken. A fcepticifm like this, founded in pride and indolence, is equally fubverfive both of fpeculation and of action. We can apply to no branch of human learning which is fecure from illufion, or exempt from controverfy; nor engage in any plan of life with undeviating judgment, and uninterrupted fuccefs. So true is the fentiment of the Roman poet:

" Nunquam quifquam ita bene fubducta ratione ad vitam fuit,
" Quin res, ætas, ufus, femper aliquid apportet novi;
" Aliquid admoneat: ut illa, quæ te fcire credas, nefcias,
" Et quæ tibi putaris prima in experiundo repudies."
                                        TERENT.

But as difappointments in life often furnifh the beft leffons of wifdom, fo thofe in philofophy may frequently be applied to the promotion of fcience. In experimental purfuits, which are not undertaken at random, but with confiftent and rational views, we neceffarily form a preconception of the induction to be eftablifhed. If the trials fucceed in which we are engaged, our end is obtained, and for the moft part we reft fatisfied. But if the proofs fail, fome unexpected phænomena often occur, which awaken our attention, fuggeſt new analogies, and excite us perhaps to the inveſtigation of other propoſitions of more importance than the antecedent ones.   The very intereſting and comprehenſive diſcoveries of Dr. Black, concerning the nature of calcareous earths, and alkaline ſalts, in their different ſtates of mildneſs and cauſticity, originated from an incident of this kind.*   And many ſimilar examples might be adduced from the records of philoſophy.   But whether ſuch be the fortunate event or not, a negative truth may be of as much value as a poſitive one; and conſequently, ſucceſs or diſappointment may prove equally uſeful in experimental reſearches.†

To deduce the general characters of a body from one ſingle property of it, individually conſidered, ſeems contrary to the rules of philoſophizing: and the young experimenter ſhould be cautious both of admitting and of forming ſuch analogies.   Yet they are ſometimes ſo ſtrong as to force conviction even againſt the evidence of ſenſe, and of general opinion. The diamond was held by chemiſts, in the time of Sir Iſaac Newton, to be apyrous, and could not be ſuſpected, from any of its known qualities, to be of an inflammable nature.   Yet this vigilant philoſopher did not heſitate to conſider it as an *unctuous coagulum*, ſolely from its poſſeſſing a very high degree of refractive power on the rays of light.   For this power he

---

* See Eſſays Phyſical and Literary.

† See the Author's Philoſophical, Medical, and Experimental Eſſays, vol. i. fourth edit.

found to depend chiefly, if not wholly, on the ful-
phureous parts of which bodies are compofed. Late
experiments have confirmed this opinion, and fully
proved that diamonds confift almoft entirely of pure
phlogifton; fince they are capable of being volatilized
by heat in clofe veffels, of pervading the moft folid
porcelain crucibles, and of being converted into
actual flame.

The accuracy of this inference is a ftriking proof
of the importance of judicious and comprehenfive
analogies, and of the advantages refulting from the
mode of reafoning by induction. For, to ufe the
words of Sir Ifaac Newton, " though the arguing
" from experiments and obfervations by induction is
" no *demonftration* of general conclufions, yet it is
" the beft way of arguing, which the nature of things
" admits of; and may be looked upon as fo much
" the ftronger, by how much the induction is more
" general." This improved fpecies of logic was firft
recommended and introduced into phyfics by Lord
Verulam, who at a very early period of life faw the
futility of Ariftotle's fyllogyftic fyftem, which, proceeding on the fuperficial enumeration of a few particulars, rifes at once to the eftablifhment of univerfal
propofitions. *Duæ viæ funt, atque effe poffunt, ad
inquirendam et inveniendam veritatem. Altera a
fenfu et particularibus advolat ad axiomata maxime generalia, atque ex iis principiis, eorumque immota veritate judicat et invenit axiomata media; atque hæc via
in ufu eft. Altera à fenfu et particularibus excitat*

*axiomata, afcendendo continenter et gradatim, ut ultimo loco perveniatur ad maxime generalia; quæ via vera eft, fed intentata.**

It is obvious that the force of this inductive method of reafoning muft depend on the advancement which has been made in the different branches of phyfics. Indeed, it prefuppofes a ftore of particular facts, gradually accumulated, but fufficiently ample, and fit for reduction into their proper claffes. Time and obfervation will be continually diminifhing the number, and confequently enlarging the boundaries of thefe claffes, by difcovering other relations between them, and pointing out the connection of phænomena, deemed at firft diftinct and independent. But it muft be remembered that every acceffion to knowledge renews the doubts and difficulties that refult from ignorance, becaufe it prefents frefh objects to our inveftigation, and further *defiderata* to our wifhes. It is this endlefs progreffion of fcience, which, by gratifying curiofity with perpetual novelty, and animating ambition with profpects of higher and higher attainments, fometimes gives the attachment to it an undue afcendancy over every other principle of the mind. But having expatiated in another Effay,* on the folly of fuch extravagant ardour in the purfuits of knowledge, I fhall now clofe thefe reflections with the following lines from Milton:—

---

* Bacon, Nov. Organ. lib. i. Aphor. 19.

* On Inconfiftency of Expectation in Literary Purfuits.

" . . . Apt the mind, or fancy, is to rove
" Uncheck'd, and of her roving is no end;
" Till warn'd, or by experience taught, fhe learn,
" That not to know at large of things remote
" From ufe, obfcure and fubtle, but to know
" That which before us lies, in daily life,
" Is the prime wifdom; what is more is fume,
" Or emptinefs, or fond impertinence,
" And renders us in things that moft concern,
" Unpractis'd, unprepared, and ftill to feek.''

PAR. LOST, book viii.

A

TRIBUTE

TO THE MEMORY OF

CHARLES DE POLIER, ESQ;

ADDRESSED TO THE

LITERARY AND PHILOSOPHICAL SOCIETY OF

MANCHESTER.

OCTOBER 30, 1782.

AT a meeting of the LITERARY *and* PHILOSO-PHICAL SOCIETY *of* MANCHESTER, *the following refo-lution paſſed unanimouſly :*—

" *The Members of the* LITERARY *and* PHILOSOPHICAL SOCIETY, *lamenting, with heartfelt concern, the death of their late much honoured brother* CHARLES DE POLIER, *eſq: unanimouſly reſolve, that* DR. PERCIVAL *be requeſted to draw up a grateful and reſpectful Tribute to his Memory, to be inſerted in the Journals of the Society, with a view to record his diſtin-guiſhed merit, and to prolong the influence of his bright example.*"

NOVEMBER 13, 1782.

AT a meeting of the LITERARY *and* PHILOSO-PHICAL SOCIETY, *it was reſolved unanimouſly,*

" *That the Thanks of the Society be returned to* DR. PER-CIVAL, *for his Tribute to the Memory of* CHARLES DE POLIER, *eſq; and that he be d ſired to print the ſame.*"

A

TRIBUTE

TO THE MEMORY OF

CHARLES DE POLIER, ESQ;

ADDRESSED TO THE

LITERARY AND PHILOSOPHICAL SOCIETY OF MANCHESTER.

THE contemplation of moral and intellectual excellence affords the most pleafing and inftructive
exercife to a well-conftituted mind. By exalting our
ideas of the human character, it expands and heightens
the principle of benevolence; and at the fame time is
favourable to piety, by raifing our views to the
Supreme Author of all that is fair and good in man.

The wife and the virtuous have ever dwelt with
delight on the meritorious talents and difpofitions of
their fellow-creatures : and an amiable philofopher
drew from this fource fuch fweet confolations, under
the toils and diftreffes of life, that he warmly recom-
mends the practice to our imitation. " *When you*

" *would recreate yourfelf,*" fays M. Antoninus, " re-
" *flecton the laudable qualities of your acquaintance ;*
" *on the magnanimity of one, the modefty of another,*
" *or the liberality of a third.****" Generous meditation ! which every one prefent may indulge ; and by
indulging, affimilate to his own nature the various
perfections of others; transfufing, as it were, into his
breaft, the virtues which he contemplates.

Can we engage ourfelves in fuch an exercife, without the moft lively recollection of our late honoured
and beloved colleague ? His image prefents itfelf
before us ; and we inftantly recognife the agreeable-
nefs of his form, the animation of his countenance,
the vigour of his underftanding, and the goodnefs of
his heart. How graceful was his addrefs; how
fprightly, entertaining, and intelligent, his converfation ! What rich ftores of knowledge did he difplay; what facility in the ufe, what judgment in the
application of them ! Few have been the fubjects
of difcuffion in this Society, which his obfervations have not enlightened: and what he could not
himelf elucidate, he has enabled others to do, by
the pertinency of his queries, and the fagacity of
his conjectures. So quick was his penetration, fo
enlarged his comprehenfion, fo exact the arrangement
of his intellectual treafures! Learning, with fome,
is the parent of mental obfcurity ; and the multiplicity of ideas which have been acquired by fevere
ftudy, ferve only to produce perplexity and confufion.

* M. Antonin. lib. vi.

But Mr. de Polier's thoughts were always ready at command: and he engaged with perfpicuity on every topic of difcourfe, becaufe he faw, at one view, all its relations and analogies to thofe branches of knowledge with which he was already acquainted. With fuch felicity of genius, he was continually making large acceffions to his ftock of fcience, without laborious refearches, or feclufion from the focial enjoyments of life.

Of his abilities as a writer, he furnifhed us with a ftriking proof, in the Differtation he delivered laft winter;* which is equally diftinguifhed by the juftnefs of its fentiments, and the purity of its diction; and fully difplays his perfect attainment both of the idiom and embellifhments of the Englifh language.

But Mr. de Polier had merits, more eftimable than thofe, which he derived from the vivacity of his fancy, the elegance of his tafte, or the powers of his underftanding. And his friends will cordially unite with me in teftifying, that, if honoured for his *intellectual*, he was beloved for his *moral* endowments. His heart was open to every generous fympathy; and the fenfibility of his nature fo enlivened all his perceptions, that the ordinary duties of focial intercourfe were performed by him with a warmth, almoft equal to that of friendfhip. Nor was this the artificial deportment of unmeaning courtefy; but the generous effufion of a heart, which felt for

---

* On the pleafure which the mind receives from the *exercife* of its faculties, and particularly that of *tafte*.

all mankind. In fuch *philanthropy*, politenefs has its true foundation : and of this joint grace of nature and education, " which aids and ftrengthens virtue " where it meets her, and imitates her actions where " fhe is not," our lamented brother was a bright example. So engaging were his manners, and at the fame time fo fincere his difpofition, that we may apply to him with *honour*, what Cicero meant as a *reproach*; that he was qualified, *cum triftibus feverè, cum remiffis jucundè, cum fenibus graviter, cum juventute comiter vivere.* Thefe powers of pleafing flowed from no fervile compliances, nor ever led him into criminal indulgences. As a companion, he was convivial without intemperance, and gay without levity or licentioufnefs. His converfation was fprightly and unreferved; but, in the moft unguarded hours of mirth, exempt from all indecency and profanenefs: and the fallies of his wit and pleafantry were fo feafoned with good humour, that they gave delight, unmixed with pain, even to thofe who were the objects of them. If the coarfer pleafures of the bottle be banifhed from our tables; or if rational converfation, and delicacy of behaviour, with the fweet fociety of the fofter fex, be now fubftituted in their room, this happy revolution has been rendered more complete by the influence of Mr. de Polier.

Yet though URBANITY, according to the moft liberal interpretation of that term, was the *characteriftic* of our excellent colleague, he poffeffed other endowments, of more intrinfic value : and I could enlarge, with pleafure, on his nice fenfe of rectitude, his inviolable integrity, and facred regard to truth. Thefe moral virtues were, in him, founded on no fictitious principle of *honour*, but refulted from the conftitution of his mind; and were ftrengthened by habit, regulated by reafon, and fanctioned by religion: for, notwithftanding the veil which he chofe to caft over his *piety*, it was manifeft to his intimate friends; and may be recollected by others, who have marked the ferioufnefs with which he difcourfed on every fubject relative to the being and attributes of God. Defective indeed muft be the character of that man, who can difcern and acknowledge, without venerating, the divine perfections; and partake of the bounties of nature, yet feel no emotions of gratitude towards its benevolent Author. *A little philofophy,* fays Lord Verulam, *may incline the mind to atheifm; but depth in philofophy will bring it about again to religion.**

I have thus attempted to draw a rude fketch of the features of our late honoured friend. A fuller delineation might furnifh a more pleafing picture to ftrangers; but to the members of this fociety, a few outlines will fuffice to revive the image of the beloved original. This image, I truft, will be long and for-

---

* The noble author fubjoins a juft reafon for this obfervation: "For while the mind of man," fays he, "looketh upon *fecond caufes* "fcattered, it may fometimes reft in them, and go no farther: but "when it beholdeth the chain of them linked together, it muft "needs fly to Providence and Deity."

BACON's Effay on Atheifm.

cibly impreffed on our minds; and that every one
here prefent may adopt the language of Tacitus, on
a fimilar occafion: " *Quicquid ex Agricola amavimus,*
" *quicquid mirati fumus, manet, manfurumque eft in*
" *animis hominum.*"   " Whatever in Agricola was
" the object of our love and of our admiration, re-
" mains, and will remain, in the hearts of all who
" knew him."

Having taken a fhort view of the character of Mr.
de Polier, curiofity and attachment concur in prompt-
ing us to extend the retrofpect; and we become folicitous to know fomething of his connections and education; and to trace the leading events of a life, in
the conclufion of which we have been fo deeply interefted.   But our friend was no egotift; and the zeal
with which he entered into the concerns of others,
precluded the detail of his own.   I muft content
myfelf, therefore, with prefenting to the fociety the
following brief memoirs.

Charles de Polier Bottens was the fon of the Rev.
—— de Polier Bottens, Dean of the Cathedral
Church of Laufanne, Prefident of the Synod of the
Pais de Vaud, Member of the Society of Arts and
Sciences at Manheim, and citizen of Geneva.   He
was born at Laufanne, in the year 1753; and received the firft part of his education in the public
fchools of that city.   As foon as he had acquired a
fufficient knowledge of the claffics, he was fent to an
academy near Caffel, in Germany; from whence,
after a refidence of two years, he was removed to

the univerfity of Gottingen.   In this celebrated feat
of learning, he paffed three years; and being then
inclined to a military life, he obtained a lieutenant's
commiffion in the Swifs regiment of D'Erlach, in the
French fervice.   But he foon refigned his commiffion,
and returned to Laufanne, where he had a command
given him in one of the provincial regiments of dra-
goons.   In this fituation, his connection commenced
with the Earl of Tyrone; who offered him the tuition
of his eldeft fon, Lord le Poer, on terms equally
honourable and advantageous.   But before the engagement was completed, propofals were made to
him by the Duke of Saxe Gotha, to become governor to the hereditary prince, with an annuity for life
of twelve hundred rix-dollars, an apartment at court,
and the poft of chamberlain, or rank of colonel.
Thefe propofals, however, he declined in favour of
Lord Tyrone.   And he executed the important truft
affigned to him with fuch judgement, tendernefs, and
fidelity, as induced that refpectable nobleman to commit three of his children to his fole direction.   Thefe
amiable youths he brought to England in the fummer of 1779, and fettled them at the fchool of a
clergyman in Manchefter, who is eminently diftinguifhed by his virtues and abilities.

    At this period our firft acquaintance with Mr. de
Polier was formed.   By the laws of hofpitality he
was entitled to our attention as a ftranger.   But his
perfonal accomplifhments, and the charms of his con
verfation, foon fuperfeded the ordinary claims of

cuſtom, and converted formal civility into eſteem and friendſhip.   He became our companion in pleaſure, our aſſiſtant in ſtudy, our counſellor in difficulty, and our ſolace in diſtreſs.   Amuſement acquired a dignity and zeſt by his participation, and he ſoftened the auſterity of philoſophy whenever he joined in the purſuit.   The inſtitution which now celebrates his memory, owes to him much of its popularity and ſucceſs; and ſo long as it ſubſiſts, his name will be revered as one of its founders and moſt ſhining ornaments.

About the middle of laſt winter he was attacked by a complaint, which at firſt gave no diſturbance to the vital functions.   But being aggravated by the fatigues of a long journey to Holyhead, and of a voyage from thence to Dublin, at a time when he laboured under the _Influenza_, the malady rapidly increaſed after his arrival in Ireland, and put a final period to his valuable life on the 18th of October 1782*.   The vigour of his faculties, and the warmth of his affections, continued even to the hour of his diſſolution.   And the amiableneſs of his behaviour in the cloſing ſcene of trial and ſuffering through which he paſſed, gave ſuch completion to his character, that we may apply to him what the poet has ſaid of Mr. Addiſon:

> - - - " He taught us how to live ; and, oh! too high
> " The price of knowledge, taught us how to die!"†

---

* At Curraghmore, near Waterford, the ſeat of the Earl of Tyrone.
† Tickell's Poems on the death of Mr. Addiſon.

On this affecting event, I cannot exprefs your feelings and my own, in terms fo forcible as thofe of the
animated hiftorian, whom I have before quoted. *Si
quis piorum manibus locus; fi, ut fapientibus placet,
non cum corpore exftinguuntur magnæ animæ; placide
quiefcas, nofque ab infirmo defiderio, ad contempla-
tionem virtutum tuarum voces, quas neque lugeri neque
plangi fas eft! Admiratione te potius temporalibus
laudibus, et fi natura fuppeditet, fimilitudine decore-
mus!** " If there be any habitation for the fhades
" of the virtuous; if, as philofophers fuppofe,
" exalted fouls do not perifh with the body; may
" you repofe in peace, and recall us from vain regret
" to the contemplation of your virtues, which allow
" no place for mourning or complaint! Let us
" adorn your memory rather by a fixed admiration,
" and if our natures will permit, by an imitation of
" your excellent qualities, than by temporary
" eulogies.†

* Tacit. Vit. Agricolæ.

† See Mr. Aikin's Tranflation of the Life of Agricola.

AN

APPENDIX;

CONTAINING

SUPPLEMENTARY REMARKS,

AND ILLUSTRATIONS.

AS the Socratic mode of discussion admits not of interruption by Notes, the author has chosen to insert in this place such additional REMARKS *and* ILLUSTRATIONS, *concerning the subject matter of the Discourse on* TRUTH, *as further reading or reflection have suggested to his mind. He has also annexed a few supplementary Notes to the other* DISSERTATIONS.

SOCRATIC DISCOURSE.

SUPPLEMENTARY REMARKS AND ILLUSTRATIONS.

I. TRUE AND FALSE HONOUR.*

THERE is a principle of HONOUR which feems to be, in fome meafure, diftinct from that of virtue; and originates from the affociation of certain ideas of propriety, or pride, with rectitude of conduct. Amongft the ancient Greeks and Romans, virtue and honour were deified; and a joint altar was confecrated to them at Rome; but afterwards each of them had feparate temples; fo connected, however, that no one could enter the temple of honour without paffing through that of virtue.

The genuine principle of honour, in its full extent, may be defined, a quick perception and ftrong feeling of moral obligation, particularly with refpect to probity and truth, in conjunction with an acute fenfibility to fhame, reproach, or infamy. But in different characters, thefe two conftituent parts of the principle are found to exift in proportions fo widely diverfified, as fometimes to appear almoft fingle and detached. The former alway *aids and ftrengthens virtue;* the latter may, occafionally, *imitate her actions,*† when

---

* See page 8.

† " Honour's a facred tie, the law of kings,
" The noble mind's diftinguifhing perfection,
" That aids and ftrengthens Virtue where it meets her,
" And imitates her actions where fhe is not:
" It ought not to be fported with."   ADDISON's Cato

fashion happily countenances, or high example prompts to rectitude. But being connected, for the most part, with a jealous pride,
and capricious irritability, it will be more shocked with the *imputation*, than with the *commission* of what is wrong. And thus it
will constitute that spurious honour, which, by a perversion of the
laws of association, *puts evil for good, and good for evil;* and, under
the sanction of a name, perpetrates crimes without remorse, and
even without ignominy. To this empirical morality *duelling* owes
its rise, which, with fatal confidence, pretends to cure the indeco-
rums of social intercourse, whilst it destroys the lives of individuals,
subverts the peace of families, and violates the most sacred laws of
the community. It is astonishing that a practice, which originated
in the dark ages of ignorance, superstition, and disorder, should be
continued in this enlightened period, though condemned by the
polity of every state, and utterly repugnant to the spirit and precepts of Christianity. The ancient Germans, Danes, and Franks
were used to decide criminal questions of fact, in the last resort,
by combat. But this method of trial, about the close of the fifth
century, was restrained to the following conditions :—1. That the
crime, for which it was instituted, should be capital. 2. That it
should be certain that the crime had been perpetrated. 3. That
the accused, by common fame, should be supposed guilty. 4. That
the matter should not be capable of proof by witnesses. A custom
thus regulated appears wise and equitable in comparison with modern duelling, which has seldom any object, but the redress of
fantastic wrongs, or the display of resentment, that often subsists
before its execution. Is there a man of probity and humanity, and
many of this character, I am persuaded, have been seduced by the
illusions of false honour, who, if not prohibited by law, would think
himself authorized to call forth his antagonist, place him as a mark,
and appoint a ruffian to fire a pistol at him, because, in the heat
of argument, or in the unguarded hours of convivial mirth, he has
committed some trifling offence, or verbal incivility And is it
not adding the most egregious folly to injustice, to undertake himself this opprobrious office, at the hazard of his own life, and to the
ruin, perhaps, of his dearest connections? For, I presume, it now
forms no part of the creed of the duellist, that Divine Providence
will interpose, on such occasions, to preserve the injured, and to
punish the aggressor.

The military fpirit which a long war has revived amongft the inhabitants of this country, and which the armed affociations, eftablifhed in different places, cannot fail to fofter and fupport, may, perhaps, contribute to multiply challenges, and to extend the practice of fingle combat. Courage is fo effential to the character of a foldier, that it becomes magnified in his eftimation, far beyond its real defert; and he is not only in danger of miftaking its true nature, and proper object, but of acquiring a contempt for every virtue, which, in his perverted judgment, ftands in competition with it. Like Achilles, *jura negat fibi nata ; nihil non arrogat armis.* Reafon and religion fhould, therefore, exert their united authority to check the influence of fuch baneful errors: and law fhould rigoroufly punifh, with difgrace and infamy, the man who can facrifice humanity to pride, and juftice to the fpecious counterfeit of gallantry.

I fhall clofe this fection with the following paffage, from the celebrated Commentaries of Sir William Blackftone :—" Exprefs " malice is, when one with a fedate, deliberate mind, and formed " defign, doth kill another; which formed defign is evidenced by " external circumftances difcovering that inward intention; as lying " in wait, antecedent menaces, former grudges, and concerted " fchemes to do him fome bodily harm. This takes in the cafe of deli- " berate duelling, where both parties meet, avowedly with an intent " to murder; thinking it their duty as gentlemen, and claiming it " as their right, to wanton with their own lives, and thofe of their " fellow-creatures, without any warrant or authority from any " power, either human or divine, but in direct contradiction to the " laws both of GOD and man: and therefore, the law has juftly " fixed the crime and punifhment of murder, on them and on their " feconds alfo."*

II. FALSE MAXIMS OF MORALITY.†

THE hiftory of Lord Herbert, of Cherbury, admirably exemplifies the folly and danger of adopting FALSE MAXIMS of MORALITY. From the variety of inftances which offer themfelves in the memoirs of this romantic nobleman, I fhall felect the fol-

* Book iv. chap. 14.   † See page 9.

lowing:—During his abode at the Duke of Montmorency's, about twenty-four miles from Paris, it happened one evening, that a daughter of the Dutchefs de Ventadour, of about ten or eleven years of age, went to walk in the meadows with his lordfhip, and feveral other gentlemen and ladies. The young lady wore a knot of riband on her head, which a French chevalier fnatched away, and faftened to his hatband. He was defired to return it, but refufed. The lady then requefted Lord Herbert to recover it for her. A race enfued; and the chevalier finding himfelf likely to be overtaken, made a fudden turn, and was about to deliver his prize to the young lady, when Lord Herbert feized his arm and cried out, " I give it you." ' Pardon me,' faid the lady, ' it is he who gives ' it me.' " Madam," replied Lord Herbert, " I will not con-" tradict you; but if the chevalier do not acknowledge that I con-" ftrain him to give the riband, I will fight with him." And the next day he fent him a challenge, " being bound thereunto," fays he, " by the oath taken when I was made knight of the bath."

He relates, alfo, three other fimilar cafes to fhew, *how ftriftly he held himfelf to his oath of knighthood.* " This oath," fays the ingenious editor of Lord Herbert's life, " is one remnant of a fuper-" ftitious and romantic age, which an age calling itfelf enlightened " ftill retains. The folemn fervice at the inveftiture of the knights, " which has not the leaft connection with any thing holy, is a piece " of the fame profane pageantry. The oath being no longer fup-" pofed to bind, it is ftrange mockery to invoke heaven on fo " trifling an occafion." And it would be more ftrange, if each knight, like the mifguided Lord Herbert, fhould think himfelf obliged to cut a man's throat, whenever a young lady lofes her top-knot!

Thefe religious engagements are fo often mifapplied, that it cannot be unfeafonable to enter into a brief difcuffion of their true nature and obligation. A vow may be defined, *a devout promife made to God, refpecting either the performance or omiffion of fome voluntary act;* and is often accompanied with an imprecation of divine vengeance on the infraction of it. The only legitimate ufe of fuch an engagement is, to increafe our abhorrence of what is evil, and to confirm our refolution in the more arduous purfuits of virtue. It cannot, therefore, be applied to the neglect of any antecedent duty, or to the accomplifhment of any impious or immoral purpofe. Were it otherwife, thefe arbitrary ties might be made a plea for violating every law, whether human or divine. Even prudence, in certain cafes, is of fufficient force to fuperfede the validity of a vow. Thus, if the fuperftitious parent of a numerous and helplefs family were, in fome preffing danger, to invoke the affiftance of heaven, by the moft folemn avowal of his refolution to give all his fubftance to the church, or to the poor; fuch an abfurd intention has not the nature of an engagement, and is void in itfelf: for, we are affured, that the execution of it could never prove acceptable to a wife and benevolent Deity, with whom alone the contract was made. But this reafoning does not extend to rafh and injurious bargains, or to promifes of a focial natnre, which have been confirmed by an oath: for, as the maintenance of faith is of the higheft importance in the commerce of life; to add impiety to the breach of it, muft certainly be deemed an aggravation of the offence: and in fuch inftances, *the good man changeth not, though he fware to his own hurt.*

III. FEALTY TO MAGISTRATES.

THE COMMANDS of the MAGISTRATE, or of the LEGISLATURE, are not binding, when they oppofe the known and acknowledged obligations of morality; and the younger Cato has been juftly cenfured, for engaging in the execution of what he himfelf deemed a violent and moft oppreffive fentence againft Ptolemy, king of Cyprus. This prince was brother to the king of Egypt, and reigned by the fame right of hereditary fucceffion. He was in full peace and amity with Rome, and was accufed of no practices, nor fufpected of any defigns againft the republic. But the infamous Clodius, who was then tribune, propofed and obtained the law, from motives of private pique and revenge. To give a fanction to it, Cato was charged with its fulfilment; and undertook the commiffion, though contrary to all his ideas of juftice and rectitude. I believe no moralift of the prefent times will admit the validity of Cicero's apology for the mifconduct of his friend: " The commiffion," fays

* See page 9.

he, " was defigned not to adorn, but to banifh Cato; not offered,
" but impofed upon him. Why then did he obey it? For the
" fame reafon, that he *fwore to obey* other laws, which he knew to
" be unjuft, that he might not expofe himfelf to the fury of his
" enemies, or by a fruitlefs pertinacity, deprive the republic of his
" fervices."—Orat. pro Sexto.

The conduct of Scipio Africanus, in the deftruction of the brave
Numantines, is equally reprehenfible; for it is confeffed, by Lu-
cius Florus, that the Romans commenced hoftilities againft that
people, without even a pretence to render them juftifiable: and
the horrid barbarities, exercifed in the fiege of Numantia, excite
peculiar indignation, from the unparalleled fortitude and vigour which
the inhabitants difplayed in the defence of their liberties. Such bra-
very, exerted in a caufe fo noble, merited the patronage, and
fhould have called forth the clemency, not the refentment of Scipio.
But the Romans appear to have entertained no confiftent ideas concerning the privileges of other nations, or the common rights of
mankind. They proudly arrogated to themfelves the government
of the world, and the maxim, *regere imperio populos,** was the
plea for every conqueft. This principle pervades the writings of
all their poets and hiftorians: and even the philofophical Tacitus,
in delivering the memoirs of Agricola, expreffes not the flighteft
difapprobation of the numerous and deftructive expeditions into
Britain. Yet he has, inadvertently, put into the mouth of Galgacus,
one of the chieftains of our warlike anceftors, fuch fentiments as
may be deemed a ftigma on his venerable father-in-law, for obedience to imperial mandates, founded on cruelty and injuftice.
Raptores orbis, poftquam cuncta vaftantibus defuere terræ, et mare
ferutantur: fi locuples hoftis eft, avari; fi pauper, ambitiofi. Quos
non oriens, non occidens fatiaverit: foli omnium, opes atque inopiam,
pari affectu concupifcunt. Auferre, trucidare, rapere falfis nomi-
nibus, imperium; atque ubi folitudinem faciunt, pacem appellant.†
" Thefe plunderers of the world, after exhaufting the land by
" their devaftations, are rifling the ocean: ftimulated by avarice, if

---

* " Tu regere imperio populos Romane memento,
" Hæ tibi erunt artes) pacifque imponere morem,
" Parcere fubjectis, et debellare fuperbos." Virg.

† Tacit. Vit. Agric.

"their enemy be rich; by ambition, if poor; unfatiated by the eaft,
"and by the weft; the only people who behold wealth and indi-
"gence with equal avidity: to ravage, to flaughter, to ufurp under
"falfe titles, they call empire; and when they make a defert, they
"call it peace."*

Modern conquefts have been founded on claims equally invalid
and tyrannical with thofe of the Romans. It is a fatire on human
reafon, and ftill more difgraceful to the moral feelings of mankind,
to review the principles on which the Spaniards affected to eftablifh their rights to the extenfive dominions in the new world.
Their generals were inftructed to notify, with great formality, to
the innocent and ignorant natives of the weftern hemifphere, that
St. Peter had fubjected the univerfe to the jurifdiction of the Roman
Pontiff; and that this lord of the whole creation had made a grant
of the iflands, of the *Terra Firma*, and of the ocean, to the Catholic
Kings of Caftile. To thefe monarchs they were required to fubject themfelves; and if they refufed, the moft exemplary vengeance
was denounced againft them. They were threatened to be defpoiled
of their wives and children, to have their country ravaged, and to
be themfelves fold for flaves.†

Inftances like thefe afford the moft irrefragable evidence, that
fealty to magiftrates muft always be regarded as a conditional obligation; and that implicit obedience to their commands may
involve us in high degrees of guilt and infamy. Yet a very diftinguifhed hiftorian and moralift has caft a reflection on certain fea-
officers, under the protectorate of Oliver Cromwell, who refigned
their commiffions from fcruples of confcience relative to the Spanifh
war, in 1656; which the hiftorian himfelf acknowledges to have
been highly impolitic, and a moft unwarrantable violation of treaty.
"They thought," fays Mr. Hume, "no command of their fuperiors
"could juftify a war, which was contrary to the principles of na-
"tural equity, and which the civil magiftrate had no right to
"order. Individuals they maintained, in refigning to the public
"their natural liberty, could beftow on it what they themfelves
"were poffeffed of, a right of performing lawful actions; and could

* Aikin's Tranflation of the Life of Agricola.
† See Herrara, Dec. I. lib. vii. cap. 14; alfo Robertfon's Hiftory of America, note 23.

" inveft it with no authority o commanding what is contrary to
" the decrees of heaven. Such maxims, though they feem reafon-
" able, are perhaps too perfect or human nature, and muft be re-
" garded as one effect, though of the moft innocent and even
" honourable kind, of that fpirit, partly fanatical, partly republican,
" which predominated in England." That *maxims which feem
reafonable, and a fpirit of the moft innocent and even honourable kind*
fhould be deemed *too perfect for human nature*, participates of Machiavelian policy. It muft be acknowledged, however, that individuals cannot often be fully competent to decide of the juftice or
injuftice of foreign wars; and that the officers of the ftate are
bound to obey the commands of lawful authority, when they are
not oppofite to the clear dictates of honour and equity. But whenever the mind has fufficient evidence of the improbity, oppreffion,
or tyranny of public meafures; no one, under fuch conviction, can
voluntarily abet or aid them, in confiftence with duty to himfelf,
to his country, and to mankind. At the commencement of the late
conteft with America, the Earl of Effingham found himfelt in this
diftrefsful predicament; as appears from his letter of refignation
addreffed to Lord Barrington; wherein he expreffes his feelings in
the following terms:—" Your lordfhip is no ftranger to the con-
" duct which I have obferved in the unhappy difputes with our
" American colonies. The King is too juft and too generous not
" to believe, that the votes I have given in Parliament have been
" given according to the dictates of my confcience. Whether I
" have erred or not, the courfe of future events muft determine.
" In the mean time, if I were capable of fuch duplicity as to be any
" way concerned in enforcing thofe meafures of which I have fo
" publicly and folemnly expreffed my difapprobation, I fhould ill
" deferve what I am moft ambitious of obtaining—the efteem and
" favourable opinion of my fovereign.

" My requeft, therefore, to your lordfhip is this, that after having
" laid thofe circumftances before the King, you will affure his ma-
" jefty, that he has not a fubject who is more ready than I am, with
" the utmoft cheerfulnefs, to facrifice his life and fortune in fupport
" of the fafety, honour, and dignity of his majefty's crown and
" perfon. But the very fame principles, which have infpired me
" with thefe unalterable fentiments of duty and affection to his ma-
" jefty, will not fuffer me to be inftrumental in depriving any part

" of his people of thofe liberties, which form the beft fecurity for
" their fidelity and obedience to his government. As I cannot,
" without reproach from my own confcience, confent to bear arms
" againft my fellow-fubjects in America, in what, to my weak dis-
" cernment is not a clear caufe; and as it feems now to be finally
" refolved that the 22d regiment is to go upon American fervice,
" I defire your lordfhip to lay me in the moft dutiful manner at his
" Majefty's feet, and humbly beg that I may be permitted to retire.

" Your lordfhip will eafily conceive the regret and mortifica-
" tion I feel at being neceffitated to quit the military profeffion,
" which has been that of my anceftors for many generations, to
" which I have been bred almoft from my infancy; to which I have
" devoted the ftudy of my life; and to perfect myfelf in which, I
" have fought inftruction and fervice in whatever part of the world
" they were to be found.

" I have delayed this to the laft moment, left any wrong con-
" ftruction fhould be given to a conduct which is influenced only
" by the pureft motives. I complain of nothing; I love my pro-
" feffion, and fhould think it highly blameable to quit any courfe
" of life, in which I might be ufeful to the public, fo long as my
" conftitutional principles, and my notions of honour, permitted me
" to continue in it." Sept. 12, 1775.

In the prefent hoftilities between the Swedes and the Ruffians,
difquietndes are faid to have arifen in the minds of fome of the
Swedifh officers, concerning the legality of the war   " The 14th
" article in the form of government, prefented by the king, and
" agreed to by the diet, after the revolution of 1772, exprefsly de-
" termines, ' that the king cannot carry on an offenfive war, with-
" out the confent of the ftates affembled.' Neverthelefs the hoftile
" difpofitions of Ruffia againft Sweden, at the period of fitting out
" the armaments, have been fufficiently proved, fo as not to render
" it doubtful, whether the prefent war on our part is more *offenfive*
" than *defenfive*.   On this account fcruples have arifen in the
" minds of fome officers ferving in the army in Finland, ' whether
" the officers, who, from the mere will of the king, without the
" previous confent of the diet, and even without the knowledge of
" the ftates, allow themfelves to be employed in the war, which
" has every appearance of being OFFENSIVE on our part, at leaft,
" in the prefent campaign, do not render themfelves refponfible to

" the nation affembled, and punifhable fooner or later, for having
" acted contrary to their oath.' Yielding to thefe fcruples, five offi-
" cers applied for difmiffion, and their example was foon followed
" by feveral others.*"

IV. FALSE OPINIONS CONCERNING FRIENDSHIP.§

MANY of the ancients appear to have entertained very enthufiaftic notions of FRIENDSHIP; and to have fuppofed,
that it fuperfedes, in particular circumftances, both wifdom and
prudence, and every fpecies of moral obligation. When Bloffius,
the bofom companion of the elder Gracchus, was fummoned
before the fenate of Rome, after the tumult which proved
fatal to that tribune, he was interrogated whether he had always
obeyed the commands of Gracchus? " Yes," anfwered Bloffius,
" moft punctually, for fo I thought it my duty to do. And, if it
" had been poffible for him to defire me to fire the capitol, I fhould
" not have fcrupled to comply, from my full confidence in his
" rectitude."† The folly and criminality of fuch a blind facrifice
of reafon and judgment to the will of another, are too obvious to
need any comment. Connections, of this fervile nature, merit not
the honourable appellation of friendfhip. And we may juftly adopt
the opinion, which Cicero has delivered concerning them: *Si omnia
facienda fint, quæ amici velint, non* AMICITIÆ *tales fed* CONJURA-
TIONES *putandæ funt.*‡

Not lefs foreign to the true obligations of this amiable and venerable paffion, was the exclamation of Themiftocles: " God for-
" bid, that I fhould fit upon a tribunal, where my friends were not
" more favoured than ftrangers!" The letter of King Agefilaus,
to one of the Spartan judges, which Plutarch has preferved, is a
ftill more ftriking proof of the practical influence of the fame falfe

* General Evening Poft, Sept. 2, 1788.

§ See page 13.   † Plut. Vit. Gracchi.   ‡ Cic. de Off.

- - - - - - - - " The friendfhips of the world
" Are oft *confederacies* in vice."   ADDISON's Cato.

opinion; becaufe this prince was a man of probity and equity, virtues which belonged not to the Athenian ftatefman. " If Nicias " be innocent," fays he, " acquit him, for the fake of juftice; but, " if he be guilty, acquit him, for the fake of my attachment to " him."* The Roman moralift, whom I have fo lately quoted, very forcibly objects to the interference of friendfhip, in the magifterial functions: yet, by a ftrange delufion, he permits an advocate to give a *plaufible colouring* to the offence, with which his friend is charged; and to place the fact in the moft advantageous, though it fhould be a *falfe* light.† In his treatife *ac Amicitia*, he remarks, that, " in cafes, which affect the life, or good fame of a " friend, it may be allowable to deviate a little from what is *ftrictly* " *right*, in order to comply with his defires; provided, however, " that our own character be not injured by it." Such loofe and erroneous maxims certainly merit animadverfion : and I fhall relate the following incident, which occurred feveral centuries before the period of Cicero, as an antidote to them. Chilo, the Lacedæmonian, one of the fages of Greece, who is celebrated for the fentence, KNOW THYSELF, which he caufed to be written at Delphos in letters of gold, is faid to have addreffed himfelf to his friends, when on his death-bed, in terms to this effect:—" I cannot " through the courfe of a long life, look back with uneafinefs upon " any fingle inftance of my conduct, unlefs, perhaps, on that which " I am going to mention; wherein I confefs, I am ftill doubtful " whether I acted properly or not. I was once appointed judge, " in conjunction with two others, when my particular friend was " arraigned before us. Were the laws to have taken their due " courfe, he muft inevitably have been condemned to die. After " much debate, therefore, with myfelf, I adopted this expedient. " I gave my own vote according to my confcience, but, at the fame " time, employed all my eloquence to prevail with my affociates to " abfolve the criminal. Now I cannot but reflect upon this act " with concern, from an apprehenfion that there was fomething of " perfidy, in perfuading others to go counter to what I myfelf " efteemed right."‖

---

* Plut. in Vit. Agefilai.   † Cic. de Off. lib. ii. 14.

‖ See fome judicious obfervations on this fubject in Fitzofborne's Letters.

Tully's falfe ideas, concerning the privileges of friendfhip, betrayed him on feveral occafions into meannefs, and even immorality of conduct. In one of his letters, he earneftly folicits Atticus to be guilty of prevarication in his defence. It feems that he had written an invective oration againft an eminent fenator, fuppofed to be Curio. This piece was defigned only for the entertainment of a felect party; but had fallen into the hands of his enemies, and been publifhed by them. He wrote, therefore, to his friend in the following terms: *Percuſſiſti autem me de oratione prolata; cui vulneri, ut ſcribis, medere, ſi quid potes.* —— *Et quia ſcripta mihi videtur negligentius quam cæteræ, puto poſſes probare non eſſe meam.** " You have fhocked me with the news that my oration " is made public. Heal the wound, if you poffibly can. —— " As it is written more negligently than my other orations, I think " you may prove it *not to be mine.*" It is remarkable, that Tully fhould have made a requeft of this nature to Atticus, who is faid to have had fuch an abhorrence of deceit, that he never uttered a falfehood himfelf, nor could pardon it in another. Cicero's letter to Lucceius, requefting him to write the hiftory of his life, " and not " to reject the generous partiality of friendfhip, *but to give more* " *to affection than to truth,*" is too well known to be recited here.†

But, extravagantly as many of the ancients have eftimated friendfhip, a modern writer of diftinguifhed eminence has rated it ftill higher; and does not hefitate to affert, that all the difcourfes

---

* Ep. ad Attic. iii. 12.

† In the intercourfe of friendfhip the Romans do not appear to have difplayed much delicacy of fentiment. The paffages which I have quoted from Cicero, evince the truth of this obfervation. Horace affords a further confirmation of it in the clofe of his beautiful addrefs to Grofphus, Ode XVI. lib. ii. And Pliny m one of his familiar epiftles (Ep. XIX. lib. i.) difgraces an act of the moft exalted generofity, by the infult to amity which accompanies it. "Born," fays he to Romanus Firmus, " in the fame town, educated in the fame fchool, and living " with you from early youth in habits of ftrict connection, I feel the ftrongeft " motives to promote the advancement of your fortune and dignity. I fend you, " therefore, three hundred thoufand fefterces, (2421l. fterling) to elevate you from " the rank of decurio to that of a Roman knight." But he then adds, " From " my knowledge of your character, it is unneceffary to admonifh you to behave " in your new ftation, thus conferred by me, with the modefty which becomes " my beneficiary. For that honour fhould be folicitoufly preferved, in which the " reputation of a benefactor is involved." *Ego ne illud quidem admoneo, quod admonere deberem, niſi te ſcirem ſponte facturum, ut dignitate à me data quam modeſtiſſime, ut a me data, utare. Nam ſolicitius cuſtodiendus eſt honor, in quo etiam beneficium amici tuendum eſt.*

on the fubject, which are handed down to us, appear to him flat and low, in comparifon with the fenfe which he entertains of it. "This bond," he fays, "diffolves every antecedent obligation; "and the fecret which I have fworn not to reveal to another, I "may, without perjury, communicate to him, who is not *another*, "but *myfelf*."* If the author of the *Internal Evidence of Chrifti-anity*† had confined himfelf to fuch unwarrantable ideas of friend-fhip, when he divefts it of the fanction of our Divine Lawgiver, there could be no difficulty in acquiefcing in his decifion. But an affection fo congenial to the principles of our religion, when properly governed, and judicioufly directed, feems to merit, and I truft is not deftitute of, evangelical fupport. Benevolence is, indeed, the great law of the Gofpel difpenfation; but it muft have its commencement in the more confined and partial chari-ties: and the man who has felt not the appropriated regard of a fon, a brother, a hufband, or a friend, cannot have a heart capable of being expanded with philanthropy. Even piety itfelf originates from the filial relation and we learn to transfer to the Deity that gratitude and veneration, with which the tender offices and wifdom of our parents firft infpired us. It is not the object of Chriftianity to overturn, but to regulate the œconomy of the human mind: and if benevolence muft have its foundation in private affection, the divine law, which directs the former, necef-farily inculcates the latter.

That our Saviour himfelf experienced the tendereft fympathies of frien fhip, may, I think, be juftly deduced, both from his ftrong attachment to John, the favourite difciple, and from the expreffions of peculiar endearment, with which he performed the miracle of raifing Lazarus from the dead. On this affecting occafion the Evangelift relates, that *Jefus wept*: and fo fenfible were the Jews of the anguifh of his foul, that they cried out, *Behold how he loved him!** And if Christ gave fuch a decifive proof of perfonal at-tachment and friendfhip, the hiftory of the Gofpel no lefs clearly evinces, that his difciples felt an affection of the fame tender and peculiar kind to their Divine Mafter. In the pathetic converfation which paffed previous to the fufferings and death of Jesus, when

* See Montaigne's Effays, book i. chap. 27.   † Soame Jenyns, efq.
* John, chap. xi. ver. 35, 36. See fome admirable reflections on this fubject in the Notes to Mr. Melmoth's Tranflation of Lælius.

be prophetically, but tenderly, charged them with their future defection, Peter, in the warmth of his regard, replied, *though I should
die with thee, yet will I not deny thee.* The bitter repentance of
this Apostle, subsequent to the misconduct which his great Master
had predicted, affords a further display of the force of his friendship: and CHRIST himself afterwards honoured him with the
kindest and most explicit acknowledgment of it. *So when they
had dined, Jesus saith to Simon Peter, Simon, son of Jonas, lovest
thou me, more than these? He saith unto him, Yea, Lord, thou
knowest that I love thee. He saith unto him, Feed my lambs. He
saith unto him again the second time, Simon, son of Jonas, lovest
thou me? He saith unto him, Yea, Lord, thou knowest that I love
thee. He saith unto him, Feed my sheep. He saith unto him the
third time, Simon, son of Jonas, lovest thou me? Peter was grieved
because he said unto him the third time, lovest thou me? And he said
unto him, Lord, thou knowest all things; thou knowest that I love
thee. Jesus saith unto him, Feed my sheep.*†

In the interesting passage here recited, that lively, reciprocal,
and peculiar regard, which constitutes friendship, is not only recognised, but appealed to and authorized as a generous and animating principle of action. And if the great Founder of our religion
has no where expressly ordained it as a duty, it is probably, because
this virtue is of *special*, and not of *universal* obligation; depending
on particular relations, and contingent circumstances, which human
power can seldom influence or command. It may be added, too,
that the divine law presupposes the existence of such affections as
are purely natural and spontaneous; and directs its precepts, not to
their production, but solely to their government and regulation.
Hence we find not in the whole compass of the scriptures, one explicit injunction to parents to love their children : yet, surely, this
very essential moral office is not to be excluded from the catalogue
of evangelical graces, notwithstanding the silence of sacred writ
concerning it. And the same plea may be extended to friendship,
with due allowance for its rarer occurrence and more partial obligation. The Christian, therefore, in perfect consistency with his
faith, may admire and imitate the examples of generous amity,
which history and observation exhibit to his view. *Peradventure
for a good man,* says the Apostle, *some might even dare to die.*

† John, ch. xxi. ver. 15, 16, 17.

And the facrifice of our own eafe, intereft, or life itfelf, for the advantage of another, with whom we are connected by ftrong and peculiar ties, may not only be juftifiable, but highly honourable and meritorious. Let it be remembered, however, that the privileges of friendfhip are fubordinate to the rights of fociety; and that no attachment, merely perfonal, can warrant the violation of juftice, fidelity, or truth.

The ideas which have been entertained of VALOUR, and the LOVE of our COUNTRY, are ftill more licentious than thofe above recited concerning FRIENDSHIP. It fhould feem, that the underftanding is dazzled by the fplendour which ufually accompanies thefe virtues; and that they are eftimated by the rarity of their occurrence, or by the elevated ftation of their poffeffors, rather than by the ftandard of intrinfic merit or public utility. Juftice and probity are flightly regarded, as the *ordinary* duties of focial life, equally incumbent on all ranks of men: and he who practifes them, appears to have no claim to more than common approbation. But great exertions of courage or patriotifm, as they exceed the demands, fo they proportionably excite the admiration of our fellow-citizens. This admiration kindles in the mind an enthufiafm which often fufpends, and fometimes fuppreffes, the calmer principles of humanity, equity, and truth; and the hero or patriot is indulged in all the privileges which he affumes; nothing being judged criminal that promotes the perfonal glory of the one, or the ambitious views of the other. The hiftory of all ages confirms the truth of thefe obfervations: but they are more particularly applicable to the records of antiquity; which, for the moft part, celebrate the deeds of warriors and ftatefmen with unqualified applaufe, and without the leaft difcrimination of right and wrong.

V. DUPLICITY OF CHARLES I.*

CONSULT Clarendon, vol. i. p. 22; Rufhworth, vol. i. from p. 119 to 127; Hume's Hift. 4to. vol. i. p. 103, ed. 1754. "He " had promifed to the laft Houfe of Commons a redrefs of this reli- " gious grievance; but he was too apt, in imitation of his father, to

* See page 54.

" confider thefe promifes as temporary expedients, which, after the
" diffolution of the parliament, he was not any further to regard."
Id. p. 156. See alfo the Life of the Lord-Keeper Williams, p. 143;
Whitlock, p. 10; the Petition of Rights; Harris's Hiftory; Sidney's
State Papers, vol. ii. p. 665, &c.   Rapin fays, " Charles made fre-
" quent ufe of mental refervations, concealed in ambiguous terms,
" and general expreffions, of which he referved the explication to a
" proper time and place. For this reafon the parliament could
" never confide in his promifes, wherein there was always either
" fome ambiguous term, or fome reftriction that rendered them ufe-
" lefs. This may be faid to be one of the principal caufes of his
" ruin; becaufe giving thereby occafion of diftruft, it was not poffi-
" ble to find any expedient for a peace with the parliament. He was
" thought to act with fo little fincerity in his engagements, that it
" was believed there was no dependence on his word. The parlia-
" ment could not even refolve to debate on the king's propofitions,
" fo convinced were they of his ability to hide his real intentions
" under ambiguous expreffions." Rapin's Hift. vol. ii. p. 570.
The following paffage is taken from the works of an hiftorian,
who is acknowledged to have been very partial to King Charles.
" *Malé pofita eft lex, quæ tumultuariè pofita eft*, was one of thofe
" pofitions of Ariftotle," fays he, " which hath never fince been
" contradicted; and was an advantage, that being well managed,
" and ftoutly infifted upon, would in fpite of all their machinations,
" which were not yet firmly and folidly formed, have brought them
" to a temper of being treated with. But I have fome caufe to
" believe, that even this argument, which was unanfwerable for the
" rejecting that bill, was applied for the confirming it; and an opi-
" nion that the violence and force ufed in procuring it rendered it
" abfolutely invalid and void, made the confirmation of it lefs con-
" fidered, as not being of ftrength to make that act good, which
" was in itfelf null. And I doubt this logic had an influence upon
" other acts of lefs moment."—Clarendon's Hift. vol. ii. p. 30.
Rapin makes the following obfervation on this paffage:—" Let
" the reader judge after this, if we may boaft of King Charles's
" fincerity, fince even in paffing acts of parliament, which are the
" moft authentic and folemn promifes a king of England can make,
" he gave his affent, merely in an opinion that they were void in
" themfelves, and confequently he was not bound by this engage-

" ment." I have inferted thefe references and quotations, not
merely to authenticate the charge againft King Charles, but to fhew,
from his unhappy fate, how delufive, dangerous, and inf mous, is
the following political obfervation of Machiavel:—" It has appeared
" by experience, that thofe princes who have made light of their
" word, and artfully deceived mankind, have all along done great
" things, and have at length got the better of fuch as proceeded
" upon honourable principles."

VI. DISPUTATION.*

POLEMIC fkill is a dangerous qualification; and, if not governed
by charity, wifdom, and integrity, may betray the poffeffor
either into intemperate zeal, or abfolute indifference for truth.
Every object affumes an importance, in our eftimation, proportioned
in fome degree to the labour and attention which we beftow upon
it: and the fame enthufiafm that dignifies a butterfly or a medal to
the virtuofo and the antiquary, may convert controverfy into quixo-
tifm; and prefent, to the deluded imagination of the theological
knight-errant, a barber's bafon, as Mambrino's helmet.* The real
value of any doctrine can only be determined by its influence on the
conduct of man, with refpect to himfelf, to his fellow-creatures, or
to GOD: and it has been well obferved, by a writer of diftinguifhed
abilities, that fome kinds of error and fuperftition are fo intimately
connected with truth and virtue, as to render the feparation of them
impracticable, without doing violence to both. It is better, therefore, according to our SAVIOUR's excellent advice, to let a few
tares grow up with the wheat, (if they be of fuch a nature, as to
fuffer the wheat to grow along with them,) than to endanger the
deftruction of the wheat by rooting up the tares.§

Bigotry may be affociated with truth, as well as with error: and
this temper of mind is always unfavourable to piety and philanthropy, whatever be the principles on which it is founded. Erafmus
afferts, that moft of the reformers with whom he was acquainted,
became worfe men in confequence of the revolution which they

* See page 61.

* See Don Quixote.   § See Prieftley on the Sacrament, p. 64.

accomplifhed. I know not whether this fact will be admitted e.
his authority: but certain it is, that the fury of zeal, and the acri-
mony of difputation, are neither confonant to the religion of nature,
nor to the meek and peaceable fpirit of the Gofpel

But polemic fkill is fometimes employed in the defence of opinions, which are known or believed to be falfe: and by this practice,
the underftanding either becomes the dupe of its own impofitions,
or acquires that indifference to truth which conftitutes incurable
fcepticifm, and fometimes terminates in the moft fatal depravity.
For he who has learned to be regardlefs of right and wrong, in fentiment or in principle, can have no folicitude about the like diftinctions in his difpofitions or behaviour. Such moral apathy gives full
fcope to every irregular defire, and vicious propenfity; and if it be
affociated with great intellectual endowments, a character may be
formed, at once the glory and the difgrace of human nature. Salluft
defcribes Cataline as *fubdolus, varius, cujuflibet rei* SIMULATOR ac
DISSIMULATOR. And I am inclined to believe, that the remarkable
portrait of SERVIN, which the Duke of Sully has drawn, owes fome
of its moft diftinguifhing features to the caufe here alluded to:—"Let
" the reader reprefent to himfelf a man of a genius fo lively, and an
" underftanding fo extenfive, as rendered him fcarcely ignorant of
" any thing that could be known; of fo vaft and ready a comprehen-
" fion, that he immediately made himfelf mafter of whatever he
" attempted; and of fo prodigious a memory, that he never forgot
" what he had once learned. He poffeffed all parts of philofophy and
" the mathematics, particularly fortification and drawing. *Even*
" *in theology he was fo well fkilled, that he was an excellent preacher,*
" *whenever he had a mind to exert that talent; and an able difputant*
" *for and againft the reformed religion, indifferently.* He not only
" underftood Greek, Hebrew, and all the languages which we call
" learned, but alfo all the different jargons, or modern dialects.
" He alfo accented and pronounced them fo naturally, and fo per-
" fectly imitated the geftures and manners, both of the feveral
" nations of Europe, and the particular provinces of France, that
" he might have been taken for a native of all or any of thefe
" countries; and this quality he applied to counterfeit all forts of
" perfons, wherein he fucceeded wonderfully. He was, moreover,
" the beft comedian and greateft droll, that perhaps ever appeared.
" He had a genius for poetry, and had written many verfes. He

" played upon almoſt all inſtruments, was a perfect maſter of muſic,
" and ſung moſt agreeably and juſtly. *He likewiſe could ſay maſs;*
" *for he was of a diſpoſition to do, as well as to know, all things.*
" His body was perfectly well ſuited to his mind, he was light,
" nimble, dextrous, and fit for all exerciſes: he could ride well;
" and in dancing, wreſtling, and leaping, he was admired. There
" are not any recreative games that he did not know; and he was
" ſkilled in almoſt all mechanic arts. But now for the reverſe of
" the medal: here it appeared, that he was treacherous, cruel,
" cowardly, deceitful; a liar, a cheat, a drunkard, and a glutton;
" a ſharper in play, immerſed in every ſpecies of vice, a blaſ-
" phemer, an atheiſt. In a word, in him might be found all the
" vices contrary to nature, honour, religion, and ſociety; the truth
" of which he himſelf evinced with his lateſt breath; for he died,
" in the · flower of his age, in a common brothel, perfectly cor-
" rupted by his debaucheries, and expired, with a glaſs in his hand,
" curſing and denying GOD."*

VII. INDISCRIMINATE PLEADINGS OF LAWYERS.†

THE Roman orators engaged in the defence of their clients or
dependents, in the courts of judicature, without fee or reward: and, under ſuch circumſtances, it might be ſuppoſed, that
their pleadings would be regulated by the pure principles of juſtice
and rectitude. But the fact was often far otherwiſe, through the
influence of ambition, the pride of victory, the connections of party,
and the future expectation of gifts or legacies. Hortenſius ſupported the cauſe of the infamous Verres: and Cicero ſeems to have
formed a deſign of undertaking that of Cataline, when he was
brought to trial on account of his cruel and ſcandalous oppreſſions
in Africa: for, in a letter to Atticus, he ſays: " It is my preſent inten-
" tion to defend Cataline. We have judges to our mind; yet ſuch as
" pleaſe the accuſer himſelf. I hope, if he be acquitted, it will in-

" cline him to ferve me in our common petition." Indeed, this
celebrated orator does not fcruple to declare, that it is the bufinefs
of an advocate not fo much to deliver what is *true* as what is ufeful
to his client; the difcovery of truth being the office of the judge,
and not of the pleader! a fentiment which he juftifies on the authority of Panætius the Stoic, (De Officiis, ii 14.) In one of his orations
he fays, " That man is much miftaken, who conceives he has an
" authentic fpecimen of our opinions in thefe judicial pleadings:
" they are the fpeeches of the caufes, and of the times, not of the
" men or the advocates."—Pro. A. Cluentio. Quinctilian, though
he lays it down as a rule, that an orator fhould be a good man, (*ora-
torem effe virum bonum, dicendi peritum,*) allows, notwithftanding,
very confiderable latitude to the art of pleading, as will appear
from the clofe of the firft chapter of his twelfth book. Modern
lawyers have carried the licenfe of the bar to its utmoft extent: and
a judge, in his charge to the jury, at the affizes for the county and
city of Worcefter, declared it to be " the duty of every counfel,
" upon all occafions, and without referve, to take the brief which
" fhould be firft offered him."—See Notes to Juftification, a poem.
It is probably on this ground a celebrated hiftorian has afferted,
that the gentlemen of the long robe " govern their confciences by
" rules peculiar to themfelves, and entirely oppofite to the ideas
" which prevail with honeft men of other profeffions."—Macaulay's
Hift. of England. It fhould feem, that the father of Sir Matthew
Hale entertained the like fentiments: for Bifhop Burnet relates, that
he quitted the bar, becaufe he difapproved of the common mode of
giving colour in pleadings, which he thought a culpable deviation
from truth. It is recorded alfo, of Sir Matthew Hale himfelf, that
whenever he was convinced of the injuftice of any caufe he would
engage no farther in it than to explain to his client the grounds
of that conviction. His biographer fays, that he abhorred the practice of mifreciting evidences, quoting precedents or books falfely or
unfairly, fo as to deceive ignorant juries, or inattentive judges; and
that he adhered to the fame fcrupulous fincerity in his pleadings,
which he obferved in the other tranfactions of his life. For he ufed
to fay, " it was as great a difhonour as a man was capable of, that
" for a little money he was to be hired to fay or do otherwife
" than he thought."*

* See Britifh Biography, vol. v. p. 383.

According to the laws which now fubfift, no counfellor can maintain an action for his fees, or fo much as demand them, without
doing wrong to his reputation.* He is liable alfo to a year's imprifonment, and to be condemned to perpetual filence in the courts,
if detected in the practice of deceit or collufion.†

ON

HABIT AND ASSOCIATION.

SUPPLEMENTARY REMARKS AND ILLUSTRATIONS.

I. REV. SIMON BROWNE.*

THE conjectures, concerning the caufe of Mr. Browne's very
extraordinary infanity, having been read, in the former edition
of this work, by one acquainted with the real circumftances of the
cafe, I have been favoured with the communication of the following
interefting particulars:—" Mr. Browne and another minifter were
" walking together, near Hampftead, in a part of the road infefted
" by a notorious footpad. His companion faid, fuppofe the footpad
" fhould attack us, what fhall we do?· It will be a fhame, replied
" Mr. Browne, for two perfons, fo ftout as we are, to be robbed by
" one man. Soon afterwards, the footpad appeared; and, whilft
" the other minifter amufed him with the delivery of his money,

✳ See Blackftone's Commentaries, book iii. chap. 3.
† Statute Weftm. I. 3 Edw. I. ch. 28. Blackftone's Commentaries, b. iii. ch. 3.
* See page 78.

" Mr. Browne got behind him, took him in his arms, threw him
" down, and held him faſt, but did not ſtrike him. The companion
" ran for aſſiſtance, and ſoon returned. Mr. Brown roſe up; but
" on detaching himſelf from the robber, found that he had preſſed
" him to death. The ſhock of this event, with his previous agita-
" tion of mind, affected his brain ſo forcibly, that he thought God
" had taken away his ſoul from him; and that he did it, judicially,
" for his neglect of the divine rule of our Saviour, *If any man
" take thy cloak, let him have thy coat alſo.*"

II. INFLUENCE OF SCENERY ON ASSOCIATION.*

IN the life of the Hon. Robert Boyle, drawn up by himſelf, we are
informed, that " curioſity led him to thoſe wild mountains,
" where the firſt and chiefeſt of the Carthuſian abbies does ſtand
" ſeated; where the devil, taking advantage of that deep raving
" melancholy, ſo ſad a place, his humour, and the ſtrange ſtories
" and pictures he found there of *Bruno*, the father of that order,
" ſuggeſted ſuch ſtrange and hideous thoughts, and ſuch diſtracting
" doubts of ſome of the fundamentals of Chriſtianity; that, though
" his looks did little betray his thoughts, nothing but the forbid-
" denneſs of ſelf-diſpatch hindered his acting it. But after a tedi-
" ous languiſhment of many months, in this tedious perplexity, at
" laſt it pleaſed God, one day he had received the ſacrament, to
" reſtore unto him the withdrawn ſenſe of his favour."—Boyle's
Works, 4to. vol. i. p. 23.

III. LUDICROUS ASSOCIATIONS.†

THE author of the Critique on the former edition of this work,
in the Engliſh Review for September 1784, has related the
the following curious fact:—" Some years ago, a reſpectable cler-
" gyman, an inhabitant of London, took country lodgings at a

---

* See page 89.   † See page 92.

" small diſtance from the capital. While at theſe lodgings, he
" uſually roſe early, walked into the fields, and drank warm milk.
" In one of his morning walks, it ſtruck him that he would try if
" he could milk a cow; he immediately ſquatted down, in imitation
" of the dairy-maids, and began to exerciſe his fingers after their
" manner. In the midſt of his operations, two of the damſels
" arrive in the field, and perceiving a grave clergyman in ſo ludi-
" crous a poſture, burſt into an immoderate fit of laughter, accom-
" panied with ſome jocular reproaches. Struck with the ridicule of
" his ſituation, the clergyman hurried to his lodgings in the utmoſt
" confuſion; and ſo ſtrong is the impreſſion, which this inconſider-
" able incident has made upon his mind, that ever ſince he fancies
" theſe women, or ſome of their companions, are conſtantly follow-
" ing him wherever he goes, ſinging ballads relative to the event
" which has ſo much affected him, and expoſing him, in a variety
" of ways, to the laughter of his neighbours. In every other re-
" ſpect he poſſeſſes the moſt perfect clearneſs and ſolidity of under-
" ſtanding, diſcharges the duties of his office as formerly; and, as
" he is a man of wit and learning, is conſidered by his acquaint-
" ance as a valuable and an agreeable companion." The author
of this article has added, that M. Paſchal believed a gulph was before him, and a ſcreen placed to guard him from the view of it.

IV. SECT OF QUAKERS.*

THE genius and manners of the French ſeem peculiarly unfavourable to the principles and habits of the ſect called Quakers.
Yet this reſpectable community has lately planted a colony, and
" obtained a civil eſtabliſhment, amongſt our gay and volatile
neighbours. During the aſſembly of the NOTABLES, a memorial
was preſented to the Couut de Vergennes, by one of the heads of
their ſociety, ſtating that, " In the northern provinces of France,
" there are many hundred dutiful ſubjects, who, though they are
" neither Roman Catholics nor Proteſtants, yet worſhip GOD in

* See page 101.

" the fame temples with Jefus and his Apoftles, viz. in the inward
" of their fouls; and purfue, in reverent filence, the doctrine of
" Christ only, without any mixture of human innovation." The
Proteftants, it is faid, oppofed the petition of the Quakers for the
free exercife of their religion; and ftrongly folicited, that they alone
might be included in the plan of toleration. But juftice and found
policy prevailed in the king's council; and the Quakers obtained
liberty of confcience, not only for themfelves, but, agreeably to their
prayer, for every fect, which maintains peace and good order.
Decent places of burial are affigned to them; they are confirmed
in all their rights of poffeffion and inheritance; and the edict of the
king provides, that whenever a child is born, belonging to one who
does not believe in the neceffity of baptifm, it fhall only be required
of the father or mother to notify fuch birth to the magiftrate.

ON

INCONSISTENCY OF EXPECTATION.

I. COMPLAINTS OF LITERARY MEN.*

MR. GRAY, in one of his letters to Mr. Mafon, thus expreffes
himfelf:—"A life fpent out of the world has its hours of
" defpondence, its inconveniences, its fufferings, as numerous and
" as real, though not quite of the fame fort, as a life fpent in the
" midft of it. . . . . As to myfelf, I cannot boaft, at prefent, either of
" my fpirits, my fituation, my employments, or fertility. The days
" and the nights pafs, and I am never the nearer to any thing, but
" that one to which we are all tending; yet I love people that leave

* See page 117.

" some traces of their journey behind them, and have strength
" enough to advise you to do so while you can."—Letter xxviii.
vol. iv. p. 25. To Dr. Wharton, Mr. Gray writes in the following
terms:—" You flatter me, in thinking that any thing I can do,*
" could at all alleviate the just concern your loss has given you;
" but I cannot flatter myself so far, and know how little qualified I
" am, at present, to give any satisfaction to myself on this head,
" and in this way; much less to you. I by no means pretend to
" inspiration; but yet I affirm, that the faculty in question is by no
" means voluntary; it is the result (I suppose) of a certain dispo-
" sition of mind, which does not depend on one's self, and which
" I have not felt this long time. You, that are a witness how sel-
" dom this spirit has moved me in my life, may easily give credit
" to what I say."—Letter xxxii. vol. iv. p. 45.

II. LOVE OF SCIENCE, THE RULING PASSION.†

IN the Biographical Dictionary, vol xii. under the article EULER,
it is recorded of BOERHAAVE, that when lying on his death-
bed, he anxiously counted his pulse, to ascertain whether he could
live to see a publication, which he expected from the press.

M. EULER, in 1735, solved, in three days, a very extraordinary
problem. But the violent and unremitting efforts which it cost,
occasioned a fever, which endangered his life, and deprived him of
the use of his right eye. Annual Register, 1785, p. 10.

* Dr. Wharton had requested Mr. Gray to write an epitaph on his son.

† See page 122.

ON THE ALLIANCE OF

NATURAL HISTORY WITH POETRY.

I. YELLOW VISION IN JAUNDICE.*

THIS obfervation I regarded as a vulgar error, and have endeavoured to fhew, in the Differtation now referred to, that it is
neither confirmed by experience, nor confonant to reafon; but two
inftances have lately occurred in the circle of my practice, which
clearly evince that the opinion has fometimes a foundation in fact,
and that conclufions drawn, even from a very general induction,
may be fallacious: for my obfervations were made with attention,
during a courfe of near twenty years. The patients now alluded
to, were men of middle age, who had lived intemperately, whofe
malady had proved obftinate, but whofe eyes were not tinged with
bile, in an extreme degree: yet they were uniform in their teftimony, that all white objects affumed a yellow caft; and that this
hue was deepeft on their rifing from bed in a morning.

* See page 145.

AN

INQUIRY

INTO THE

PRINCIPLES and LIMITS of TAXATION,

AS A BRANCH OF

MORAL AND POLITICAL PHILOSOPHY.

AN INQUIRY

*Principles and Limits of Taxation.**

M AN has a natural right to life, liberty, and
property. Life is the gift of GOD, and held
under his difpofal and authority: Liberty is effential
to the perfection of a rational, a moral, and an accountable agent: and Property refults from the exertion of thofe powers and faculties, which theDeity has
beftowed, which duty calls forth into action, and which
are neceffary to well-being, and even to felf-preferva-
tion. Thefe feveral rights involve the lawfulnefs of
their fupport, and the guilt of their invafion. An
attack upon his life or liberty will juftify a man, in the
defence of them, even to the deprivation of the life or
liberty of his enemy; and the invafion of his property

---

* This little tract was written for difcuffion in the Literary and
Philofophical Society, at a period when taxation was a fubject peculiarly interefting to the inhabitants of Manchefter, on account of
a recent duty on the cotton-manufactory; which was afterwards
repealed, through the candour and wifdom of Parliament. It was
ballotted for infertion in a former volume of the Society's Memoirs,
but was then withdrawn by the author, and has fince been revifed
and enlarged. An Appendix is added, at the end of the Inquiry,
containing fupplementary notes and illuftrations.

will warrant his reprifals on the property of the invader. But the ability of an individual would frequently be inadequate to the defence or protection of his rights; nor could he judge, with impartiality, concerning the punifhment due to the violation of them. In a ftate of fociety, therefore, individuals give up to the civil magiftrate, as their reprefentative, the right of protection and punifhment. This right becomes a public one, and is to be defended by the collective power and united expence of the community. From thefe principles flow the duty of allegiance, the authority of laws, and the claims of revenue. To refift the attack of foreign enemies, fleets and armies muft be provided; to fupport domeftic peace, to adminifter diftributive juftice, and to regulate the police of cities and diftricts, civil officers of various ranks and denominations are to be maintained and remunerated; and confiderable funds will be required for the encouragement of fcience, the advancement of arts, and the extenfion of commerce. Thus multiplied and complicated are the juft and neceffary charges of government.

The *moral obligation* to pay taxes refults from the ALLEGIANCE due to the fovereign power, for the PROTECTION which it affords to life, liberty, and property; and for the energy which it exerts in the promotion of order, induftry, virtue, and happinefs.

This obligation is common to the fubjects of every government; but under the happy conftitution of Great-Britain, where fubfidies are never claimed by

the fupreme magiftrate without the confent of parliament, we become bound, by a VOLUNTARY COM-
PACT, made by our delegates, to contribute to the
public exigencies, in fuch proportions, and according
to fuch modes, as they have deliberately enacted.

And, by the refufal to grant fuch contributions,
or by the evafion of them, we not only injure the
public weal, but, indirectly, INVADE the PROPERTY
of our FELLOW-CITI ENS, who muft bear the bur-
den of additional impofts, in confequence of our
contumacious exemption.

The validity of thefe feveral obligations is equally
clear and forcible. And as man is deftined, by his
intellectual powers and moral propenfities, no lefs
than by his wants and weakneffes, for a ftate of fociety, the obligations are not merely voluntary, or of
pofitive inftitution; but fo far as they are effential to
that focial ftate, originate in the law of nature, which
can be deemed no other than the will of GOD. Yet,
though government, in this fenfe, is of divine authority, it is fo conftituted by its adaption to the interefts and felicity of its fubjects. The rights of the
people, therefore, are not only antecedent to, but
included in, thofe of the magiftrate; and confequently
there can never fubfift a legitimate competition between them. Yet the hiftory of the world is one
continued feries of fuch competitions; and experience
hath fully evinced, that they have generally fprung
from the arrogance, the ambition, and the defpotifm
of rulers. To vindicate the facred and unalienable

rights of the people, is, in reality, to subferve the true ends of government. A good citizen, under every legal, equitable, and well-adminiftered polity, with duty and gratitude, will *render unto Cæsar, the things that are Cæsar's.* But the decifion, concerning the *things that are Cæsar's,* refts not on the unftable foundation of arbitrary will; and the appeal may with confidence be made to the principles of reafon, of juftice, and of patriotifm. On thefe principles, I fhall endeavour to explain the limits of the feveral *moral obligations,* laid down in the three foregoing propofitions. (A.)*

I. ALLEGIANCE is due for the PROTECTION of the fovereign power. But protection may be paid for at too high a rate: for, in every convention, a juft proportion fhould be preferved, between the price and the value of the commodity. " If, to purchafe " a fword for my defence againft a thief, I muft empty " my purfe, intereft will lead me rather to make a " compofition with the plunderer; or prudence will " dictate fome other lefs chargeable means of fecu- " rity."† Lord Herbert of Cherbury relates, in his travels through Savoy, that " though the Duke had " put extreme taxations on his people, infomuch that " they paid him not only a certain fum for every horfe, " cow, ox, or fheep that they kept; but afterwards " for every chimney; and, finally, every perfon by the

---

* The capitals refer to the notes in the Appendix, which is placed at the end of the Effay.

† Abbé Raynal.

" pole, which amounted to a piſtole or fourteen
" ſhillings a head or perſon, yet he wanted money;
" at which I did not ſo much wonder, as at the pa-
" tience of his ſubjects."‡   After the cruel expulſion
of the Moors from Spain, by which that kingdom
was deprived of more than half a million of induſtrious
inhabitants, new contributions were impoſed on the
poor and indolent natives, to ſupply the unavoidable,
though unexpected deficiency of the royal revenue,
reſulting from that impolitic meaſure.   This fertile
country has indeed been deſolated by the oppreſſive
laws and rapacious exactions of its government. The
number of the people has been reduced, within the
ſpace of a few centuries, from twenty to ſeven millions; and the produce of corn, formerly furniſhing
not only a full ſupply for internal conſumption, but
alſo a large exportation to other parts of Europe, is
now inſufficient for its own diminiſhed population.
Every manufacture, and even neceſſary of life, is
charged with an impoſt of fourteen *per cent.* on the
firſt, which is repeated on each ſubſequent, ſale.*
Philip II. attempted to lay the ſame burthenſome duty
on his ſubjects in the Netherlands; and the attempt,
it is well known, was one principal cauſe of the glorious revolution, which freed the United Provinces
from his tyranny.

Protection may be very unduly or unequally dis-
penſed; and the ordinary benefits of the ſocial union
not participated, in any reaſonable degree, by the

Life of Lord Herbert.   * Lord Kaims.

bulk of the community, Great lords may be fuffered to tyrannize over their tenants or vaffals, whilft the country is, at the fame time, made a prifon to its inhabitants, by the fevereft prohibitions of emigration. At the beginning of the fixteenth century, there fubfifted in Ruffia no other flaves except prifoners of war. A new arrangement took place after the conqueft of Cafan and Aftracan. Thefe beautiful and fertile provinces fo powerfully attracted the peafantry, that a rigorous law enfued, in 1556, which confined them all to their own glebe: and they were thus at once divefted of property and perfonal liberty.* Similar revolutions have occurred in the other northern ftates; and the confequences have been penury, wretchednefs, and a degradation of the human fpecies. In France, the tax called the *Taille* ufed to be levied on men, who, being without any other property than their neceffary utenfils, and fubfifting folely on their daily wages, could not be compelled to payment, even by violence itfelf. Every collector, who was conftrained to undertake the levy of the tax, had authority to call upon the four perfons in the diftrict, whofe proportion of the *Taille* was the greateft, to fill up all deficiencies; and they were thus forced, by the fale of their effects, or by imprifonment, to expiate the negligence of the collector, or the poverty of their neighbours; notwithftanding they had themfelves difcharged their own fhare of the impoft.†

---

* Abbé Raynal.

† Life of Turgot, by the Marquis de Condorcet.

In fuch cafes, and in others which might be fpecified, the principles are fubverted, on which the claim to allegiance is founded : and taxes may then be enforced by penalties, but will no longer be paid from any juft fenfe of moral or political duty.

Subfidies may be perverted from their original defignation, and applied to the purpofes of ambition, oppreffion, or the eftablifhment of defpotic power. This occurred in the reign of James II. and occafioned his expulfion from the kingdom. And in that of Charles I. when fhip-money was levied under the delufive and dangerous plea of ftate-neceffity, though England then enjoyed a profound peace with all her neighbours, we venerate the intrepid patriotifm of Hampden, for the noble ftand he individually made againft its exaction. Yet the exaction had been laid with great equality; had been fo generally fubmitted to by the people, as to produce, in 1636, more than two hundred thoufand pounds; and had been folemnly authorifed by the twelve judges ; who, by their fervile decifion, to ufe the words of Lord Clarendon, " left no man any thing he might call his " own."

II. But it may be alleged, that the oppofition of Hampden was chiefly grounded on the *illegality of* fhip-money, as fubjecting the people to the arbitrary will of the prince; and that A TAX GRANTED BY PARLIAMENT is a folemn and VOLUNTARY COMPACT between the PEOPLE and their SOVEREIGN, binding the former in all cafes whatfoever. This

pofition implies the lower houfe of parliament to have
been legally and conftitutionally chofen, and not like
the packed affemblies in the reigns of Richard II. and
James II. In the former, the fheriffs were commanded to fuffer none to be returned as knights or
burgeffes, but fuch as the king's council fhould nominate:* and in the latter, the illicit practices
employed in election produced complaints from every
part of England. Yet fo fuccefsful were the arts of
the court, that James exulted in there being only
forty members, who were not entirely devoted to his
intereft.† Admitting, however, the regular election
of our reprefentatives, a little confideration will
evince, that the truft which is delegated can never be
unconditional; and that the powers vefted in them
may lofe the force of moral obligation, by palpable
abufe and unrelenting perverfion. Fear, felf-intereft,
ignorance, or corruption may predominate in their
deliberations, and prevail with them to facrifice the
deareft interefts of thofe by whom they are commiffioned. In the reign of Henry VIII. the parliament refigned both their civil and ecclefiaftical liberties
to the king, and by one act totally fubverted the
Englifh Conftitution: for they gave to the king's
proclamations the full force of a legal ftatute; and
even framed the law, as if it were merely declarative,
and intended only to explain the true extent of the
regal prerogative.‡ When the fame arbitrary mo-

* Parliamentary Hiftory.   † Burnet.
‡ Hume, vol. iv. p. 210.

narch heard that the commons made a difficulty of granting a certain fupply, which he required, he was fo provoked, as to fend for Edward Montague, a member who had confiderable influence in the houfe; and laying his hand on the head of that gentleman, then on his knees before him, imperioufly faid, *get my bill paffed by to-morrow, or to-morrow this head of yours fhall be off.* His defpotifm too well fucceeded; for, the next day, the bill was paffed.† Under the government of Edward VI. a grievous and partial tax was impofed on the whole ftock and moneyed intereft in the kingdom, with an *entire exemption of the land.* One fhilling in the pound was to be levied yearly on every perfon who poffeffed ten pounds or upwards; a fum equal to half the yearly income of all money-holders, according to the rate of legal intereft.§

In the year 1660, a perpetual excife on ale, beer, &c. was enacted, by parliament, as a *commutation* with Charles II. for the abolition of the court of wards and liveries. This court was an intolerable oppreffion on the nobility and gentry; as the king exercifed by it the wardfhip of all infant heirs; and enjoyed the benefit of their eftates, till they had attained a legal majority. He had, alfo, the abfolute difpofal both of male and female heirs in marriage; with other powers liable to great abufe. But it is evident, that thefe feudal fervices affected folely the

† See Collins's Britifh Peerage. Hume, vol. iv. p. 51.
§ Hume, vol. iv. p. 346.

proprietors of land; whereas the excife muft fall chiefly on the lower tenantry and labouring poor; and that, therefore, the alleged commutation was, in a confiderable degree, founded in fraud and injuftice. In this light it appeared to fome of the members of the houfe of commons: Mr. Annefley, in particular, urged, "that if the bill was carried, (which it was " afterwards by a majority of two voices only,) every " man who earns his bread by the fweat of his brow " muft pay excife, to excufe the court of wards; " which would be a greater grievance upon all, than " the court of wards was to a few."*

There is on record a folemn refolution,. which paffed in a committee of the houfe of commons, April 6, 1780, when no lefs than four hundred and forty-eight members were prefent, that the influence of the crown *hath increafed, is increafing, and ought to be diminifhed.* (B.)   And in the ftatute of a fubfequent feffion of parliament, for regulating the king's houfe-hold, it is enacted, that an oath be taken by the keeper of his majefty's privy purfe, that no part of it fhall be applied to the ufe of any member of the Houfe of Commons.   We are further warranted in our apprehenfions of the danger arifing from this fource, by the authority of the Baron de Montefquieu, who predicts that the liberties of England will perifh, whenever the legiflative power fhall have become more corrupt than the executive: or, as it fhould, perhaps,

---

* See Harris's Life of Charles II. vol. i. p. 396. Parliamentary Hiftory, vol. xxiii. p. 2i.

have been expreffed, whenever the executive power
fhall have acquired a corrupt afcendancy over the
legiflative.   In the reign of Charles II. if the dis-
paches of Barillon may be credited, the king of
France meditated the eftablifhment of a pecuniary
influence in the Englifh parliament.   It is alfo well
known that Charles was himfelf a penfioner to this
monarch, and received large fums of money for the
moft illicit purpofes.   When the crown egregioufly
abufes its power, the commons, on various occafions,
have thought themfelves juftifiable in withholding the
fupplies.   If they, however, unhappily countenance
and aid fuch abufes, and remain deaf to petitions,
remonftrances, and every other conftitutional claim,
the people may continue to fubmit, but cannot deem
themfelves *morally* bound by their acts: and Britons
would then lofe the glory, which Plato afcribed to the
citizens of Athens, of being at once the mafters and
flaves of the laws.

The divifion of the fovereignty of thefe realms into
three eftates, which, acting in concert, we denominate parliament, by reciprocal checks, and reciprocal
aids, gives our civil polity advantages enjoyed by no
other in Europe.   Yet it was an apophthegm of the
great Lord Treafurer Burleigh, that England could
never be ruined but by a parliament.*   And the
doctrine of its omnipotence, which fucceeded that of
the divine and indefeafible right of our kings, has
contributed to the lofs of America, as well as to the

* Blackftone,

feparation of Ireland; and may, hereafter, prove fubverfive of our liberties. For with the fpecious obfervance of every form of our Conftitution, the effence
of it may be annihilated; as occurred at Rome, under
the defpotifm of Auguftus; for the fenate retained
themfelves the image of freedom, whilft they gave a
full fanction to his ufurpation. Indeed, corporate
bodies, when they affect unlimited power, are capable
of proceeding to greater lengths than any individual.

Supreme authority is perfectly diftinct from arbitrary or abfolute power. The one is founded on
certain fundamental principles, and limited by certain
conftitutional reftrictions; whilft the other is unconditional, and without all rational controul. A juft
government is obliged to the moft fcrupulous attention to the original ends of its inftitution. Nor can
even wife and legitimate *ends* be purfued by *means*
inconfiftent with equity, becaufe no policy can ever
fuperfede the laws of morality: and this rather
dignifies, than derogates from, fovereign dominion.
For the Deity himfelf is bounded, in the exercife of
power, not only by phyfical impoffibilities, but by
the rectitude of his divine nature.

Compulfion has been faid to be the effence of government.*   But I apprehend, *compulfion* is here
miftaken for *a power to compel*; otherwife, there can
be no diftinction between government and tyranny.
The former is inftituted for the public weal, and,
when fo adminiftered as to promote its falutary ends,

* Soame Jenyns.

will have the confidence, the respect, and the *volun-tary* obedience of a great majority of its members. Whereas the latter, according to a recent definition of eastern despotism, regards " the sovereign as pos- " sessed of *all*, and the people of *no* rights." It exacts what a wise man cannot freely give, and com- mands what a good man ought not to perform. " The state of every king," says the preamble to one of our acts of parliament, " consists more assuredly in " the love of the subjects towards their prince, than " in the dread of laws made with rigorous pains."* But the love of the subject can alone be secured by a full conviction that the supreme magistracy is cor- dially interested in his prosperity and happiness. And this is best evinced by a reluctance to impose unne- cessary burthens; by equity and impartiality in the assessment and collection of them; and by a readiness to participate in the sacrifice of private interest to public good. The Roman emperor, Marcus Aure- lius, sold the furniture of the imperial palace, to- gether with his own vestments, and those of the empress, ather than levy a new tax on the people!†

III. In support of the moral obligation to pay taxes, it is justly urged, that by our refusal to grant such contributions, we not only injure the common- wealth, but cast upon others that debt, which we

* See Blackstone's Commentaries, vol. iv. p. 17.

† Aul. Gell.

ought to difcharge ourfelves. A venerable philofopher has, in a very appofite manner, illuftrated this
argument by the following analogy. " What fhould
" we think of a companion, who having fupped with
" his friends at a tavern, and partaken equally of the
" joys of the evening with the reft of us, would
" neverthelefs contrive, by fome artifice, to fhift his
" fhare of the reckoning upon others, to go fcot free?
" If a man, who practifed this, would, when detected,
" be deemed and called a fcoundrel; what ought he
" to be called, who can enjoy all the ineftimable
" benefits of public fociety, and yet contrive to evade
" paying his juft fhare of the expence, and wrongfully
" throw it upon his honefter, and perhaps poorer,
" neighbours?"*   But fuppofe the fhare to be unjuft, or partially demanded; is the impofition to be
fubmitted to without complaint or remonftrance?
The plea of equity, which authorizes one to withhold
a public fubfidy, if well-founded, muft be clearly dis-
cernible by the underftanding of his neighbour, and
ought alike to direct his conduct.   Should he, therefore, through the want of patriotifm, or the fear of
penalty, acquiefce in oppreffion, he defervedly incurs
both the blame and the fuffering.   Mr. Hampden
withftood the affeffment of fhip-money, in oppofition
to the unanimous opinion of the twelve judges; and,
in vindication of the unalienable rights of his fellow-
fubjects, expofed himfelf, for the trifling fum of

---

* Franklin's Political and Mifcellaneous Pieces, p. 69.

twenty fhillings, to the indignation and rigorous perfecution of the Court.

I am fenfible that pride, refentment, faction, and felf-intereft fet themfelves in oppofition to the ftate; and that men fo actuated may falfely affume the motives and principles of the confcientious and the good. Penalties, therefore, are wifely₂ annexed to the infringement of the laws of revenue: and authority is properly exerted, in the ordinary courfe of government, to awe the refractory into fubmiffion. But it muft ftill reft with the people, ultimately, to decide concerning the moral force of that obligation to pay any particular tax, which is antecedent to the penalty incurred by difobedience; becaufe fueh decifion can be referred to no other tribunal, without the moft egregious folecifm. And where can the cafe be fhewn, in which the judgment and determination of the many hath not received its commencement in the judgment and determination of the few, and even of an individual? The right, therefore, muft be admitted to fubfift in both; though the exercife of it can only be juftified on extraordinary occafions. (c.) Nor can danger be apprehended to a well-governed fociety from this doctrine. For oppreffion muft be manifeft and heavy, before it will be generally refifted; and partial offences, unfupported by public opinion, will be readily prevented by a vigilnat police, or compenfated by pecuniary mulcts. The refufal of Mr. Townfend, a very refpectable magiftrate in London, to pay his

affeffment to the land-tax, is within the memory of
every gentleman prefent. He grounded this refufal
on the arbitrary proceedings of the Houfe of Commons, relative to the Middlefex election; and the
confequent illegality of an impofition, levied on a
county in which the people were not duly reprefented. His conduct, on this occafion, was influenced
by no fordid motives, and proceeded folely from a
patriotic zeal to fecure the rights of election. Yet a
jury of Middlefex men gave a verdict againft him,
without fcruple or hefitation: and their decifion was
reafonable and proper, becaufe the bonds of the ftate
are not to be rafhly loofened by every temporary
error or mifconduct of ftatefmen. Candid allowances
will and ought to be made for the paffions, prejudices, and imperfections incident to our governors,
provided their general conduct evinces wifdom and
rectitude. Indeed there is fo much veneration for
power, fo great a fear of prefent fuffering, and fuch
habitual regard to the forms of civil jurisdiction in
the bulk of the people, that maxims of paffive obedience are not neceffary to their fubjection; whilft
they are highly injurious to their rulers, of which
the hiftory of the Stuarts affords the fulleft evidence;
(D:) for the temptations to abufe power are, at all
times, greater than thofe of oppofition to it; .and the
abufe is attended with more permanent evils to fociety. An equitable and well-eftablifhed legiflature
can, therefore, be under no neceffity of inflicting
heavy penalties on breaches of the laws of revenue;

and punifhments of a different nature are feldom, if
ever, to be juftified. We read with horror, that in
the empire of Japan, death is inflicted on the fmug-
gler; and our fentiments of equity and humanity
are almoft equally fhocked with the account given by
M. Neckar, that more than three hundred men of
the province of Bretagne alone are annually configned to flavery in the gallies of France, for carrying on an illicit commerce in the two articles of falt
and tobacco. The truth is, this political crime makes
little impreffion on the moral feelings of the mind,
till its nature, extent, and confequences have been
examined and recognized by reafon. And to fuch
inveftigation the generality of men have neither leifure nor ability to apply themfelves. Turpitude in
human actions is marked either by the grofs defect
of good principles, or the prevalence of bad ones.
Fraud, difhonefty, perfidy, and cruelty, neceffarily
involve in them a confcioufnefs of guilt; and, therefore, indicate a mind devoid of rectitude, or overborne
by the predominance of malignant paffions. But the
retention of what is the acknowledged property of
the individual, before it is claimed by the ftate, though
at all times culpable, and deferving of punifhment
in ordinary cafes, when the nature of the obligation
is not fufficiently underftood, implies no high degree
of criminality.* And he who avails himfelf, without
the fcruples which he ought to feel, of the carelefsnefs

---

* On this fubject confult Montefquieu, Beccaria, Blackftone,
Lord Kaims, Dr. Adam Smith, &c.

or miftake of a tax-gatherer, to evade the propor-
tional payment exacted from his neighbours, would
blufh to take advantage of the tradefman who, by
fimilar careleffnefs or miftake, hath omitted in his bill
fome part of the debt which is owing to him. But,
when invafion threatens a country, or public calamity
calls forth the exertions of every member of the ftate,
the fentiments of the mind being reverfed, breach of
allegiance, under fuch circumftances, would be deemed
almoft equal to the crime of parricide. We may
illuftrate this obfervation by a cafe in military fervice,
with refpect to our feelings, fomewhat parallel. No
one, but the officer on guard, would punifh the *fleep-
ing centinel* with feverity, during the feafon of peace.
But, on fome critical and very important conjuncture in time of war, the fame offence would merit
death, in the eftimation of the moft humane fpectator.
To eftablifh a fcale of crimes, with exact precifion, fo
as to affign to each its due degree of punifhment, is
beyond the extent of human ability; and can be accomplifhed only by the omnifcient Searcher of hearts.
But the penal laws of government fhould be founded
on a like difcrimination, fo far as it is practicable,
clear, and obvious; and, in all doubtful cafes, fhould
incline more to mildnefs than feverity. For it is juftly
obferved, in the preamble of the ftatute before referred to, " that laws made for the prefervation of
" the commonwealth without great penalties are
" more often obeyed and kept, than laws made with
" extreme punifhments."

I have thus endeavoured, with great brevity, to trace the origin, to explain the principles, and to determine the extent of a duty, which, though effential to the being of fociety, and of equal importance to the governors and governed in every community, has not hitherto, I believe, received a fpecific denomination in any language. Nothing tends more to the eftablifhment of juft authority, than the free and temperate inveftigation of the reafons on which it is founded. And, from what has been advanced, I prefume, it may be inferred, that a *tax* can be of no *moral obligation*, when the claim to allegiance is abfolutely forfeited; that it is of *imperfect* obligation from mere general allegiance; and that to give it *full* and *complete* validity, it fhould be A LEVY MADE ON THE COMMUNITY BY LAWFUL AUTHORITY; ACCORDING TO PRESCRIBED FORMS; IN AN EQUITABLE MODE AND PROPORTION; AND FOR THE PUBLIC WEAL.

In Britain, the LAWFUL AUTHORITY, competent to impofe a fubfidy, can only be that of the King, Lords, and Commons, in Parliament affembled. The King is reprefentative of the majefty of the people; from them he derives his dignity; to their deputies, his minifters and counfellors are amenable; and his prerogatives* confift only in a difcretionary power of doing good. And if the regal office be a delegation, the peerage, which flows from it, muft participate of its nature. The three eftates, therefore, though in

* Locke; Blackftone.

different modes of truft, feverally and collectively, act in behalf of, and are virtually refponfible to, the community, who poffefs, and frequently exercife, towards each of them, the right of petition and remonftrance. But much circumfpection is required in applying practically the ideas of REPRESENTATION to the regal and ariftocratical branches of our Conftitution. Thefe indeed are delegates, but in a qualified fenfe, and fhould be reforted to only, in this view, on preffing emergencies. For the Commons are the deputed guardians of the people's rights; commiffioned by them to act according to, and to exprefs, their united fuffrage; and renewing their truft and accountablenefs, on every fucceffive election. It is derogatory, therefore, of their importance and dignity, and muft tend to diminifh their due weight in the fcale of government, to transfer the peculiar functions with which they are invefted to the Peers, or to the Throne. (E.)

Of the FORMS prefcribed in paffing a money bill, the moft effential to its moral validity, becaufe moft interefting to the liberty of the fubject, is, that it fhould originate folely in the Houfe of Commons. For the Lords, being a permanent hereditary body, created at pleafure by the King, are fuppofed to be more liable to be influenced by the crown; and when once influenced, to continue fo; than the Commons, who are freely elected, and only for a limited time, by the people.* This privilege forms the great con-

* Blackftone.

ftitutional check on the executive branch of administration, and every good citizen fhould watch over it
with unremitting and jealous attention; extending his
diligent and patriotic obfervation even to turnpikes,
parifh-rates, and impofts collected, not for the exigencies of government alone, but for private and
local benefit.

To APPORTION the taxes, with all poffible IMPAR-
TIALITY, is effential to their having the full force
of moral obligation.   Yet this is the moft arduous
office of the financier; and, when a kingdom is under
the preffure of accumulated debts, can perhaps be
accomplifhed only by fuch a modification of the whole
fyftem of revenue, as fhall compenfate the unavoidable
exceffes in fome cafes by equitable exemptions in
others.   Impofts on articles of provifion have often
been fo improvidently laid, as to occafion great diftrefs
amongft the poor: and, as they are the chief con-
fumers, becaufe the moft numerous order of the ftate,
the difproportion attending fuch exactions is an injuftice equal to the cruelty of the exactions themfelves.
" Previous to all the laws of fociety, man had a right
" to fubfift: and is he to lofe that right by the
" eftablifhment of laws?   To fell the produce of the
" earth to the people at an exorbitant price is, in re-
" ality, to deprive them of it.   To wreft from them
" by a tax, the natural means of preferving life, is to
" affect the very principle of their exiftence."*   But
I would not be underftood to object to the impofition of

* Abbé Raynal.

moderate duties on the neceffaries of life. When judicioufly planned, and gradually laid on articles which are cheap and plentiful, they promote induftry, ingenuity, and fobriety; and are paid cheerfully, becaufe imperceptibly, as they are confounded with the value of the commodity itfelf. (F.) During the impofts of the Sforzas on the harvefts and markets of the Piedmontefe, the fkill and enterprifing fpirit of that people were roufed to the higheft exertion; and their fabrics of filk and cotton were then worked with fuch elegance and expedition, by the invention of machinery, as precluded all competition. The gentlemen engaged in the manufactures of Manchefter will find thefe obfervations perfectly confonant to their own experience; yet they are of dangerous tendency, and admiffible only within certain reftrictions. For both art and activity are not only bounded in their extent, but are precarious in their duration, and dependent on a variety of unforefeen contingencies. And, though the moderate preffure of wants, which may be gratified without much difficulty, ftimulates to exertion; yet neceffity creates defpair, the parent of idlenefs, profligacy, and mifery. Under fuch circumftances, the productive labourres of the ftate will be confiderably diminifhed in number, and will be compelled to raife the price of induftry to a height fubverfive both of trade and commerce. It muft be remembered, alfo, that thefe working members are incident to the feverity of feafons, as well as to the fluctuation and inftability of thofe manual arts which depend on

fafhion, local conveniencies, or foreign materials;
and that they are often plunged into fufferings which
call for public aid, and ought to fuperfede exaction.
Befides, there is,at all times, and in every place, a numerous clafs of poor, who, from a want of fkill, of health,
and of that energy which originates from the united
powers of nature and education, are barely qualified
to earn from day to day a fcanty fubfiftence.   Yet
thefe are, equally with ourfelves, the commoners of
the earth, and have a juft claim to fome portion of
the good things of life.   May we not alfo add, that
there muft be *hewers of wood* and *drawers of water;*
and, that to execute the meaneft and moft fubordinate offices is effential to complete the aggregate of
human induftry and happinefs.   A wife polity, therefore, will not, by a rigid fyftem of finance, promote
the extinction of fuch men; but will treat them with
proper indulgence, will encourage their marriages,
and, by well-planned inftitutions, render their pofterity virtuous, active, and ufeful citizens.   The penury
and depopulation of Spain have been proved, by
Uftariz, to arife, not from emigrations to America
and the Weft-Indies, but from the oppreffive laws
of revenue which prevail in that country.   When
Lord Molefworth refided in Denmark, the collectors
of the poll-tax were obliged to accept of old feather-
beds and other neceffaries, inftead of money, from
the inhabitants of a town, which once raifed 200,000
rix-dollars for Chriftian IV. on twenty-four hours'
notice.   In Holland, manufactures have long been in

a declining ftate. It has been calculated, that one third of every man's income is paid in fubfidies. Bread, I am informed, is taxed at from twelve to fifteen *per cent.* and in towns much higher; malt liquor at fifteen *per cent.* and butchers' meat at twenty *per cent.* Nothing could counteraft fuch heavy duties on the lower orders of the people, but the extreme frugality and perfevering induftry, which charafterize the inhabitants of the United Provinces.

The EQUITY of an impoft; and, confequently, its moral validity, is very materially affefted by the MODE of ASSESSMENT. For the time expended, the vexation occafioned, and the indignity fuftained by it, may be equivalent to a manifold, and therefore, difproportional payment. Hearth-money, which was granted to Charles II. his heirs and fucceffors for ever, was abrogated in the year 1688, by an aft of William and Mary; of which the following is the preamble, " That it is not only a great oppreffion " upon the poorer fort, but a badge of flavery upon " the whole people; expofing every man's houfe to " be entered into, and fearched at pleafure, by per- " fons unknown to him."* The excife, from its firft inftitution to the prefent time, has been odious to the people of England. It extends to a very numerous detail of commodities, the lift of which, fays Sir William Blackftone, no friend to his country would wifh to fee farther increafed. Yet it has been greatly increafed fince the time of this excellent

* Lord Kaims's Sketches, vol. ii. p. 354.

judge, and, I believe, with additional vexations and severities. The officers concerned in this branch of revenue are authorized to enter and to search the houses of persons, who deal in exciseable articles, at all hours of the day, and, in many cases, of the night also. And the proceedings, under suspicion of transgression, are so summary and sudden, that, in a very short space of time, a man may be convicted in the penalty of many thousand pounds by two commissioners, or justices of the peace, or even by the same number of magistrates in the smallest corporate town, to the total exclusion of the trial by jury, and without regard to the common law of the land.*

This mode of assessment might, perhaps, be rendered more consonant to the principles of British liberty, and to the ordinary proceedings of legal administration. There seems to be no sufficient reason for the exclusion of a jury, nor for deciding in a way so unusually sudden and summary. Appeals also should be admissible in all cases to the quarter-sessions, or to some public and respectable tribunal: and the persons prosecuted should be allowed counsel for their defence, together with full costs of suit, and even damages, if judgment be awarded in their favour. Nor does it seem equitable, provided no perjury has been practised, nor malignant intention manifested, that, when the plaintiff is nonsuited, the officer of revenue should recover treble costs. These alterations in the statutes of excise would not occasion any

---

* See Blackstone; Burn's Justice of the Peace; &c.

delay of confequence to the revenue; and they might obviate abufes, which, by creating murmurs and dis-content, diminifh the veneration due to the laws. (G.)

In the Highlands of Scotland, it is faid by Lord Kaims, that the excife upon ale and fpirits defrays not the falaries of the officers who levy it. The people, therefore, are burthened with a contribution, which adds to the expence of government, and withdraws from ufeful labour many induftrious hands. This laft confideration feldom enters into the eftimate of the financier: yet the magnitude of it will be ap-parent from the late obfervations of M. Neckar, who computes that the tax-gatherers in France amount to two hundred and fifty thoufand perfons; thirty-five thoufand of whom devote their whole time to the bufinefs. The enforcement of imposts by oaths may be fuppofed rather to increafe, than to diminifh, their moral validity : yet it is a practice that, on tri-vial occafions, feems to participate of impiety; and, on all occafions, is conducted with fo much carelefs-nefs and irreverence, as tends to the moft pernicious confequences. A million of perjuries are fuppofed, by a very able calculator, to be annually committed in this kingdom.* (H.)

In the definition of a tax, which has the full force of a moral obligation, it has been laid down as its ultimate and moft important conftituent, that it is a levy made for the PUBLIC GOOD: and it is the fpe-cial duty of the fupreme power to keep this facred

* Price on the American Revolution, p. 82.

end in view, in the exaction of every fubfidy. The confidence and veneration of the people would thus be fecured; and a refpectful fubmiffion would be paid even to the errors of government, as unavoidable confequences of human frailty; and as only temporary grievances, which better information would redrefs. In the application, alfo, of the national funds, the like rigid attention to wifdom and rectitude fhould be uniformly maintained. How often has it been urged to me, fays M. Neckar, can you refufe to afk the king for a thoufand crowns, to relieve fuch a perfon whofe misfortunes are known to you? Will the royal exchequer be the poorer for it? Forget, I have replied, this royal exchequer, which you confider only as an accumulated mafs of money, without having examined its fource: a thoufand crowns are the amount of the land-tax of two villages; and I leave you to judge whether the perfon for whom you folicit has a juft claim to the labour and contributions of their inhabitants. It is a violation (obferves the fame honeft financier, in another part of his work, with which I fhall now conclude) —It is a violation of the moft facred of all depofits, to employ the facrifices of a whole nation in inconfiderate prodigalities, ufelefs expences, and undertakings foreign to the good of the ftate.

AN

APPENDIX

TO

THE INQUIRY

CONCERNING THE

PRINCIPLES OF TAXATION,

CONSISTING OF

SUPPLEMENTARY NOTES AND ILLUSTRATIONS.

ADVERTISEMENT

IN the following Notes the Author has not deemed it necessary to confine himself strictly to the subject of Taxation; but has touched upon various other topics, relative to political œconomy, and to the foundation of civil government. As these are intimately connected with and illustrate each other, he trusts the reader will excuse the latitude he has taken in this Appendix.

APRIL 1, 1789.

AN

APPENDIX

PRINCIPLES OF TAXATION,

CONTAINING

SUPPLEMENTARY NOTES AND ILLUSTRATIONS.

———

NOTE (A) PAGE 235.

PROPERTY NOT THE MERE CREATURE OF CIVIL SOCIETY.

A Learned Friend, of diftinguifhed rank both in the Church, and in the republic of letters, to whom I communicated the Inquiry concerning the Principles of Taxation, " regards property " as very much the creature of civil fociety, and the fupreme ma- " giftrate as authorized to apply the whole of the property of every " individual to the ufe of the whole community."*

Notwithftanding the deference and refpect I feel for the decifion of one, whom I know to be a very able judge of the fubject of legiflation; yet I am ftrongly inclined to controvert the doctrine advanced, which, by *leaving nothing that a man may call his own,* (to adopt the expreffion of Lord Clarendon,) feems to fubvert the intereft we have in fociety itfelf

I. A defire of poffeffion, and tenacioufnefs of what is attained, are manifefted in the earlieft ftages of life. They are modifications of one and the fame principle, which grows with our growth, is in- dependent of fociety, and fubfifts in as full force among favages as

* A fimilar opinion is advanced by Puffendorf.

in the moſt cultivated nations. The like principle is common even to the brutes. The beaſt of prey aſſerts an excluſive right to his den, and to the proviſions he has ſtored for himſelf, or for his off-ſpring. The cock drives every invader from his dunghill; and the rooks puniſh with ſeverity the marauders that come to pilfer their neſts. But to enter into a diſcuſſion of the origin of property would exceed the limits of a note. Suffice it to obſerve, that we can clearly deduce it from the neceſſities, the deſires, the affections, and other active energies of man. Of theſe energies, civil ſociety is the *conſequence*, and not the *cauſe;* and its office is to regulate them, to augment their vigour, and to afford more complete ſecurity in whatever is acquired by them. If, therefore, the powers of his nature be man's excluſive right, every thing reſulting from them muſt be equally appropriate: and the juſt claim of government extends only to an equivalent to the benefits enjoyed under it.

II. Juſtice, fidelity, and veracity, imply in their exerciſe the ſocial ſtate: but their obligation is independent of and pre-ſuppoſed by the political union; and conſtitutes its only rational and legiti-mate bond. Is property, more than thoſe moral virtues, the crea-ture of civil ſociety? All of them may ſubſiſt without government: for if only two men dwelt together on a deſert iſland in a ſtate of perfect equality, each would have his appropriate rights of poſſeſſion; and the claim to juſtice, fidelity, and veracity, would be reciprocal.

III. The ſocial union is a combination of numbers, for mutual aſſiſtance, comfort, improvement, and protection. If every indivi-dual concur in the public acts of ſuch a community, at the firſt view, there might ſeem to be no violation of private rights. It ſhould be remembered, however, that the circumſtances and opinions of thoſe individuals may vary in the lapſe of time; and that the rights of poſterity, alſo, are involved in their deciſions. The preſent inha-bitants of Denmark are now enſlaved by the raſh ſurrender of their liberties, which was made in 1660. Beſides, the public acts of a community, if large, muſt neceſſarily be acts only of the majority: and a majority may, indeed frequently does, as the hiſtory of all nations evinces, commit violence on the rights of the minority.

Fanaticiſm, like that which ſubſiſted amongſt the Anabaptiſts of Munſter, about two centuries ago, may induce the civil magiſtrate to order every man to bring forth his gold, ſilver, and precious effects, to be depoſited in a public treaſury, and to be diſpenſed, for common ufe. But this would be an act of power, not of juftice or legitimate authority.

IV. Grants of money, in almoft every country, are made on exprefs conditions, and as voluntary facrifices of private rights to public good.

*Whenever the public good requires the involuntary facrifice of the good of an individual, great attention is paid, in all juft and moderate governments, to do as little violence as poffible, and to make full recompence for the injury fuftained. This feems to be an unequivocal acknowledgment of the exiftence of private pro-perty, in the ftricteft fenfe of the word.

V. As every man has a natural right to life, he muft have the fame natural right to the means of fupporting life. On this prin-ciple, the Athenians feem to have confidered that fhare of a man's property, which is neceffary to his fubfiftence, as abfolutely exempt from taxation. Thus a rent of five hundred meafures of corn was affeffed in the yearly contribution of a talent; a rent of three hun-dred paid half a talent; a rent of two hundred paid one-fixth of a talent; and a land of a lower produce paid no fubfidies at all. In the early days of Rome, feven acres were the utmoft extent of landed property, which a Roman citizen was allowed to hold. This portion was, probably, not more than adequate to the fupply of a family.

VI. There is a fpecies of acknowledged property appertaining to ftates, over which they exercife an exclufive power of difpofal, which bears a clofe analogy to private poffeffions. It confifts in crown-lands, public buildings, highways, fortifications, &c. Can public levies to a confiderable extent be, like this, regarded as the abfolute right of the civil magiftrate?

VII. But it may be urged, that the greateft part of property, whether perfonal or real, is enjoyed by *inheritance* under the au-thority of *laws;* and that the laws, being the creatures of civil fociety, render property itfelf equally fo. The argument, however, is a fallacy. Law does not conftitute the right to property; but only recognizes, fanctions, and regulates the exercife of it. What a man has acquired by art or induftry, without violation done to others, is at his abfolute difpofal; and may, if not applied to his own ufe, be given to his children, his relations, or friends. Nor

---

* *Dominium eminens:* tranfcendental property.

can there be any definite time for the reftriction of fuch transfer; and confequently it will have equal validity at the hour of death as in the prime of life, provided the donation be voluntary, and made with a found mind. It has indeed been faid, that in a ftate of nature, a man's right to a particular fpot of ground arifes from his ufing and wanting it, and confequently ceafes with the ufe and want; fo that at his death the eftate reverts to the community, without any regard to the laft owner's will.* But this prefuppofes what is in itfelf a contradiction, that man in *community* is a *folitary* animal, labouring and living only for himfelf: whereas the truth is that he labours and lives more for his family and his 'dependents, than for himfelf; that his attachments to them ftimulate his faculties, and give energy to his exertions; and that to deprive him of the future end he feeks in his acquifitions, is the fame wrong in kind, and much greater in degree, becaufe more injurious to his beft and ftrongeft feelings, than it would be to deprive him of the prefent ufe of them. A father may leave an infirm widow, and numerous helplefs orphans, for whom he anxioufly toiled, and toiled with fuccefs. Is it equitable that they fhould be caft on the public for fupport? If it be not, the law, which guarantees to them their father's poffeffions, only confirms, and does not inftitute, their right, which is founded in nature, reafon, and juftice.

VIII. The difpute, perhaps, about the right of the fupreme ma‑giftrate to the entire property of the whole community, is rather verbal than fubftantial. For, admitting it to fubfift, it can only be exercifed, when rights of the whole community, ftill dearer than thofe of property, are in the moft imminent hazard, fuch as life, liberty, and religion. There muft then be a juftifying plea for fuch exercife of power: and the ultimate decifion, concerning this jufti‑fying plea, muft reft with the people.

* Paley's Moral Philofophy, vol. i. p. 222, 8vo.

NOTE (B) PAGE 240.

INFLUENCE OF THE CROWN.

THE refolution, that "the influence of the crown hath increafed, "is increafing, and ought to be diminifhed," was moved by Mr. Dunning; who explained his meaning to be, not the influence of the virtues of the fovereign, or the juft rights of his prerogative, but that which arofe from corruption, and other undue practices.

Sir Fletcher Norton, the Speaker of the Houfe, obferved, " that " it would be criminal in him to remain filent on this occafion. He " declared, in the moft direct terms, that the influence of the crown " had been increafing of late to an alarming degree. No man had " a higher veneration for monarchy than he had: he meant that fpe- " cies of it eftablifhed in this country; a monarchy limited by law. " Such a government required no affiftance, but what was derived " from the conftitution and the laws. The powers, vefted in the " executive part of government, were ample and fufficient for all " the purpofes of good government; and, without any further aid, " much too ample for the purpofes of bad government. And he " thought himfelf bound, as an honeft man, to fay, that the influ- " ence of the crown had increafed much beyond the ideas of a " monarchy ftrictly limited in its nature and extent."—See New " Annual Regifter, 1780, p. 148.

Sir William Blackftone, fpeaking of the ancient prerogatives of the crown, and of the bounds fet to them, at the revolution, fays, " though thefe provifions have, in appearance and nominally, re- " duced the ftrength of the executive power to a much lower ebb " than in the preceding period; if, on the other hand, we throw " into the oppofite fcale (what perhaps the immoderate reduction " of the ancient prerogative may have rendered, in fome degree, " neceffary) the vaft acquifition of force, arifing from the riot act, " and the annual expence of a ftanding army; and the vaft ac- " quifition of perfonal attachment, arifing from the magnitude of " the national debt, (now, 1788, augmented one hundred millions) " and the manner of levying thofe yearly millions that are appro- " priated to pay the intereft; we fhall find that the crown has,

" gradually and imperceptibly, gained almoſt as much in influence,
" as it has apparently loſt in prerogative."—Commentaries, b.
" iv. ch. 33.

Mr. Hume obſerves, that, " on a moderate computation, there
" are near three millions a year at the diſpoſal of the crown. The
" civil liſt amounts to near a million; the collection of the taxes
" to another; and the employments in the army and navy, toge-
" ther with eccleſiaſtical preferments, to above a third million: an
" enormous ſum, and what may fairly be computed to be more than
" a thirtieth part of the whole income, and labour of the kingdom."
—Eſſay vii. vol. i. p. 49, 8vo. edit. But Mr. Hume's remarks were
firſt publiſhed in 1742; ſince which period, the national debt has
been more than doubled. The army has been increaſed, and eccleſiaſtical preferments have been conſiderably augmented in value.
An immenſe patronage has alſo been eſtabliſhed in the Eaſt-Indies.
That of America has indeed been loſt; but, in a comparative view,
it was of ſmall eſtimation.

The influence of the crown may be conſidered in two points of
view: firſt, as it reſpects the exerciſe of the royal prerogative;
ſecondly, as it affects the freedom and independence of parliament.
In the firſt, we muſt regard the exerciſe of every branch of the royal
prerogative, as no other than *a diſcretionary power to do good;* and
conſequently that every appointment to civil or military offices,
except of perſons known or believed to be beſt qualified for their
execution; every diſtinction of rank conferred on thoſe who are
not of adequate deſert; and every reward given, but for real ſervices to the ſtate; is a violation of a truſt repoſed in the ſupreme
magiſtrate. In the ſecond point of view, we are to conſider each
individual, compoſing the two branches of the legiſlature, as under
a ſacred obligation to weigh attentively all queſtions that relate
to the public intereſt, and to vote upon them agreeably to his honeſt and ſerious conviction. If he deviate from this rule, he betrays
his truſt, and forfeits the character of patriotiſm, probity, and honour: and if the CROWN have ſeduced him, by office, titles, or
pecuniary reward, the double guilt is incurred, of violating its own
duty, and of inciting another to a correſpondent violation.

What then is juſt and honourable influence? In the ſovereign,
it is to ſtimulate to exertion, and to excite ſteadineſs in duty, by
well-grounded reſpect, gratitude, and attachment. In the ſubject,

it is to feel thefe principles in all their force, but with a proper attention to their true object; to difcriminate between the perfonal and official capacity of the fupreme magiftrate; and whenever a competition fubfifts between their refpective interefts, to regard himfelf as the beneficiary of the public, and as thus bound, by an additional obligation, to fulfil the duties of his ftation, either as a military commander, a magiftrate, or a legiflator. This diftinction the Emperor Trajan nobly maintained. on the appointment of Suberanus, to be captain of the Prætonian guard. Prefenting him with a fword as the badge of his fealty, he faid, " Let this be drawn " in my defence, if I rule according to equity; but if otherwife, it " may be employed againft me."* With the fame magnanimity he would have addreffed a præfect of the treafury, or of the city. " I " have invefted you with a poft of high dignity, authority, and " emolument; becaufe I have confidence in your talents and your " virtues. Manifeft your fenfe of the favour, by your zeal in my " fervice; always remembering, however, that my fervice implies " only that of the commonwealth." Prince Kaunitz, the minifter of the Imperial Court of Vienna, is applauded by M. Neckar, for his impartiality, integrity, and dignity of character, in the choice of perfons to fill up the great offices of ftate. He relates, that having perfuaded the Emprefs Maria Therefa, to beftow the conduct of the war department on a general of great ability, but whom he had juft reafon, as an individual, to diflike; the commander, affected by fo generous an action, earneftly wifhed for a reconciliation. Prince Kaunitz, however, declined all his advances; obferving that he had only done his duty, in caufing his fovereign to pay due regard to merit; but that in the direction of his private intimacies or connections, he was fubject to no controul, and might, in perfect confiftence with duty, indulge an entire freedom of choice. This fact well illuftrates the true application and extent of influence.

* Plinii Epiftolæ.

NOTE (C) PAGE 245.

DOCTRINE OF PASSIVE OBEDIENCE.

MR. Hume has very facetioufly imputed *Toryifm* to Socrates; becaufe, by declining to make his efcape out of prifon, he fanctions the doctrine of paffive obedience and non-refiftance. But the truth is, this venerable philofopher difdained to fave the fhort remnant of his days by an ignominious flight; by practifing the arts of corruption; or by involving the minifters of juftice in the guilt of betraying their truft. He does not appear to have treated the tumultuous affembly, which fat in judgment upon him, with *paffive* deference. " Be not offended, Athenians," he faid; "it is im- " poffible, that any one fhould long preferve his life, who arraigns, " with intrepidity, your licentioufnefs and injuftice!"

In the admirable arguments for fubmiffion to the laws, which Plato has put into the mouth of his mafter, in the dialogue entitled CRITO, the obligation of the *focial compact* appears to be ex- prefsly and forcibly pleaded. Very able writers have contended for and againft this alleged foundation and bond of civil fociety. It has been condemned, as built on the chimerical fuppofition, that " favages have been called out of caves and deferts, to deliberate " and vote upon topicks, which the experience, the ftudies, and " the refinements of civil life alone fuggeft."* But the fuppofition involves in it no fuch abfurdity. Savages could never affemble to- gether or live in community, without fome common principles of harmony and agreement. And each individual feeling their influ- ence, and yielding to their authority, a focial compact was thus eftablifhed, without deliberation or formal defign, by laws which refult from the original conftitution of human nature. The vene- ration of age; refpect for fuperior talents or virtues; a fenfe of juftice, of veracity, and honour; a regard to common intereft; the defence againft, or invafion of, common enemies; fubftantiated thefe laws. They were voluntarily acquiefced in by all; they became confirmed

---

* See Paley's Principles of Moral and Political Philofophy, book vi. chap. iii. p. 516, 4to.

by time, improved by experience, and enlarged by the progreſſive advancements of ſociety.

It is ſaid, that " if by virtue of a compact, the ſubject owes obe-" dience to government, he ought to abide by the form of govern-" ment which he finds eſtabliſhed, be it ever ſo abſurd or incon-" venient. He is bound by his bargain."* This objection will appear to have no validity, when it is recollected, that it is not an ordinary bargain or contract, in which two parties are ſuppoſed, of oppoſite intereſts; but an union of partnerſhip, in which all are equally concerned, though with various truſts and deſignations. To the firſt and neceſſary laws of this union, which conſtitute the eſſence of government, ſubmiſſion is abſolutely due. Governors, who are the organs of adminiſtration, are equally ſubject to them with the governed. And as theſe governors repreſent the majeſty and authority of the whole, it is evident that the whole, or a ma-jority of the whole, (which can alone act,) are ſuperior to their re-preſentatives; and may enlarge, circumſcribe, or new-model the authority which they delegate, as they ſhall deem moſt expedient. The public good, however, requires that government ſhould poſſeſs ſtability, becauſe revolutions are uſually attended with much preſent ſuffering and evil. Civil magiſtrates, therefore, are inveſted with powers and prerogatives adequate to extraordinary emergencies: and the policy of this is ſo clear and rational, as to command ge-neral acquieſcence, or implied conſent.

It is further alleged, that, " if every man has a right to ſurrender " his independence on bargain, (whether expreſs or implied,) he " muſt have an equal right to retain it."† This is a fallacy: for as man is by nature a ſocial being, ſociety is eſſential to his im-provement and happineſs. But ſociety cannot ſubſiſt without civil polity; that is, without ſuch laws and regulations, as are neceſſary to guard againſt imperfection and depravity; and man being alſo rational as well as ſocial, he is bound not to withhold his conſent from what is conducive to his intereſt and felicity.

Government is aſſerted to have been " at firſt§ either patriarchal " or military; that of a parent over his family, or of a commander

---

* Idem, p. 421.

† Diſquiſition on Government and Civil Liberty, by Soame Jenyns, eſq. A very excellent anſwer to this Diſquiſition, appeared in 1782; printed for Debrett, in Piccadilly.   § Paley's Moral Philoſophy, p. 399.

" over his army." When the offspring of the patriarchs had attained the age of difcretion, and the capacity of judging and acting for themfelves, it is evident that their fubmiffion to paternal authority muft have been voluntary; and it could only be voluntary, on terms of reciprocal benefit and comfort. Such terms, though not expreffed, muft be underftood; and confent, on implied terms, is in its nature a tacit compact. When two or more patriarchal families united together, the compact was probably exprefs, and not implied.

If government was at firft military, this pre-fuppofes compact: for no individual could have fufficient force to compel numbers to fubmit to his authority, and combine for its extenfion. Their union with him, and fubjection to him, muft have been by choice and agreement. A civil polity was, therefore, conftituted antecedent to conqueft; and I prefume, conqueft will not be deemed a legitimate foundation of any government.

Every juft government feems to include, in its conftitution, the three following acts of the community:—1. A compact to unite together, to be governed in their common interefts by common laws. 2. An agreement refpecting the perfons to be intrufted with the framing and the adminiftration of the laws. 3. A reciprocal agreement between the governors, thus conftituted, and the governed.* At the glorious revolution in 1688, thefe feveral acts may juftly be faid to have taken place. For the Prince of Orange, in his declaration, invites and requires all the peers of the realm; all gentlemen, citizens, and other commons, of all ranks, to come and affift him in the execution of his defign, to re-eftablifh the conftitution of the Englifh government. The convention, which affembled on this ever-memorable occafion, depofed the fupreme magiftrate, *exprefsly* becaufe he had broken the *original contract;* and appointed another, on certain ftipulated terms, declarative of the reciprocal duties of king and people: and reducing the contract, as Sir William Blackftone obferves, before built on theory and natural law, to a plain certainty. The fame learned judge remarks, that the original contract is now comprehended in the coronation oath, and in that of allegiance.†

* Confuit Hachefon's Syftem of Moral Philofophy, vol. ii. p. 227.
† See Blackftone's Commentaries, book i. p. 233.
N. B. Thefe notes and illuftrations were written before the revolution in France, an event that confirms many of the principles that have been advanced.

When Maria Therefa afcended the throne of Hungary, in 1740, fhe took the ancient oath as follows:—" If I, or any of my fuc-" ceffors, fhall at any time infringe upon your privileges; *by virtue* " *of this promife,* you and your defcendants fhall be allowed to " defend yourfelves, and fhall not be treated as rebels." It fhould feem that the two laft Kings of Pruffia regarded the privileges of their fubjects as conferred, not confirmed, by virtue of the coronation oath; and therefore they declined the ceremony of a coronation; probably becaufe, according to ufage, it would have obliged them to an explicit declaration of the duties owing to their fubjects. Baron Bielfield, in one of his letters, thus expreffes himfelf:— " Frederick I. of Pruffia, had good reafons for *fubmitting* to that " ceremony; but his fucceffors receive the crown from the hands of " Providence, and not from their fubjects. They content them- " felves with adminiftering the oath of fidelity to the troops, to the " nobility and to the people."*

Mr. Hume argues againft the original contract with much acute- nefs: yet he candidly acknowledges, that the confent of the peo- ple, where it has place, is the *beft and moft facred foundation of government.* But the converfe to the beft and moft facred can never be, in any degree, good or facred. If full confent render government moft legitimate, the entire want of it, or abfolute force, muft conftitute the moft unjuft tyranny. A fcale may thus be formed between thefe extremes, by which the degree of legitimacy in every civil eftablifhment may be eftimated.

In the Effay on Taxation, I have adopted the expreffion SOCIAL UNION, as more comprehenfive than any other, becaufe it involves in it all the *rights* and *duties*, that reciprocally belong to the indi- viduals of which it is compofed. The obligation to it is antecedent to compact, confent, or expediency. It is the ordinance of GOD, manifefted in the conftitution of our nature. For no man has the moral, though he may have the phyfical power, to withdraw him- felf entirely from the intercourfe of his fellow-creatures; as it would be, in a great degree, the extinction of being, fo far as relates to virtue and intellectual improvement, which are the chief objects of

The Count Boulainvilliers, who ridicules the notion of an ORIGINAL CONTRACT, although himfelf a republican, had he lived at this period, would have feen the doctrine eftablifhed in his own country, as well as in that of America.

* See Tower's Life of the King of Pruffia, vol. i. p. 82, 115.

it. Civil polity is a confequence of the focial union, the mode of which is regulated by temporary expediency, and confirmed by compact or confent. But no original compact or confent can give permanent validity to what is inconfiftent with the fundamental principles of the SOCIAL UNION. *Salus populi fuprema lex.*

━━━━━◆━━━━━

NOTE (D) PAGE 246.

THE DOCTRINE OF NON-RESISTANCE MERELY SPECULATIVE.

IN the year 1760, James I. thus expreffes himfelf, in his fpeech to both houfes of Parliament:—"As it is atheifm and blafphemy, " in a creature, to difpute what the Deity may do; fo it is pre- " fumption and fedition, in a fubject, to difpute what a king may " do, in the height of his power. Good Chriftians," he adds, " will be content with GOD's will, revealed in his word; and good " fubjects will reft in the king's will, revealed in his law."[*] The king's fpeech is now always fuppofed, by Parliament, to be the fpeech of the minifter. How cruel would it have been on King James's minifters, fays Mr. Horace Walpole, if that interpretation had prevailed in his reign!

Thofe who adopt the doctrines of indefeafible right, and abfolute dominion, deceive both their fovereign and themfelves; and fanction tyranny by fpeculative principles, which it is not in human nature to carry into practice. *The judgment and decree of the Univerfity of Oxford, paffed in the convocation, July 21, 1683, againft certain pernicious books, and damnable doctrines, deftruc- tive to the facred perfons of princes, their ftate and government, &c.* was fully contravened, in its moft effential point, by the conduct of her own members at the revolution. The decree was drawn up by Dr. Jane of Chrift-Church, who was afterwards one of the four delegates from the Univerfity to offer their plate to the Prince of

<hr>

[*] See King James's Works. Rapin's Hiftory, vol. ii. p. 178.

Orange, when on his march to London: and in 1710, it was burnt by the common executioner, in obedience to the order of the Houfe of Peers.*

When the great Lord Ruffel was condemned, on account of the Rye-houfe plot, in 1683; Dr. Tillotfon and Dr. Burnet were both anxioufly affiduous in their endeavours to perfuade his Lordfhip, that "the Chriftian religion abfolutely forbids the refiftance of au-" thority; and that it is not lawful, on any pretence whatfoever, to "take up arms againft government." The impreffion they made on the mind of their noble friend may be collected from the follow-ing paffage in his fpeech. "For my part, I cannot deny, but I "have been of opinion, that a free nation like this might defend "their religion and liberties, when invaded and taken from them, "though under pretence and colour of law. But fome eminent and "worthy divines, who have had the charity to be often with me, "and whom I value and efteem to a very great degree, have offered "weighty reafons to perfuade me, that faith and patience are the "proper ways for the prefervation of religion; and the method of "the Gofpel is to fuffer perfecution, rather than to ufe refiftance. "But if I have finned in this, I hope GOD will not lay it to my "charge, fince He knows it was only a fin of ignorance."†

The paffages in the New Teftament, wherein obedience to ma-giftracy is fo emphatically inculcated, are juftly fuppofed to have been particularly addreffed to the Gaulanites, a wild and deluded party, the followers of Theudas, a native of Gaulan in Upper Ga-lilee. This fanatic, in the tenth year of JESUS CHRIST, "which "was the laft of Auguftus, excited his countrymen the Galileans, "and many others of the Jews, to take arms and venture upon all "extremities, rather than pay tribute to the Romans. The princi-"ples he infufed into his party were, not only that they were a free "nation, and ought to be in fubjection to no other; but that they "were the elect of GOD, that He alone was their Governor, and "that therefore they ought not to fubmit to any ordinance of "man. And though he was unfuccefsful, infomuch that his party, "in their very firft attempt, were entirely routed and difperfed: "yet fo deeply had he infufed his own enthufiafm into their hearts, "that they never refted, till in their own deftruction they involved

---

* Birch's Life of Tillotfon, p. 189. † Idem, p. 116.

" the city and temple."* It muſt be recollected, alſo, that the
followers of JESUS had long a prepoſſeſſion that the Meſſiah was
to enjoy a temporal kingdom and authority; and that, under his
dominion, Judea was not only to recover her independency, but
even to ſubvert the Roman power. Hence the ſeducing queſtion
propoſed to our SAVIOUR, *Is it lawful to pay tribute to Ceſar, or
not?* And St. Paul delivers this expreſs injunction, *Render, therefore,
unto all their dues: tribute to whom tribute is due; cuſtom, to whom
cuſtom; fear, to whom fear; honour, to whom honour.* But though
it be true that CHRIST's *kingdom is not of this world; that every
ſoul is to be ſubject unto the higher powers;* and that *whoever reſiſteth the power, reſiſteth the ordinance of GOD;* yet we are at the
ſame time aſſured, that *rulers are not a terror to good works, but to
the evil;* that *they are miniſters of GOD to us for good;* and that
for this cauſe we pay tribute. From hence, I think, it is clearly to
be inferred, that magiſtracy is the ordinance of GOD, for the good
of ſociety; but that the duty of allegiance is exactly proportionate
to its adaption to the great ends of its inſtitution.

It is curious to obſerve, how conſonant the law of England, relative to the diſputed titles of our ſovereigns, is to the maxim of the
great Apoſtle of the Gentiles, *the powers that be are ordained of
GOD.* The 11th ſtatute of Henry VII. recites, that " the ſubjects
" of England are bound, by the duty of their allegiance, to ſerve
" their prince and ſovereign lord, *for the time being,* in defence of
" him and his realm againſt every rebellion, power, and might,
" raiſed againſt him. And that whatſoever may happen in the for-
" tune of war againſt the mind and will of the prince, *as in this
" land,* ſome time paſt, it hath been *ſeen;* it is not reaſonable, but
" againſt all laws, reaſon, and good conſcience, that ſuch ſubjects,
" attending upon ſuch ſervice, ſhould ſuffer for doing their true
" duty and ſervice of allegiance." " This," ſays Sir Michael
Foſter, " putteth the duty of the ſubject upon a rational and ſafe
" bottom. He knoweth that protection and allegiance are reci-
" procal duties. He ſeeth the fountain from whence the bleſſings
" of government, liberty, peace, and plenty, flow to him; and there
" he payeth his allegiance."†

* Percy's Key to the New Teſtament.

† See Sir Michael Foſter's Diſcourſes on the Crown Law, folio, p. 399.

Having made the foregoing quotation from the works of this excellent judge, I am tempted to add a few more paſſages, on the ſubject
of government, from the ſame invaluable diſcourſe. Some learned
men " ſeem not to have ſufficiently attended to the nature and ends
" of civil power, whereof the regal dignity is a principal branch;
" they ſeem to have conſidered the crown and regal dignity merely as
" a DESCENDABLE PROPERTY; or an eſtate or intereſt veſted in the
" poſſeſſor, for the emolument and grandeur of himſelf and heirs, in
" a regular invariable courſe of deſcent. And therefore, in ques-
" tions touching the ſucceſſion, they conſtantly reſort to the ſame
" narrow rules and maxims of law and juſtice, by which queſtions
" of mere property, the title to a pig-ſtye or a lay-ſtall, are governed.
" If I could conceive of the crown as an inheritance of *mere pro-*
" *perty,* I ſhould be tempted to argue in the ſame manner. But
" had they conſidered the crown and royal dignity, as a deſcend-
" able OFFICE, as a TRUST for millions, and extending its influence
" to generations yet unborn; had they conſidered it in that light,
" they would ſoon have diſcovered the principle upon which the
" right of the legiſlature to interpoſe in caſes of neceſſity is mani-
" feſtly founded: and that is the SALUS POPULI, already men-
" tioned upon a like occaſion."*—" All the rights and powers for
" defence and preſervation belonging to ſociety are nothing more
" than the natural rights and powers of individuals transferred to
" and concentering in the body, for the preſervation of the whole.
" And from the law of ſelf-preſervation, conſidered as extending
" to civil ſociety, reſulteth the well-known maxim, *ſalus populi ſu-*
" *prema lex.*

" I think the principles here laid down muſt be admitted, unleſs
" any one will chooſe to ſay, that individuals in a community are, in
" certain caſes, under the protection of the primitive law of ſelf-
" preſervation; but communities, compoſed of the ſame individuals,
" are, in the like caſes, excluded. Or, that when the enemy is at
" the gate, every ſingle ſoldier may and ought to ſtand to his arms,
" but the *garriſon* muſt ſurrender at *diſcretion.*"†

* Sir Michael Foſter's Diſcourſes on the Crown Law, folio, p. 404.

† Id. p. 382, 383.

ADVANTAGES OF THE BRITISH GOVERNMENT.

THOMSON, whofe authority may be quoted, as a moralift and philofopher, has admirably defcribed the Britifh conftitution, in the fecond canto of his Caftle of Indolence:

" Whereas the knight had fram'd in Britain land
" A matchlefs form of glorious government,
" In which the fovereign laws alone command;
" Laws 'ftablifh'd by the public free confent,
" Whofe majefty is to the fceptre lent."

Under this view of our conftitution, loyalty in a Briton is a rational and patriotic principle. It is not a blind and fervile attachment to the perfon or family of the monarch; but a reverence for him, as the minifter of law and juftice, and the patriarch of his people. If, however, his private and public virtues happily merit confidence and efteem, fubjection will be accompanied with cordial fatisfaction; and obedience performed with promptitude, zeal, and love. This warmth of loyalty ought to be peculiarly encouraged in a free ftate; becaufe it may often be found neceffary to counteract the infidious arts of faction, or the enterprizing fpirit of ariftocratic ambition.

It is a common obfervation, adopted even by fome republican writers, that an abfolute monarchy is the beft of all forms of government, provided a fucceffion of wife, virtuous, and patriotic fovereigns be infured. But, admitting the fuppofition, however improbable it may be, I am perfuaded it is effential to the higheft interefts of the people, that they poffefs a fhare in the adminiftration; and that the calm of defpotifm, even under a Titus or an Antoninus, would be lefs favourable to moral and intellectual improvement, than the agitations which occafionally arife in our mixed fyftem of polity. Thefe agitations diffufe the love of our country, kindle the ardour of ambition, animate the fpirit of enterprize, and call forth into public exertion many talents which might otherwife have remained in obfcurity.

" This is true liberty, when free-born men,
" Having to advife the public, may fpeak free ;
" Which he who can and will deferves high praife,
" Who neither can nor will may hold his peace:
" What can be jufter in a ftate than this ?"*

Thefe high and important privileges infpire a veneration for the dignity of the human character, and a difdain of whatever tends to the degradation of our fpecies. And the enthufiafm of liberty, thus roufed, extends itfelf beyond our country: we learn to regard ourfelves as citizens of the orld, and become affertors of the equal and unalienable rights of all mankind.

It is to the influence of this magnanimous principle, that we may reafonably afcribe the noble efforts, which have been lately made, towards accomplifhing the abolition of flavery and the African flave trade. " A flave, or a negro," fays Judge Blackftone, " the mo-
" ment he lands in England, falls under the protection of the laws;
" and, fo far, becomes a freeman. This fpirit of liberty is rooted
" even in our very foil."* But I truft it is not to be *locally* cir-
cumfcribed; that it is deeply implanted in our minds; and that, according to the affertion of Fortefcue, *Angliæ jura IN OMNI CASU libertati dant favorem.*† In the cafe of Somerfet, the negro, de-
cided in 1772, it was the judgment of the Court of King's-Bench, that the mafter could not recover his power over his fervant, by fending him abroad at pleafure. And the Chief Court of Jufticiary in Scotland, in 1778, made an award againft John Wedderburn, in favour of Jofeph Knignt, an African, " that the dominion affumed
" over this negro, under the law of Jamaica, BEING UNJUST, could
" not be fupported, in this country, to *any* extent: that, therefore,
" the defender, had no right to the negro's fervice, for any fpace
" of time; nor to fend him out of the country againft his confent."‡
So explicit a condemnation of the fervitude of the negroes, by very high legal authority, clearly implies a condemnation equally ftrong of that infamous traffic from which it originates; exclufively of every confideration, relative to the barbarity with which it is conducted.

* Milton, motto to the Areopagitica, tranflated from Euripides.
* Comment. book i. chap. i. p. 12.
† De laud. leg. Ang. cap. 42.—" One nation there is in the world that has, for the direct end of its conftitution, political liberty." Montefquieu's Spirit of Laws, vol. i. p. 215.
‡ Millar on the Origin of Ranks, edit. 3d, p. 361.

From the report of the Lords of the Committee of Council, concerning the prefent ftate of the trade to Africa, and particularly the trade in flaves, it appears that this traffic is frequently carried on by *kidnapping*, and bears a clofe analogy to *piracy.* The former is defined by Judge Blackftone, " the forcible abduction or ftealing " away of man, woman, and child, from their own country; and " felling them into another." By the Jewifh law, this was a capital offence: *He that ftealeth a man, and felleth him, or if he be found in his hand, fhall furely be put to death:* Exodus xxi. 16. By the civil law, alfo, the crime termed *Plagium* was capital, which confifted in fpiriting away and ftealing men and children.* Piracy is an offence againft the univerfal law of fociety; a pirate being, according to Sir Edward Coke, *hoftis humani generis.* And, by ftatute 8 Geo. I. the trading with known pirates, or furnifhing them with ftores or ammunition, is deemed piracy; and all acceffaries to piracy are declared to be principal pirates, and felons without benefit of clergy.† Surely the crime of piracy, in its effence and degree, is the fame, to an enlightened mind, on the coafts of Africa as on thofe of Europe: and we condemn, with as full conviction of their enormity, the depredations of the knights of Malta on the peafants, fifhermen, and failors of Barbary, as we do thofe of the corfairs of Tunis, and Algiers, on the ftate of Italy.‖

---

* Blackftone's Comment. book iv. chap. xv.

The extent of this crime, as practifed on the coaft of Guinea, overpowers the fenfe of its enormity, and of the miferies produced by it. Of thefe miferies we may form an eftimate, by the following affecting account of the fufferings of a few natives of another part of the globe, on being forced away from their country, their families, and friends. Chriftiern IV. king of Denmark, fent three fhips to make difcoveries on the coaft of Greenland. The commanders of thefe veffels carried off feveral of the natives, who, when firft captured, " rent the air with " their cries and lamentations. They leaped into the fea ; and when taken again " on fhip-board, for fome time refufed all fuftenance. Their eyes were conti- " nually turned towards their dear country, and their faces always bathed in tea rs " Even the countenance of his Danifh majefty, and the careffes of the court and " people, could not alleviate their grief. One of them was perceived to fhed tears " always when he faw an infant in the mother's arms; a circumftance from " whence it was naturally concluded, that he had left his wife with a young child " in Greenland."—See Encyclop. Britan. Art. Greenland.

† Blackftone's Comment. book iv. chap. 5.

‡ Howard on Lazarettos, p. 58.

Servitude is founded, by thofe civilians who deem it lawful, on voluntary compact, on captivity, on debt, and on the power of the magiftrate in the punifhment of crimes.

Slavery, founded on *voluntary compact*, muft in itfelf be void; becaufe man, being an accountable creature, has not in himfelf a right to difpenfe with that accountablenefs, or to vield up his will and conduct to the abfolute difpofal of another. Befides, every compact implies reciprocal and proportionate benefit. But what benefit can he derive from an act which divefts him of all the capacities for property, all the rights of a citizen, and all the honourable diftinctions of a rational being? *Captivity* cannot itfelf be juftified, except as the confequence of *lawful* war: and the prifoners, though they may properly be compelled to work for their own maintenance, or perhaps, in fome fpecial inftances, to make compenfation for damages fuftained, owe no farther fervices to their captors, and have a natural right to be reftored to liberty, when fuch obligation has been fulfilled, or whenever there fhall be a ceffation of war. In the cafe of *debt*, alfo, the claim to fervitude is limited, extending only to the retribution of the creditor; and never involving in it any right over pofterity. As a *punifhment* for crimes, flavery may fometimes be deemed both reafonable and politic; but, in its duration and feverity, it muft be exactly proportionate to the offence: and as moft punifhments are intended for reformation, no lefs than for example, the benefit of the flave and of the public is to be the fole ftandard of its meafure. How little applicable are thefe canons to the juftification of flavery, as it formerly fubfifted in Europe; or to the practice of tranfporting flaves from the coaft of Africa to our colonial poffeffions! But the authority of the Holy Scriptures is pleaded. To the Jewifh laws and cuftoms we owe no obedience; and the evangelical code will affuredly be found repugnant to flavery, in its doctrines, its precepts, and the example of its Divine Founder. We are therein taught, that all mankind are equally the children of one common Father, redeemed by the fame Saviour, and joint heirs of glory and immortality. We are commanded *to love our neighbours as ourfelves; and to do unto others, as we would they fhould do unto us*. And our Divine Mafter was himfelf *meek and lowly in fpirit, condefcending to men of low eftate*, and *continually going about to do good*. Converted fervants, indeed, *under the yoke*, are enjoined *to count their own mafters worthy of all honour.* This, however, can only mean all reasonable honour: and the *believing masters* are at the same time instructed *not to despise their servants, because they are brethren; but rather to do them services, because they are faithful and beloved partakers of the benefit.* 1 Tim. vi. 1, 2. Several of the injunctions of scripture, regarding submission, are to be considered as *prudential*, not as *moral*, precepts. *If a man smite thee on the right cheek, turn to him the left also: And, if any man take thy cloak, let him have thy coat also.* Such a rule could relate only to the particular circumstances and situation of those to whom it was delivered: and the command to bear injury, oppression, or injustice, can, in no instance, give a sanction to the commission of those crimes.

St. Paul addresses an epistle to Philemon, a native of Colosse in Phrygia, in behalf of Onesimus his slave, who had robbed and run away from him, but was afterwards converted to the Christian faith at Rome. The Apostle says, *I beseech thee for my son Onesimus, whom I have sent again: thou, therefore, receive him that is my own bowels, not now as a servant, but above a servant, a brother beloved, specially to me; but how much more unto thee in the flesh and in the Lord!** Servitude, under such circumstances, is *virtually* annihilated: and it was by the spirit of meekness and brotherly love, that Christianity was adapted to promote a gradual abolition of the cruel bondage, in which more than two-thirds of the Roman empire were held at the time of its promulgation.

NOTE (F) PAGE 252.

TAXES ON THE NECESSARIES OF LIFE.

AT Tobolski, in Siberia, the price of provisions is so extremely low, that it seems to encourage both idleness and debauchery in the inhabitants; for the labour of one day furnishes sufficient

---

* It has been conjectured, that Onesimus received his freedom, and was afterwards bishop of Berœa in Macedonia. "When Ignatius wrote his epistle to the "Ephesians, about the year 107, their bishop's name was *Onesimus*; and Grotius "thought him to be the same for whom Paul interceded with Philemon."— Lardner's History of the Apostles. Bishop Watson's Theological Tracts, vol. ii. page 297.

fupport for a whole week, and every additional exertion fupplies the means of riot and excefs.* Sir Wm. Temple, in his comparifon between the people of Ireland and the Netherlands, afcribes the lazinefs of the former to the like caufe. " For men," fays he, " naturally prefer eafe before labour, and will not take pains if they " can live idle; though, when by neceffity they have been inured to " it, they cannot leave it, being grown a cuftom neceffary to their " health and very entertainment."† But in Siberia and in Ireland, the inhabitants having never feen or tafted the enjoyments procured by induftry, and being in a ftate of oppreffion, from which they have not the power to free themfelves, they are deftitute of adequate incitements to exertion: whereas in the provinces of America, though the price of labour is very high, and the neceffaries of life ftill more cheap and plentiful than in the countries above-mentioned, induftry fubfifts in its full energy. The evils flowing from high wages and the cheapnefs of provifions are chiefly obferved in our great manufacturing towns, and in the diftricts immediately dependent upon them. In the kingdom at large, fuch confequences are not experienced; yet the country working poor are fuppofed to conftitute three-fourths of the whole body of labourers: fo that the adoption of a maxim, which is juft and falutary with refpect to the ingenious but profligate inhabitants of towns, may prove injurious to the more fober, orderly, but lefs active inhabitants of the country; who are alfo the great fources of population. For it appears, from Mr. Howlet's calculation, that, at Dunmow in Effex, two hundred and fixty poor families have four hundred and fixty children; whereas one hundred and fixteen families, of the ranks above them, have only one hundred and twenty children.

NOTE (G) PAGE 256.

STATUTES OF EXCISE.

IT is the complaint of an enlightened French ftatefman, M. Turgot, that the eftablifhed rule of finance, in all doubtful cafes, is to make the decifion in favour of the revenue: and that, by the

* Lord Kaims's Hiftory of Man, vol. ii.
† Account of the Netherlands, ch. vi.

complication of laws, almost every case is rendered doubtful. M
Neckar also observes, that when the taxes are immoderate, when
they even exceed certain limits, exactness is augmented in proportion to the difficulty of collection: it becomes necessary to give
greater authority to the collectors; to be insensible to complaints;
to venerate the science of finance; and to honour all the professors
of it, without distinction.

As the finances of the kingdom are now said to be in a flourishing
state, and as the annual collection of more than fifteen millions bears
so large a portion to the whole capital stock and income of the
community; it may be hoped that the legislature will engage in a
thorough revision of the laws of revenue, with a view, not merely
to their productiveness, but to their equity and consistency with the
rights of the people. Tacitus records the justice of an edict of
Nero, commanding the prætor of Rome, and similar officers in the
provinces, to receive complaints against the publicans, and to redress the wrongs committed by them on the spot.* Let us compare this with the conduct of Frederic II. king of Prussia, whose
tax-gatherers supported the double office of exciseman and judge;
so that if a tenant did not pay his assessment on the very day appointed, the collector put on the magisterial robes, and fined the
delinquent in double the sum.†

A very judicious writer‡ on the subject of taxes remarks, " that
" though vexation is not, strictly speaking, expence, it is certainly
" equivalent to the expence, at which every man would be willing
" to redeem himself from it." This important consideration pleads
strongly for a revisal of the excise laws; by which six millions and
a half, a sum equal to two-fifths of the whole revenue of the state,
are raised chiefly from the arts and industry of the people. It is
said, that the number of informations tried in one year amounted
nearly to five thousand; but the actual forfeitures only to seven
thousand pounds. A fuller proof can hardly be adduced that frivolous and vexatious suits are often instituted, even under the
present just and lenient government. What oppression, therefore,
may be dreaded from a farther extension of an uninterrupted system
of excise, if power and long usage shall hereafter silence the
public voice against it!

* Annal. xiii. 51.   † Towers's Life of the King of Prussia.
‡ Smith on the Wealth of Nations, book v. ch. ii. part ii.

NOTE (H) PAGE 256.

OATHS.

IN the edict of the Grand Duke of Tuscany, for the reform of Criminal Law, of which the benevolent Mr. Howard has favoured me with a copy, it appears that the number of oaths are greatly diminished; and that they are administered with the utmost solemnity and reverence. As this tract is not published, I shall transcribe the following paragraphs from it :—

" In consequence of the foregoing regulations, instead of the " warning to declare the truth, which it was for the judge in the " process to give the witness, previous to his taking his oath, the " said officer shall represent to him, that the laws, both human and " divine, make it the duty of every man not to attest a falsehood, " nor to declare himself ignorant; he is likewise to remind him, " not only of the importance of that obligation, but also that he is " liable to be obliged to confirm by oath, at the request either of " the accused, the plaintiff, or the injured party, whatever he is " about to declare, in reply to the simple queries that are to be put " to him."

" And we order that, in whatever case and circumstance it may " be permitted to administer an oath, let it be to whom it will, and " on any occasion whatsoever, the judge or public officer carrying " on the trial, before he administers the said oath, shall represent to " the person the obligation that accompanies it, explaining to him " its meaning and importance; and to the end that it may make a " greater impression, we abolish the simple formality of touching a " leaf of the bible only, instead of which the person shall kneel " down, and swear before a crucifix. When the person who is " about to swear, is of a religion different from ours, he shall take " his oath in the form the most respected and dreaded by those of " his own persuasion, the great importance of the undertaking " having previously been represented to him."

Mr. Howard, in his Observations on Foreign Prisons, informs us, that, in *La Prison Ordinaire*, at Bern, a serious exhortation is hung up, concerning the awful nature of an oath, together with the forms of those which are to be taken. He transcribes the one following: " My deposition, which has now been read to me, I confirm before

" the face of God omnipotent, omniscient, and true, to contain the
" truth, as I desire that God may be my help, at the end of my
" days." The same excellent author speaks, with much approbation, of the mode of administering oaths in Scotland; and asserts
that perjury is not frequent in that country. But I know not how
to reconcile this observation with what Lord Kaims, a late respectable judge of the Court of Session, has delivered in his Loose Hints
on Education:—" Custom-house oaths," says his Lordship, " now-
" a-days, go for nothing; not that the world grows more wicked,
" but because no person lays any stress upon them. The duty on
" French wine is the same in Scotland and in England. But as we
" cannot afford to pay this high duty, the permission, under-hand,
" to pay Spanish duty for French wine, is found more beneficial to
" the revenue than the rigour of the law. The oath however
" must be taken, that the wine we import is Spanish, to entitle us
" to the ease of the Spanish duty. Such oaths, at first, were highly
" criminal, because directly a fraud against the public; but now
" that the oath is only exacted for form's sake, without any faith
" intended to be given or received, it becomes very little different
" from saying in the way of civility, *I am, Sir, your friend, or your*
" *obedient servant*. And in fact, we every day see merchants deal-
" ing in such oaths, whom no man scruples to rely upon in the
" most material affairs."

Such Machiavelian sentiments, offered by a learned judge, must
surprize and shock every well-informed and well-principled mind.
But I shall make no other comment on them, than that they irrefra-
gably evince the corrupting influence of the present multiplication
of oaths on the moral opinions as well as practices of mankind.

ADDITIONAL NOTE, PAGE 247, LINE 16.

TURPITUDE MARKED BY THE GROSS DEFECT OF
GOOD PRINCIPLES, &c.

THE distinction of *positive* and *negative* turpitude is of considerable importance in ethics. Yet there may subsist great apathy,
or defect of good principle, in a mind virtuous as to its general
constitution. The people of Hindostan are remarkable for the gen-

tlenefs of their difpofitions, the foftnefs of their manners, and the force of their attachments in love; yet they feem to be devoid of compaffion and generofity. They are faid to be unaffected by the diftreffes, the dangers, or even the death, of a fellow-creature. "An " Englifh gentleman was ftanding by a Hindoo, when a fierce and " ravenous tiger leaped from a thicket, and carried off a fcreaming " boy, who was the fon of one of his neighbours. The Englifhman " expreffed fymptoms of the moft extreme horror; whilft the " Hindoo remained unmoved. What! faid the former, are you " unaffected by dreadful a fcene? The great GOD, replied the " other, would have it fo."*

* See Annual Regifter for 1752, p. 36.

BIOGRAPHICAL

MEMOIRS

OF THE LATE

THOMAS BUTTERWORTH BAYLEY, Esq;

F. R. S. &c. &c.

OF

HOPE-HALL, NEAR MANCHESTER.

" ——————— by all approv'd,
" Prais'd, wept, and honour'd, by the *friend* he lov'd."

" HEU!

" QUANTO MINUS EST RELIQUIS VERSARI,

" QÀM TUI MEMINISSE."

BIOGRAPHICAL MEMOIRS

OF

THOMAS BUTTERWORTH BAYLEY, Esq.

THE recollection of a Friend, who has finished his earthly career with distinguished honour, and recently paid the last debt to nature, is accompanied with a mixture of reverence and love, beyond what the most exalted or most beneficent actions during life inspire. We cherish the contemplation of departed excellence with pleasing sorrow; and it becomes even a grateful task, to communicate to others some participation in the feelings which occupy our minds on the mournful occasion. These reflections have been suggested by the much-lamented death of THOS. B. BAYLEY, esq; whose talents, character, and conduct have long been regarded by the public with no ordinary degree of interest. He was seized at Buxton with a disorder of the bowels, which terminated fatally on Thursday the 24th of June, 1802, at the close of the 58th year of his age. The illness was short but severe; and supported by him with exemplary ferenity and fortitude. His progenitors were perfons of fortune and great refpectability; and on his mother's fide he was defcended from the Dukenfields of Dukenfield in Chefhire; an ancient family, in the male line of which the dignity of Baronet has been tranfmitted in regular fucceffion fince the reign of King Charles II. Mr. Bayley was educated to no profeffion; but being fent to the Univerfity of Edinburgh, and placed under the fpecial care of an excellent tutor, he applied himfelf with uncommon ardour, affiduity, and fuccefs, to all thofe ftudies which were adapted to qualify him for the rank and duties of a country gentleman. Not long after he had completed his academical purfuits he was nominated to be one of his Majefty's Juftices of the Peace for the County Palatine of Lancafter. By reading, by obfervation, by attendance on the courts of judicature; and particularly by communication with a neighbouring magiftrate,* diftinguifhed for his probity, found judgment, and juridical fkill ; he acquired a very comprehenfive knowledge of the laws of his country: and becoming pre-eminent on the bench, he was in a few years appointed Perpetual Chairman of the Quarter-Seffions. This ftation, which was of peculiar importance in the populous trading diftrict where he officiated, he filled with dignity and confummate ability. His attention to the caufes brought for trial was unremitting ; his patience

* Dorning Rafbotham, Efq.

in hearing the longeſt inveſtigations, unwearied; his diſcrimination of evidence, impartial and acute; and his protection of the witneſſes from petulance or inſult was ſpirited and inflexible. The charges which he delivered to the jurymen were replete with legal wiſdom and moral inſtruction; and he pronounced the ſentence of the Court on the unhappy convicts with the moſt impreſſive ſolemnity. Indeed, on every occaſion he delivered himſelf with fluency, grace, perſpicuity, and energy.

His excellence as a Magiſtrate was not confined to the proceedings of the bench. He ſuperintended with vigilance the general POLICE, ſolicitous to diminiſh evils in their commencement, and to obviate puniſhment by the prevention of crimes. He was ſedulouſly watchful over the PAROCHIAL WORKHOUSES under his juriſdiction; which he frequently viſited, that he might make the ſtricteſt ſcrutiny into their domeſtic regulations, their comforts, ſalubrity, and the proper diſtribution of labour.

The erection of a commodious and well-ventilated GAOL and PENITENTIARY-HOUSE, at Mancheſter, was accompliſhed by him in 1787, but not without much oppoſition. Yet the meaſure was afterwards ſo highly approved, even by thoſe juſtices who were at firſt ſtrenuous againſt it, that the premiſes were ſtiled the *New Bayley*, in honour of the projector, by the unanimous vote of the whole bench of magiſtrates. Of this place of confinement, the philanthropic Mr. Howard ſpeaks in the following terms: " By the

" fpirited exertions of Mr. Bayley, and other magis-
" trates, a new prilon is building on a large fcale,
" from Mr. Blackburn's plan, in which there will be
" fingle cells and feparate apartments for faulty
" apprentices, &c. This prifon will reflect much
" credit on the good fenfe and liberality of the
" hundred of Salford, which alone defrays all the
" cofts of the building." For the improvement·in
the Courts of Affize, and the County Gaol at Lancafter, the like praife is due to Mr. Bayley. Such
indeed was the general fenfe of his fkill in the conftruction of places of confinement, that he was confulted about moft of the prifons which of late have
been enlarged or erected in this kingdom.

The ftate of the great body of the poor, in the
town and neighbourhood of Manchefter, occupied
much of the time and attention of Mr. Bayley. In
the year 1796, he took a very active part in the eftablifhment of a BOARD of HEALTH, over which
he continued to prefide, till the inftitution was deprived of his fervices by death. The firft Report of
this eftablifhment thus announces the defign of it
to the public: " To meliorate the condition of the
" indigent ; to prevent the generation of difeafes;
" to obviate the propagation of them by contagion;
" and to mitigate thofe which exift, by providing
" comforts and accommodations for the fick; are the
" profeffed objects of this undertaking." That much
good has been done by it, cannot be doubted ; and
the farther plans for the extenfion of its benefits,

which are now in contemplation, were ardently encouraged and fupported by Mr. Bayley.

The Cotton-Mills, which have been fo multiplied in
this country, as now to furnifh employment to feveral
hundred thoufand hands, very early arrefted the attention of Mr. Bayley. In the year 1784, an alarming
malignant fever was fuppofed to originate in a large
factory at Radcliffe near Manchefter. The Magistrates, therefore, requefted the Phyficians of the
town to make enquiry into its caufes, and to fuggeft
the proper means of preventing the fpreading of the
contagion. The commiffion was immediately executed; and the Medical Gentlemen thus concluded
their Memorial, addreffed to his Majefty's Juftices of
the Peace: " We earneftly recommend a longer re-
" cefs from labour at noon, and a more early dis-
" miffion from it in the evening, to all who work in
" the Cotton-Mills. But we deem (fay they) this in-
" dulgence effential to the prefent health and future
" capacity for labour of thofe who are under the age
" of fourteen; for the active recreations of childhood
" and youth are neceffary to the growth, the vigour,
" and right conformation of the human body. And
" we cannot excufe ourfelves, on the prefent occafion,
" from fuggefting to you, who are the guardians of
" the public weal, this further very important con-
" fideration; that the rifing generation fhould not be
" debarred from all opportunities of inftruction, at
" the only feafon of life in which they can be pro-
" perly improved." Since the period here alluded

to, feveral proprietors of large factories have, with
equal judgment and benevolence, adopted regulations
favourable both to health and morals.   Yet in many
of thefe works great evils ftill fubfift; and, it was the
opinion of Mr. Bayley, will continue to fubfift, till a
code of laws for their general government, framed
according to the plans which the experience of a few
fpirited individuals has proved to be practicable, wife,
and falutary, has been fanctioned by the authority of
the legiflature. On the Bill lately enacted, for the well
ordering of Apprentices in the Cotton-Mills, he was
confulted by the very refpectable Senator, who moved
and fupported it in Parliament. The claufes in general he approved; but confidered them as much too
partial and limited in their operation, to anfwer the
important and neceffary purpofes of reformation.
Indeed he was adverfe to the admiffion of apprentices
from a diftance; who, being unknown, muft in fome
meafure be unprotected. To the diffolution of family
connections alfo, even amongft the loweft orders of
the poor, which this practice tends to produce, he
was wont to urge very forcible objections. On fuch
connections the moft valuable interefts of life depend:

" Relations dear, and all the charities
" Of Father, Son, and Brother."   MILTON.

And when a parent has been induced to abandon
his offspring, and the child is placed in a fituation
which extinguifhes all the tender attachments of
affinity, the ftrongeft incentives to virtue are with-

drawn, and the mind becomes prepared for idlenefs, malevolence, and profligacy.

To counteraƌ the caufes of increafing vice and mifery, by promoting the moral and religious in-ftruƌion of the rifing generation amongft the poor, Mr. Bayley gave the moft zealous encouragement to the eftablifhment of Sunday Schools. He was a friend to the diffufion of knowledge, efpecially of that knowledge which all admit to be *prime wifdom*; and he often expreffed both furprize and concern at the error of many well-difpofed perfons, who are inimical to the extenfion of every branch of learning to the inferior claffes of the community. For his comprehenfive experience had fully convinced him, that reading, writing, and arithmetic, are not only favourable to fkill and advancement in the arts, but to fubordination, peaceablenefs, fobriety, and honefty.

More than twenty-five years ago, a few gentlemen belonging to the town and neighbourhood of Man-chefter, who had a tafte for polite literature and philofophy, formed themfelves into a weekly associ-ation, for the purpofe of converfing together on fcien-tific topics. Mr Bayley early joined this little band; and afterwards aided, both by his counfels and influ-ence, the enlargement of the original plan. Prefi-dents and other officers were eleƌed; laws were framed; and a regular inftitution eftablifhed, under the denomination of the *Literary and Philofophical Society of Manchefter*; which has publifhed five vo-lumes of Tranfaƌions, infcribed by permiffion to the

King, that have been received with much approbation
by the public. The meetings of this body Mr.
Bayley could only occafionally attend, having his
time fully occupied in other preffing and active purfuits; but he repeatedly furnifhed valuable communications.

From this Inftitution another fprung, not long
afterwards, entitled the *College of Arts and Sciences*,
for which Mr. Bayley was at great pains to obtain
the moft honourable patronage, and moft liberal fupport. It was intended to provide a courfe of fcholaftic
inftruction, compatible with the engagements of commercial life, favourable to all its higher interefts, and
at the fame time preparatory to the fyftematic ftudies
of the univerfity. To unite philofophy with art,
the moral and intellectual culture of the mind with
the purfuits of fortune, and to fuperadd the nobleft
powers of enjoyment to the acquifition of wealth,
were the objects which it profeffed to hold in view.
In the firft feffion, lectures were propofed to be delivered on practical mathematics, and on the principal
branches of natural and experimental philofophy; on
chemiftry, with a reference to arts and manufactures
on the origin, hiftory, and progrefs of arts, manufactures, and commerce; on the commercial laws and
regulations of different countries; and on the nature
of commutative juftice, of oaths, contracts, and other
branches of commercial ethics. This admirable undertaking, which was highly applauded by men of
the firft literary eminence in England and other

countries, and fo approved by Dr. Franklin, that he is faid to have left a confiderable fum of money for the eftablifhment of a fimilar inftitution in America, met with unexpected and very groundlefs oppofition in Manchefter; and for want of fufficient encouragement was foon abandoned. The effort, however, though not crowned with fuccefs, reflects honour on the memory of Mr. Bayley.

The Abolition of the Slave Trade, about fourteen years fince, became the fubject of very interefting parliamentary difcuffion. Manchefter had the honour of precedence over every other provincial town in the kingdom, in efpoufing this important caufe of juftice and humanity. Public confultations were held to promote the fuccefs of it; and no one engaged in the tranfaction with more heart-felt concern than Mr. Bayley. A petition to the Houfe of Commons was determined upon, by a numerous and moft refpectable meeting; and when it was framed and ready for fig. nature, he was the firft perfon who affixed his name to it. On taking the pen, he lifted up his hands to Heaven, and with an elevated voice exclaimed, " May " God grant his blefling on this virtuous effort in " favour of oppreffed humanity!" A profound filence enfued; one fympathetic emotion feemed to pervade the whole affembly; and every heart was in unifon with the devout afpiration.

The delightful, and it may be added, truly patriotic purfuits of Agriculture, fince on their extenfion the national profperity is far more dependent, than on foreign commerce, uniformly engaged the few leifure hours which Mr. Bayley enjoyed; and to the exercife in the open air, to which he was induced by attention to the improvements in his pleafure-grounds and farm at Hope, aided by habitual temperance, a conftitution, naturally weak and infirm, was rendered tolerably vigorous and robuft. In draining, planting, manuring, and the culture of new graffes, he had acquired no fmall degree of fkill and judgment; and the Manchefter Agricultural Society, of which he was a founder and conftant fupporter, adjudged to him many honourable premiums.

At the clofe of the American war, before peace was finally concluded with France, Government encouraged the raifing of Volunteer Corps in different parts of England. A very refpectable one was embodied at Manchefter, and Mr. Bayley was appointed by his Majefty Lieutenant-Colonel Commandant. The fame honour was again conferred upon him, on the like occafion, in 1798, a period when the country was univerfally alarmed with the apprehenfions of invafion.

In a diftrict fo immenfely populous as the Hundred of Salford, in which very confiderable viciffitudes are at times experienced in the ftate of the manufactures, affecting the prices of labour and the means of fubfiftence, violent tumults may, under particular circumftances, be expected to arife. The military force as never been employed in repreffing thefe diforders, but as an auxiliary to the civil power; and Mr. Bayley, by temperate firmnefs, and authority mixed with conciliation, was always able, in conjunction with fome of his brethren of the Bench of Juftices, to dif- perfe the mobs without the effufion of blood. On fuch alarming emergencies, his own life has been, more than once, in the moft imminent danger. Yet he fhrunk not from the expofure of it again, when public duty called him to the renewal of his exertions: and he has been known to ride into the midft of an enraged multitude, armed with ftones and bludgeons; and, when exhortations and threats availed not, has affifted perfonally in the feizure of their ringleaders; evincing, that the energy of a generous mind rifes according to the greatnefs of the exifting occafion; and that courage and intrepidity will always be ade- quate to the magnitude of the evil which is to be overcome.

Mr. Bayley married Mary the only child of Mr. Vincent Leggatt, of London; a lady whofe cheerful- nefs, good-fenfe, and maternal virtues, have endeared her to a numerous family; and whofe hofpitality, beneficence, and humanity, have rendered her a blef- fing to an extenfive neighbourhood. In the relation of hufband, father, and friend, Mr. Bayley's merits were not lefs diftinguifhed than in the offices of public life which he fuftained. The warmth of his affec- tions, and the urbanity of his manners, peculiarly qualified him for domeftic and focial endearments. In his conduct to his children, he blended together, with great felicity, authority and love. The fuavity

and playfulnefs of his mind difpofed him to participate
in all their amufements. Yet he could refume the
parental authority, whenever it was liable to injury
from familiarity or condefcenfion. The profperity
and happinefs of his intimate connections, were almoft
as dear to him as his own; and he deemed no exertions for their intereft too painful or laborious, when
the claim was important or reafonable. He had
ample means of furthering their views, by the very
numerous correfpondences which he enjoyed with
men of every rank and ftation throughout thefe
kingdoms. The powers which Mr. Bayley poffeffed of forming acquaintances, and his affiduity in
preferving all that were valuable, conftitute a remarkable trait in his character. With a perfon and addrefs truly engaging, he recommended himfelf at
once to attention and regard; and having much general knowledge, he could adapt his converfation
with eafe and propriety to the turn of mind, the
purfuits, or the occupation, of the individual with
whom he conferred. Early habits of multiplied
bufinefs had alfo trained him to all the var eties of
intercourfe. Soon after his firft entrance into the
magiftracy, he was appointed High-Sheriff of Lanca-
fhire; an office which, by its dignity and duties,
neceffarily introduced him to almoft every one of
confequence in the county. Afterwards he was
made Collector of the King's Revenue under the
Chancellor of the Dutchy; and his frequent calls to
ferve on Grand Juries; the applications to Parlia-

ment, in which at different times he was engaged;
with various circumſtances of a private nature, contributed to enlarge ſtill more the ſphere of his ſocial
relations, and conſequently to aid his capacity for
uſefulneſs both to his friends and the community.

In this ſhort biographical ſketch of a beloved friend,
it would be highly unjuſtifiable to paſs over in ſilence
his RELIGIOUS CHARACTER. The virtues and honours of a tranſitory life dwindle into inſignificance,
if they are not made to refer to a ſtate of futurity,
and to the eternal favour of GOD. This ſentiment,
at all ſeaſons, actuated the pious mind of Mr. Bayley;
and his hopes of immortality were founded on a full
confidence in the Divine Goodneſs, and a firm per-
ſuaſion of the truth of Chriſtianity. His devotion
was ſincere and fervent, but devoid either of enthuſiaſm or ſuperſtition. To the communion of the
Church of England he was cordially attached, not from
the prejudices of *early education*, but from mature
reflection and deliberate judgment. Yet though he
cheriſhed her doctrines and diſcipline, he was uniformly hoſtile to the ſpirit of bigotry, and full of
candour and benignity to other modes of faith and
worſhip. He honoured *probity* alike in the individuals of every ſect; and held the rights of conſcience and of private judgment to be inviolable. On
the awful day of reſurrection, he believed the final
enquiry will not be, What creeds have you adopted,
or what eccleſiaſtical ſyſtem have you eſpouſed; but
have you clothed the naked; have you fed the

hungry; have you miniftered to the fick; or have you ferved GOD, by doing good to your fellow-creatures, who are his offspring?

In Politics, Mr. Bayley was a Whig of the old fchool; devoted to the eftablifhed principles of the Britifh Conftitution; in fupport of which he difplayed fuch zeal and activity, during the late eventful and turbulent period, as to receive the warmeft appro-bation from his Majefty's minifters.

Such are the lineaments of an exalted character, which friendfhip has endeavoured, with powers too feeble, to pourtray. The fhades that mixed them-felves with the brighter colourings, will not, in the eye of reafon, be viewed as darkening the picture. For the condition of humanity admits not of per-fection; and almoft every excellence is occafionally blended with fome kindred defect. This conftitutes at once the trial and the triumph of virtue. In the revered man, whofe lofs is fo deeply lamented, pro-vocations fometimes excited refentful emotions, which the occafion might not perhaps entirely juftify. But thefe occurred not on the judgment-feat, nor at any feafon when duty imperioufly required felf-command. His warmth alfo was fhort-lived, and was fucceeded by the moft amiable relentings. The forgivenefs of injuries he carried almoft to the literal extent enjoined in the Gofpel, pardoning the offences of a brother, not only *feven times*, but *feventy times feven.* A verfatility of mind and of purfuits was fometimes obferved in Mr. Bayley, beyond what is confiftent with the firmnefs of purpofe, fuppofed to be characteriftic of wifdom. But let it be recollected, that in the multiplicity of concerns which occupied his attent on, new and unexpected views of things might prefent themfelves; and that pertinacity muft often have proved more injurious than a temporary difpofition to change. In the exercife of the magisterial functions, the fentence of juftice can feldom be expected to give fatisfaction to each of the parties who are the fubjects of it. He who fuffers by the award, will be inclined to complain ; and complaint, however unreafonable, may incite to condemnation. Sometimes, alfo, the decifion may be apparently rigorous and fevere; and by exceeding the moral turpitude of the offence, may ftand oppofed to the feelings of pity, and even to the fenfe of equity, in the minds of uninformed fpectators. On fuch occafions, hard is the lot of a judge, who is bound by his oath, and ftill more ftrongly by his duty to fociety, not to *difpenfe* with, but to *execute*, the laws of his country ; and whatever be the ftruggle in his heart, every foft emotion is to be controled. He muft rife fuperior to prefent obloquy, and magnanimoufly fulfil the facred obligations of his office.

The rejection of petitions for mercy to a condemned delinquent, or for the mitigation of pains and penalties, which were not unfrequently prefented to Mr. Bayley, as Chairman of the Seffions, from wellintentioned, but not well-judging, perfons, expofed him to unmerited cenfure, and often to permanent

refentment.   To render punifhments efficacious in the
correction or prevention of crimes, they mult be
known to be inevitable.   Offences otherwife would
be indefinitely multiplied; for every offender might
find advocates to plead his caufe, either from intereft
or from motives of mifplaced humanity.   When the
magiftrate, therefore, has deliberately and confcientioufly apportioned the meafure of infliction to the
atrocity of the guilt, or to the injury which it does to
fociety, he ought to remain inexorable.   At one of
the Quarter-Seffions, a memorial was delivered to the
Chairman, in behalf of a convict, who had a family
and connections poffeffing confiderable intereft in the
town of Manchefter.   When it was offered, a particular fignature was pointed out, with an intimation
that it muft carry with it irrefiftible weight.   " I love
" and refpect," faid Mr. Bayley. with fome degree of
fternnefs and vehemence, " the perfon to whom you
" refer: but it is in the ordinary intercourfe of life.
" On the bench of juftice I know neither friend nor
" enemy." His aufterity of deportment on this
occafion   was   very   unreafonably cenfured.   For
though the application might not be in itfelf improper,
yet the manner in which it was conducted implicated
a charge fufficient to excite refentment, that the
Chairman was fubject to private influence.

But why fhould the Biographer affume the language of apology, when there is fo little ground for
reprehenfion, and fo much for applaufe? The
merits and eminent fervices of Mr. Bayley will be

recorded with honour, and long remembered with gratitude. In the general fentiment of forrow for his death, his failings, which were only the frailties of human natnre, are already forgotten.

Manchefter, July 1ft, 1802.

EPITAPH.

To the Memory
of
THOMAS BUTTERWORTH BAYLEY, Efq;
of
Hope-Hall, in the Parifh of Eccles.
An active, intelligent, and upright Magiftrate;
Candid in examination, clear in judgment,
Firm in decifion, yet tempering
Juftice with Mercy;
A beneficent Patron of the Poor;
A zealous Friend, an interefting Companion;
A hofpitable Neighbour;
A lover of his Country, and of Mankind;
A good Mafter, a tender Hufband,
A kind Father,
And a devout Chriftian.
This Tablet
Is gratefully and affectionately infcribed,
by
His Mourning Relict
and
Eleven Children.

DISSERTATIO MEDICA

INAUGURALIS

DE

F R I G O R E.

QUAM,

ANNUENTE SUMMO NUMINE,

Ex Auctoritate MAGNIFICI RECTORIS,

FRIDERICI WILHELMI PESTEL,

JURIS UTRIUSQUE DOCTORIS ET PROFESSORIS JURIS PUB-
LICI ET PRIVATII IN ACAD. LUGD. BAT. ORDINARII,

NEC NON

Amplissimi SENATUS ACADEMICI *Consensu, et Nobilissimæ*
FACULTATIS MEDICÆ *Decreto,*

PRO GRADU DOCTORATUS

Summisque in MEDICINA Honoribus et Privilegiis, ritè
ac legitimè confequendis,

Eruditorum examini submittit

THOMAS PERCIVAL, ANGLUS,

REG. SOCIETAT. LOND. SOCIUS.

Ad diem vi. *Julii* MDCCLXV. *Hora* x.

Dissolve Frigus, ligna super Foco
Largè reponens.——— ——— ———
HOR. *Ode* IX.

Phœbe fave, novus ingreditur tua templa Sacerdos.

TIBULLUS.

VIRO ILLUSTRISSIMO,

JACOBO

COMITI DE MORTON,

NOBILISSIMI ORDINIS DIVI ANDREÆ EQUITI;

A SCOTIÆ PROCERIBUS AD MAGNÆ BRITANNIÆ
COMITIA ITERUM ITERUMQUE LEGATO;

REGISTRORUM ET ROTULORUM IN SCOTIA
CUSTODI SUPREMO;

REGIÆ SOCIETATIS LONDINENSIS PRÆSIDI,

ET

MUSÆI BRITANNICI CURATORI;

GENERE ET PROAVIS
CLARO;

DOCTRINA, INGENIO, VIRTUTIBUS

CLARIORI;

ARTIUM ET LITERARUM HUMANARUM

FAUTORI EXIMIO,
JUDICI OPTIMO,

Hasce Studiorum Primitias ea qua par est Observantia,

D. D. D.

THOMAS PERCIVAL.

LICEAT, Vir *Docte*, *Dissertatiunculam hanc*, juvenemque ejus *Auctorem*, qui *Laboris Academici Lauream modo adeptus*, pari timore et diffidentiâ *Templum Apollinis ingredi parat*, præsidio tuo commendare. Omnino conscius quam arduam Provinciam susceperit, te non solum consulere, sed et auxilium tuum implorare ausus est; teque non magis posse quam velle ei prodesse persuasissimum habet.

Nam nihil habet Fortuna tua majus quam ut possis, nec Natura melius quam ut velis adjuvare quam plurimos.

Perge, Vir Summe, artem Apollinæam ornare, Patriæ tuæ charus vivere, et propius propiusque ad Deos accedere Salutem Hominibus dando. Vale.

DISSERTATIO MEDICA

INAUGURALIS

DE

FRIGORE.

SECTIO PRIMA.

MAGNA eft inter Viros Doctos de natura Frigoris contentio; et adhuc etiam, an *vera*
putanda fit *fubftantia*, vel *relatio* tantum, fub judice
lis eft. Multi Philofophi in Gallia et Germania, et
imprimis inter hos Celeberrimus MUSSCHENBROEK,
pïiorem fententiam amplexi funt. Ill. autem NEW-
TONUS, aliique Anglicani eruditi, fibi ipfis perfuafum
habuerunt, Frigus nihil aliud effe quam Caloris ab-
fentiam vel diminutionem. Minimè injucundus erit
labor, nec meæ Differtationis inftituto omnino alie-
nus, hanc controverfiam breviter explorare, et quædam de hac re Auctorum placita ad trutinam revocare.

Argumenta pro Frigoris naturâ fubftantiali, à
Phænomenis aquæ glaciantis ut plurimum dedu-
cuntur.

1. In medium profertur, aquam congelatione effe expanfam; hâc faƈtâ expanfione ab introitu Frigorificæ materiæ.

Hoc argumentum omnino futile et leve eft. Aquæ enim glaciantis expanfio, à feparatione aëris in ea contenti, ut facillimè demonftrari poteft, ortum fuum ducit; quæ feparatio, tam aperta eft, ut oculis percipi poffet. Bullæ enim Aëris innumeræ femper in glacie cernuntur; et certa experimenta nos docuerunt, aquam aëre privatam per coƈtionem, vel antliâ Pneumaticâ exhauftam, expanfione valcè diminutâ glaciari.

2. Aliquid fubftantiale affirmatur aquam intrare uno eodemque momento quo congelatur, quod à parte quadam vafis oriri videatur.

In promptu eft hoc argumentum refellere. Aquæ enim faliumque concretionis ratio par atque una eft; et glaciationis phænomena eodem modo quo chryftallifationis explicanda funt. Omne vas quandam habet inæqualitatem tum caloris tum denfitatis in diverfis ejus partibus; Congelatio autem à parte frigidiffimâ incipit, illic fila glacialia formabuntur, et aeris bullæ ea præcedent.

3. Aqua facilius glaciatur in apertis quam in claufis vafis, in Aëre quam in Vacuo; quod fidem facit ampliffimam aliquid ex aëre vas intrare; nec dubium eft quin hoc, quodcunque fit, foliditate gaudeat, quum partes vafis difficulter pervadat.

Ut aciem hujus argumenti obtundamus, notan-
dum eft duo ad congelationem effe neceffaria; 1.
gradum quendam Frigoris; 2. feparationem Aëris
ex aqua. Si hæc impediatur, non facile fiet congelatio; ob eandam forfan caufam qua Acidum et Al-
kalinum in Phialâ reftè occlusâ non effervefcunt.*
Congelatio etiam Aquæ compreffione Aëris ad ejus
fuperficiem impeditur. Nam *punctum Gelandi*,
codem modo quo ipfe *articulus Aquæ Bullientis*
variatur, omni gravitatis mutatione in Æthere in-
cumbente. Prompto hoc experimento id poteft
confirmari.

EXPERIMENTUM.

Receptâ Machinâ ad aërem condenfandum con-
ftructâ, et aquâ ad dimidium impletâ; injice in eam
duas vel tres aëris atmofphæras. Tunc ejus partibus applica frigoris factitii gradum infra punctum
congelationis. Nulla glaciei concretio formabitur,
nifi frigus fit maxime intenfum; et fi ita res fe habeat, Machina certé frangetur. Attamen quamprimum aër aggregatus è vinculis emittitur, aqua in
glaciem concrefcet.

Nec facile feparatur aër, ab aquâ in vafe quodam
arctè inclusâ. Nam elafticitas Ætheris æquipon-
derat ejus gravitati. Si vero frigus valde intenfum
ad glaciem producendum applicetur, aqua profecto

---

* Vide Experiment. Reaumuri, *Mem. de l'Acad. de Sciences.*

concrefcet; interea vas nifi firmiffimum fit, ab impetu aëris fe expandentis frangetur.

De difficultate Aquam glaciandi in Vacuo obfervandum eft, Aëris prefentiam poffe fimili modo congelationem expedire, quo Cupri folutionem in Alkali Volatili adjuvat. Aër externus forfan eft *Menftruum* Aëris Mephitici ex cupro emiffi.

Sed in confeffo eft Aquam glaciari poffe tum in Vacuo, tum in vafe occlufo. Itaque fi materies Frigoris talem habeat fubtilitatem, qualis ad penetrandum corpus folidiffimum fufficiat; non intelligo quomodo partes vafis ingreffum ejus impedire poffint.

4. Hæc materies Frigoris natura gaudet falina: Nam fi Phiala aquam continens in falium folutione ponatur, aqua brevi tempore concrefcet.

Idem fal aqua miftum, pro fuo ftatu aut frigus aut calorem generare poteft. *Nitrum* fub forma Cryftallorum aquam refrigerat; exuftum autem eam calefacit. Attamen peculiares ejus qualitates mutationem hanc folummodo patiuntur, quod in priore ftatu aquam contineat, in pofteriore ea penitus privetur. Haud aliter fe habent Alkalia fixa fub effervefcentiæ et caufticitatis conditione. Eft autem incredibile hæc falia fuas impertiri qualitates Phialæ aquæ in eorum folutione immerfæ, vel ei incognitas quafdam particulas dare. Nam falia in aqua foluta vim ei fuppeditant congelationi diutius refiftendi. Facultas etiam Frigus generandi falibus non folum eft tribuenda. Quippe Camphoræ folutio peritè facta in Spiritu Vini Rectificato, quando Aëris temperies ad gradum fit 36 Thermometri FARENHEITIANI, aquam glaciabit.

5. Aqua ampullâ vitreâ contenta et ante focum pofita in vafe nive pleno, conglaciabitur fimul ac Nix regelatur.

Frigus in ipfo puncto folutionis productum hanc efficit congelationem; non debet itaque ad ullam impulfionem frigoris particularum, vi Foci, in aquam referri. Unum autem eft potentiffimum et plane invictum experimentum, quod omnia argumenta ex congelatione deducta, ad probandam *fubftantialem* Frigoris *naturam*, omnino diruit. Si portio, unciarum videlicet quatuor, Salis Ammoniaci in unciis duodecim aquæ puræ folvatur, cum utriufque temperies ad gradum 53 fupra 0 in Thermofcopio fit FARENHEITIANO, liquor in Thermometro ad gradum 33 confeftim fubfidet. Vas autem aqua plenum in Lixivio illo locatum ad glaciem formandam nequaquam refrigerabitur. At fi eadem Salis Ammoniaci portio in aquam 50°. calidam immittatur, temperies ejus ad gradum 22. reducetur, et Phiala aquæ in hanc folutionem immerfa extemplò conglaciabitur.* Si autem Sal Ammoniacum particulis quibufdam fuis frigorificis aquam revera congelat, tunc in omni aëris temperie, fufficiente falis copiâ adhibitâ, idem effici oportet. Sed res aliter longe evenit. Celeb. MUSS-CHENBROEK negat aquam uno et eodem quidem

---

* Vide Boerhavii Elem. Chem. vol. i. p. 159.

puncto Thermometri in Regionibus diverfis congla-
ciari; et hoc quafi clariffimum argumentum exiften-
tiæ Frigoris particularum adfert. Verum Ill. GEOR-
GIUS MARTINUS, teftimoniis certiffimis et experimentis luce clarioribus, hanc refellit affertionem in
Tractatu fuo de Calore fcripto. Punctum autem
conglaciationis obfervatu tam difficile eft, ut D.
MUSSCHENBROEK facillime de hac re hallucinari
poffit. Calor enim et Frigus femel alicui infinuata
corpori, diu utplurimum in illo morantur. Quarè
aëre jam difpofito ad gradum 32. in Thermometro,
nondum tamen aqua conglaciabitur. Aqua enim
quæ aëris communis gravitatem 800° et ultra fuperat, ex præcedenti qui pervaferat calore, diu manet
tepida, poftquam aër jam novam frigoris impreffionem accepit. Error etiam oriri poteft ab ipfa Thermometri pofitione. Si enim vel parieti vel alii corpori appenderis, calor infitus illis mutationem quandam inftrumenti efficiet.*

Aqua aliquando in glaciem concrefcet ex caufis
adventitiis et non facile explicandis. D. HOLMANN,
aquam in vafe claufo non congelatam invenit, licet
aër et omnia corpora circumfiftentia infra punctum
glaciationis longè fuerint. Sed quamprimum manus
fuas in veficulam impofuit, qua tectum fuit Vas,
motu excitato, aqua ftatim concrevit. In alio vafe
aquam glaciabat manu fuâ calidâ ex utraque parte
admotâ. Hæc phænomena, particulis ullis folidis
Frigoris nequaquam funt afcribenda.

* Vide Boerhav. Elem. Chem.

Ex fupra dictis verifimillimum videtur, aquæ congelationem nullo modo arguere naturam Frigoris fubftantialem. Formatio glaciei ex abfentia vel diminutione caloris oritur, pariter ac Metalli liquefacti paulo poft fufionem concretio. Nam ut Calor particulas corporum expandit, et eas à fe invicem explicat, fic privatio vel diminutio caloris eafdem condenfat arctiufque comprimit. In temperie aëris communi, aquæ prima elementa laxè inter fe cohærent; fed Frigus, i. e. caloris privatio, imminutâ vi elafticâ *Ætheris* illius, qui omnia corpora intimè pervadit, particularum aquæ coalitionem impetuofam, fecundum leges attractionis efficit, unde aër inter eas particulas pofitus expellitur.

De naturâ Frigoris fatis difputatum; ad alteram jam partem accedamus, ubi varios ejus fontes, effectus multiplices, potentiamque validam in corpus humanum, explicabimus. Primum autem ea principia Œconomiæ Animalis inveftiganda funt, quæ homines multis mutationibus vi Frigoris obnoxios reddunt.

SECTIO SECUNDA.

CORPUS humanum in tres partes a Pathologis dividitur; nempe, *Solida Simplicia*, *Humores* vel *Fluida*, et *Solida Viva*. De his fingulis feparatim dicemus.

DE SOLIDIS SIMPLICIBUS.

Multos et diverfos Morbos Pathologiæ Scriptores ad Solida Simplicia retulerunt. Iftiufmodi funt Craffitudo, Exilitas, Laxitas, Rigiditas, Fragilitas, cum multis aliis. Atqui duo tantum de his Morbis, videlicet, Rigiditas et Fragilitas, vi Frigoris attribui poffunt;* et potentia ejus etiam in his morbis generandis omnino parva et nequaquam refpicienda invenietur.

Quum autem Frigus materiam univerfam tam validè condenfat, minimè mirandum eft quod Medici fimiles ejus aftioni effectus, in Fibras corporis fimplices, tribuerint. Et quoniam Incolæ Regionum Septentrionalium plerumque funt robuftiores et firmitate corporis multo magis quam Auftrales pollen-

---

* Ingenuè etiam agnofco Frigus Exilitati favere.

tes; hæc Hypothefis tum analogia, tum experientia confirmari videtur.

At Corporis condenfatio ejufque caloris diminutio perfectè inter fe congruunt; hæc autem condenfatio nunquam ita evenit, ut oculis noftris percipi poffit, nifi corpus ad gradum frigoris longè infra naturalem ejus temperiem fit redactum. Frigus autem corpori humano æqualiter applicatum dummodo ne morbum inferat, nequaquam minuit univerfalem ejus calorem; folida ergo fimplicia minimè condenfat.* Cutis enimvero, et minima vafcula, per fuperficiem corporis fparfa, parva quadam conftrictione poffint affici; fed cum partes internæ unam et eamdem temperiem retineant, vis Frigoris ad eas certè non pervenit. Hic quoque partialis effectus ortum fuum ducere poffit, tam ex cutis fenfibilitate, quam Fibrarum mechanica condenfatione.

Quamvis Populi Hyperborei rigidiores habeant Fibras et corpora magis robufta quam Incolæ Regionum ubi foles melius nitent; hoc tamen provenire poteft à caufis, quæ licet connexæ, non ideo necef-

---

* Illa caloris æqualitas quam corpus animale in cœli temperamentis maximè diverfis retinet, admodum eft mirabilis; et aliquam *Facultatem vitalem* quæ temperat inter fe calorem externum et humanum, planè indicat. Celeb. D. ELLIS, Præfectus GEORGIÆ, Americæ Septentrionalis Provinciæ, calorem aëris in umbra ad gradum 105 Thermometri FARENHEITIANI, iftic inveniebat, cum calor ejus ipfius corporis haud excefferit gradum 97. ejufdem Thermofcopii. vid. *Phil. Tranfact. vol.* l.——Et amicus quidam meus, experimentis quibufdam a fe ipfo inftitutis, corpora ranarum æftivo tempore tribus gradibus aquâ ambientê frigidiora invenit.

fariè vel ex Frigore vel ex Calore pendent. Nationes *Torridæ Zonæ* utplurimum funt inertes et defidiofæ; et eorum cibus ex herbis recentibus potiffimum conftat. Dum Gentes Septentrioni fubjectæ, propter foli fterilitatem laborare coguntur; et per oblectamenta Venationis diverfa ad exercitium alliciuntur. Nec poffunt illi, ullo alio modo, à penetrabile frigore fe ipfos defendere, quam Corporis labore. Ad hoc quoque accedat, quod carnibus maximè vefcantur.

Pleræque autem hæ caufæ quæ corpus roborant et conftringunt, in Fibras fimplices non tam validè quam in Fibras Motrices fuas vires exerunt: Sed de hac re alibi tractandum eft.

Fragilitas alius eft effectus Frigori tributus. Hic morbus autem offibus peculiaris eft, quæ magis effe fragilia dicuntur fummâ hyemê quam tempore æftivo. Sed hæc affirmatio nequaquam fide digna eft. Offa enim tam profundè funt fita, et tam circumclufa in corpore animato partibus calidis, ut à Gelu quamvis maximè intenfo et diuturno prorfus fint tuta. Fracturæ offium certè in hyeme quam in æftate fæpius eveniunt; quæ tamen fat benè explicentur, a Terræ lubricitate, tenfione auctâ mufculorum ad prolapfionem præcavendam, et corporum rigiditate, in quæ nofmetipfos præcipitamus.

Conftat itaque Frigoris effectum in Fibras fimplices parvi effe momenti. Et hæc conclufio, operationem univerfam medicamentorum, omnefque ferè externas caufas corpus afficientes, forfan complecti poteft.

De Fluidis vel Humoribus.

Frigus in Fluida variis modis poteſt ageɾe. 1. Vaſcula conſtringendo, et inde auctam eorum preſſionem
producendo; ſed hic effectus ex ejus actione in ſolida
viva pendet. 2. Condenſationem propriam Fluidorum ipſorum efficiendo. Hæc autem condenſatio omnino perexigua eſt; nam aqua à gradu 212 ad 56°.
Thermometri FARENHEITIANI refrigerata, non
magis quam $\frac{1}{15}$ totius ejus magnitudinis denſatur.*
Quantula eſt autem ulla refrigeratio corporis humani
ab externo Frigore, huic temperiei mutationi com-
parata?

At enim Frigus ſeparationem partium Fluida
componentium efficere exiſtimetur. Qui vero hanc
ſententiam amplectuntur à vero longè aberrant. Ea
etenim animalia quæ tempus hybernum ſomno alto et
ſine ſenſu peragunt, totius ſanguinis ſtagnationem et
concretionem patiuntur ſed abſque ulla partium ſe-
paratione. Frigus minuit perſpirationem et eo modo
Fluida mutare creditur. Verum facultas quâ præditum eſt, minima vaſcula per corporis ſuperficiem
ſparſa conſtringendi, ab eorum ſenſibilitate et irritabilitate maximè oritur. Ideoque in hoc etiam caſu
agit in ſolida viva; et ſi ulla fiat mutatio in humo-
ribus, materiei obſtructæ perſpirationis, et minimè
propriæ Frigoris actioni, aſcribenda eſt.

* Vid. Boerhaav. Elem. Chem. vol. i. p. 174.

De Solidis Vivis

Sub hoc nomine, omnes corporis partes motrici vi
præditas, feu ab imperio voluntatis pendeat, feu ab
actione ftimuli cujufcunque generis, externi vel in-
terni, complectimur.* Ill. HALLERUS, qui de orbe
medico optimè meretur, propter labores ejus utiliffi-
mos in Anatomia et Phyfiologia, fumma ope nititur,
duas facultates movendi, in corpore animato, diftin-
guere. Una ab illo nuncupatur *Vis infita Mufculis,*
five *Irritabilitas ;* altera, *Vis Nervofa,* qua motus vo-
luntarius perficitur. Priorem ille affirmat nequaquam
pendere à fenfibilitate vel vi nervofa, et propriam
effe mufcularibus corporis partibus. Hypothefis
hæc à multis præclaris Phyfiologis vehementer fuit
impugnata; et imprimis ab illuftri et ingeniofiffimo
ROBERTO WHYTT, Medicinæ Profeffore in Alma
Academia Edinenfi. Sed quia omnino me abduceret
ab inftituto hujus Differtationis, hanc litem pluribus
profequi; hoc tantum notabo fenfibilitatem effe planè
diftinctam ab irritabilitate. Minime autem fequitur
eas non effe nexas, vel ex fe invicem non mutuò

---

* *Senfibilitas* huic definitioni folidorum vivorum adjici poteft. Nam
quæque pars corporis humani acutâ fenfibilitate prædita, quamvis ex
ftructura fua non apta fit ad motum, tamen eâ fympathiâ quæ per
totam Machinam animatam diffunditur, quosdam poteft motus
efficere in aliis partibus, quoties ftimulo afficitur. Sic cum leniter
titillatur cutis, convulfio ferè omnium mufculorum corporis illicò
fequitur. Nervi lacerati vel ligati fæpiffimè maxillas obferant, et
alias producunt affectiones fpafmodicas. Sedneque cutis, nec nervi
facultate movendi funt prædita.

fluere. Nec certè evicit HALLERUS ullam partem, neque nervis neque fenfu donatam, irritabilem effe.* Locus eft notatu dignus in Volumine quarto Elementorum Phyfiologiæ, quo HALLERUS agnoscere videtur Vim contractilem Mufculorum magis ex Nervis pendere, in multis infignibus exemplis, quibus non poteft animus fuum imperium exercere, quam ejus Hypothefi congruit. De Nervis differens dicit:

" Adferunt ex cerebro efficacia imperia, non volunta-
" tis, fed legum corpori animato fcriptarum quæ volunt
" ad certos nafci motus. Mufculi erectores Penis, veri
" illi quicunque funt, per Nervos accipiunt eam vim,
" quà Penem diftendunt; eaque vis non eft à volun-
" tate, neque aut imperio animæ accerfi poteft, aut
" deftrui: fed a cerebro tamen ad fpecies lubricas
" et obfervantem animæ voluptatis imaginem nafcitur.
" Adferunt ad cor in ira motus præcipites et palpita-
" tiones effecturos, non voluntatis juffu, fed tamen à
" cerebro et ab obverfante animæ infeftæ fpeciei fti-
" mulo, quô fe liberari vult, quam celerrimè. Sunt
" ergo Nervi inter animæ officia et corporis partes
" internuncii, etfi in his exemplis non voluntatis dic-
" tata perferunt."† Cum Nervi itaque in his exemplis
fint inftrumenta motus non voluntarii; cur non nobis
liceat ex analogia inferre, eos in aliis confimilibus exemplis ita fe habere? Si cor palpitatione afficiatur ex
mentis pathematis, quæ nervos ad id organum miffos

* Vid. Whytt's Phyf. Effays, p. 158.

† El. Phyf. vol. iv. p. 516, §. 111.

quodammodo perturbant; nonne verifimile eft, nervos eofdem effe caufas ejus contrâdionis per ftimulnm
calidi refluentis fanguinis? Cur autem in controverfiam me ipfum implicui, quam omninò evitare me
magis deceret?

Omnes fere mutationes in œconomia animali à
caufis cum externis tum internis oriundæ, ex fenfibilitate nafcuntur.* Attamen Scriptores Pathologici
adeo hanc veritatem ignoraverunt, ut penè omnes,
Ill. GAUBIO excepto, omninò ferè eas facultates
neglexerint. Jam inde ex quo primum cognitus eft
fanguinis circuitus, corpus humanum pro machina
tantùm hydraulica habitum eft; et Medici, omnes
ejus motus fecundum Leges Mechanicas explicare
conati funt, opus profedo vanum atque ineptum
aggreffi. Nam variæ mutationes quæ fæpiffimè
occurrunt in motu cordis et arteriarum, Sympathiæ
inter diverfas corporis partes, et validi fpafmi qui
mufculos à caufis minimis vel etiam omnino ignotis
aliquando invadunt, manifeftè demonftrant corpus
humanum legibus fubjedum effe, prorfus alienis ab
iftis mechanicis, quibus materia iners fubjicitur.

BOERHAAVIUS *caufam proximam* morborum credit
ex vitiis Fluidorum ut plurimum pendere, minimè
fecum reputans humores noftros omninò inertes effe,
et quamlibet eorum mutationem provenire, vel è
nova chemica difpofitione ultimarum fuarum particu-

---

* Irritabilitas hic comprehendit et vim infitam mufculis, et vim
nervofam; et hoc in fenfu ea voce poftea utemur.

larum ex fermentatione nata, vel à motibus virium vitalium corporis. Ita *Lentor Sanguinis* nequaquam caufa, fed Febris et Inflammationis effectus habendus eft; nam à citato impetu vaforum, qui in his morbis exftat, oritur. " Nonnunquam fanguis initio Febris " acutæ, aut etiam topicæ Inflammationis miffus, crufta " caret, habetque eandem aut in altera, aut in tertia, " aut in quarta Venæfectione."* Vid. DE HAEN, Rat. Med. pars I. cap. vi. pag. 54, Paris edit. Urina etiam tenuis et pellucida, à fœmina hyfterica excreta, non ex fanguinis tenuitate, fed à conftrictione vafculorum in renibus fecernentium, provenit. Homo enim faniffimus vel metu, vel hauftu parvo infufi Theæ fortis, urinam omninò confimilem reddet.

Robur et *Debilitas* à ftatu folidorum fimplicium multo minus pendent quam Medici Mathematici agnofcere volunt. Homines Fibris laxiffimis præditi, Iracundia vel Phrenitide permoti, Herculeis quafi viribus pollere videntur; dum metu vel mœrore etiam validiffimi fiunt debiles et inertes. Jam vero quam incredibile, quam abfurdum effet, vires in hifce exemplis auctas vel diminutas, folidorum fimplicium fubitæ mutationi attribuere? Effectus igitur

---

* Sanguinis lentor ex vafis minutis conftrictis fæpe oritur. In regionibus frigidis et feptentrionalibus, fanguis, ex hominibus qui optima valetudine fruuntur, eductus, et qui tempore hyberno venæfectione tanquam prophylactico utuntur, cruftam pleuriticam ut plurimum induit. Hoc forfan devenire poteft ex vi frigoris eodem modo quo fafcia agente. Experimentis enim probavit D. SIMSON, fanguinem è vena emiffum poft arctam in quovis membro ligaturam, femper glutinofum fore.

illi à vi nervofa in corpus variè agente omni fine
dubio nafcuntur. Et Rationi prorfus confentaneum
eft, Vinum, Corticem Peruvianum, et alia medica-
mènta roborantia, in Solida Viva omninò fere vires
fuas exerere.

Multæ et magnæ mutationes, ex ea Sympathia,
quâ præditum eft corpus humanum, proveniunt.
Hæc Sympathia nihil aliud effe videtur quam Irritabilitas magis extenfa, et ei facultati, Idiofyncrafiis
quibufdam folum exceptis, ut plurimum invenitur
aptè refpondere. Hanc autem rem liceat nobis
exemplo illuftrare. Capiant duo Homines, quorum
unus fit robuftus, alter corporis habitu mollior et debi-
lior, Pulveris Ipecacoanhæ drachmæ dimidium. Si-
mili naufea et vomitione uterque afficietur; at Homo
robuftus in Ventriculo forfan, Diaphragmate, Mus-
culis Abdominis et Œfophago folummodo male fe
habebit: alter autem ex majori fua Irritabilitate adeo
premetur, ut omnes ferè corporis mufculi nervique,
convulfiones per Sympathiam patiantur.

Nulla pars corporis humani, ventriculo excepto,
confenfum habet, tam per 'totum fyftema extenfum,
quam cutis, ut quotidiana nos docet experientia.
Hæc autem fympathia non folum ex fenfibilitate ipfi
cuti infita provenit, fed à vafis etiam minimis quæ per
ejus fuperficiem, numero ferè infinito fparguntur.
In quibufdam corporis conditionibus, hæc vafa valde
funt irritabilia; et ne unum quidem conftringitur,
quin omnia ftatim, confenfu, fimili fpafmo afficiantur.
Ex hoc evenit, quod Febres, Catarrhi, Pleuritides,

Peripneumoniæ, aliique morbi multi, à Frigore externo, pro caufis fuis prædifponentibus, concitentur.
De hac autem Frigoris vi protinus tractandum eft :.
nunc ex quibus caufis originem fuam ducit breviter
ftrictimque oftendemus.

SECTIO TERTIA.

Causæ Frigoris quatenus Corpus afficiunt.

HÆ caufæ opinionem vulgarem numero longè
fuperant; ad fequens tamen compendium re-
duci poffint.

1. Evaporatio tam ex Humo quam Veftibus
   humidis.
2. Cœlum humidum.
3. Cœlum chemicè ficcum.
4. Aër per anguftas rimas in corpus agens.
5. Frigidæ potio, corpore labore fudante.

De his diverfis Frigoris caufis fingulatim diffe-
rendum eft.

EVAPORATIO.

Tandem certiſſimis evincitur experimentis Fluida in Vapores converſa intenſiſſimum Frigus gignere. Veſtes itaque humidæ neceſſariò ſunt valde periculoſæ; quia frigus ab iis ortum corporis ſuperficiem immediatè afficit. Celeb. LIND, qui optimè de Civibus ſuis meruit ob Tractatum ingenioſiſſimum de *Scorbuto*, humiditatem exiſtimat inſignem eſſe cauſam hujus morbi. Nam in Cœli tempeſtatibus ſpuma maris undoſa, impetu procellæ ſublata, per totam navim ſpargitur, et nautæ non ſolum de die veſtibus madidis induuntur, ſed etiam ſuper ſtragula humida per noctes totas dormire coguntur.* Simile oritur diſcrimen Corpori Terræ exhalationibus expoſito. Homines qui loca demiſſa ac paluſtria accolunt, ob hanc cauſam Rheumatiſmo præcipue et Febribus Intermittentibus ſæpiſſimè corripiuntur. Hi etiam morbi frequentiores evadunt et periculoſiores, ſi anni tempeſtas admodum ſit calida. Rectè enim animadvertit doctiſſimus PRINGLE imbres crebros, tempore æſtivo in terris paludoſis maximè prodeſſe. Nam exhalationes minuunt, aquas ſtagnantes et corruptas refrigerant, vaporesque noxios et putridos præcipitant.† Vicinitas Sylvarum inſaluberrima quoque

---

* Vid. LIND on the Scurvy, p. 70.

† Diſeaſes of the Army, p. 5, 62.

merito exiftimatur. Perfpiratio enim à Foliis et
Ramis Arborum tam copiofa eft, ut fidem omnino
fuperaret, fi non experimentis Ill. HALESII tam clarè
evinceretur.* Pluvias etiam Rorefque, fub expanfa
magis latiorique fuperficie, folis et aëris actioni ex-
ponunt, et hoc modo Cœli augent humiditatem.
Nulla ferè Regio Europæa eft, quæ magnam non
fubiit Cœli mutationem intra mille et octingentos
annos; maximè, uti credibile eft, provenientem à tota
fermè excifione Nemorum, quæ hanc orbis Terrarum
plagam olim cooperiebant. GALLIA et GERMANIA,
ætate JULII CÆSARIS, trifles et algofæ fuerunt
Terræ; et in ITALIA etiam ipfa, Hyemes tam gelidæ
ac nivofæ extiterunt, ut *Tiberis* aliquando innaviga-
bilis foret. In AMERICA SEPTENTRIONALI eft
obfervatu dignum, Cœlum cujufque Provinciæ mitius
magisque falubrè fieri pro incolarum induftria in ex-
fcindendis et exurendis arboribus ibi nafcentibus.†
Europæi qui loca Americana primi occupaverunt,
omnes ferè per malignum Endemicum morbum
perierunt, qui corpora breviffimê putridâ quadam
Febris fpecie diffolvit. Id autem imprimis accidit
iis, qui loca arboribus et fruticibus obfita incole-
bant.‡ *Hybernia,* olim Paludibus Sylvifque referta,

---

* Vid. Statical Effays.

† Ill. D. FRANKLYN, uti a Familiari quodam ejus accepi, certis
fuis experimentis invenit quod, in iis Provinciis ubi arbores magna
ex parte excifæ funt, flumina ex inde quoad latitudinemque longi-
tudinemque valde minuerentur.

‡ Vid. Boerhaave Elem. Chem. vol. i. p. 620.

infaluberrima fuit. Nunc autem temporis, cum exufta fint Nemora et Paludes deficcatæ, regio eft amœna et in multis ejus agris homines longiffimâ et faniffimâ vitâ fruuntur.*

DE CŒLO HUMIDO.

Aqua vel diffufo vel diffoluto ftatu, prout cœlum fe habeat, aëri videtur ineffe. Nam multis graviffi-mifque argumentis fatis probabile redditur, quod aër fit *Menftruum* Aquæ.

1. Vis ejus diffolvens, tanquam alia menftrua, calore augetur, et frigore minuitur. Recipe Am-pullam Vitream fubere arctè occlufam, tantùmque humiditatis continentem, ut paululum obnubilet opacetque internam ejus fuperficiem. Tum ampullâ ante focum ut calefiat pofitâ, nebula quam includit aquofa brevi tempore diffolvetur, et vitrum omnino pellucidum fiet. Si autem vas, in aquam frigidam immergatur, vapor formabitur, et humoris guttulæ per latera ampullæ manabunt. Effectus hicce, Roris præcipitationi tempore vefpertino, quando aër â folis occafu frigidior devenit, maximè confimilis eft. Ambo autem falium ad faturationem folutione in aqua tepida pulcherrimè illuftrantur. Prout enim aqua refrigeratur, falis portio continuò præcipitatur; calore autem integrato, iterum refolvitur.

2. Aer veluti alia menftrua pro quantitate fua agit, uti oculis manifeftum eft, in vi ficcante ventilatorum.

* Vid. Bryan Robinfon on the Operation of Medicines, p. 122.

Hi enim nequaquam mechanicè agunt, vellendo quafi
aquæ particulas à corporibus quibus adhærefcunt,
neque enim ullum ventum, neque vel minimum etiam
flatum excitant.

3. Aëris vis folvens, previæ ejus faturationi re-
fpondet ; et in hac quoque re cum aliis menftruis
congruit. Hinc magis ficcat verno quam autumnali tempore; quod Lintei Dealbatoribus optimè
notum eft.

4. Aqua femper et in omnibus locis Terrarum
Orbis Aëri adeft. Hoc fæpè oculis ipfis per falia,
cauftica fixa, quæ ab igne aretacta et prorfus ficcata in
aëre vulgari fponte liquefcunt, manifeftè exhibeatur.
Nam Aër, qui intra ampullam, trium librarum fluidæ
capacem, continetur, tantum aquæ tenet quantum
fufficit unciam falis Tartari non folum humectare,
fed etiam aliquantulum magis ingravare: Hæc autem
aqua, quæ aëris gravitatem magis quam 850°.
fuperat, maximam partem illius ponderis quod in
ipfa aëris portione fiaticè deprehenditur, omni fine
dubio facit.* Si aër itaque omnem ferè gravitatem
ex aqua in eo volitante accipit; rectè inferri poteft
aquam effe folubilem in aëre. Nam tempeftatê diu
ferenâ et fenfibus noftris maxime aridâ aër fit femper
ponderofior, atmofphæraque gravior, ut manifeftè
ex Barometro apparet. Hoc autem nullo modo
poteft explicari, nifi aerem in eo ftatu pleniffimè aquâ
faturatum effe agnofcatur. Humiditas diffufa, gravitatem Ætheris diminuit; quia Vapor levior eft,

* Vid. Boerhaav. El. Chem. vol. i. p. 466.

et majus occupat fpatium quam aër chemicè faturatus aquâ. Eftne aër, cujus vis menftrualis frigore impreffo minuitur, et qui continet etiam multam humiditatem diffufam, fpecificè levior quam aër chemicè faturatus aquâ, magna cum copia humiditatis diffufæ conjunctâ ?

Amicus meus ingeniofiffimus ARTHUR LEE, M.D. fequentem credit obfervationem totam fere ftructuram Theoriæ hujus diruere: " Evaporatio Sp. Vini " Rectificati in Vacuo Boyleano facta, majorem " Frigoris gradum quam in vafe aperto parit. Itaque " quum Frigoris generatio ex Evaporatione pendeat, " et quoniam in hoc exemplo evaporatio augetur, " aëre interim diminuto, ritè poteft inferri aërem non " effe menftruum Vaporis à Spiritu Vini feparati."

Pone rem ita fe habere, conclufio tamen ifta minimè concedenda eft. Frigus enim intenfius ab aucta Sp. Vini Evaporatione nequaquam provenit, fed ab aëre potius per exantlationem educto cum à fluido tum à Vafe Recipiente. Nam omnibus fere notum eft ipfam exinanitionem Recipientis Antliæ Pneumaticæ, Frigus valde fenfibile gignere. Porro in hocce experimento, ut mihi videtur, evaporatio Sp. Vini reverà minuitur; extractio autem aëris majori copiâ fat bene explicat auctam Frigoris generationem.

Supputa* igitur aërem poffe diffolvere aquam, minime erit difficile, caufam iftius Frigoris explicare,

* Sequens Experimentum, fi per tempeftatem anni liceret mihi id inftituere, omnem ut opinor dubitationem tolleret, de Aëris facultate aquam folvendi. R. Salis Tartari perfecte cauftici et ab igne

quo corpus humanum à Cœlo humido femper afficitur.
Calor enim corporum noftrorum vim aëris menftru.
alem auget; et hoc modo Vapores Aquofi magis
copiosè diffolvuntur, frigufque intenfum hâc folu-
tionê ftatim oritur. At humidum Cœlum alio
quoque modo corpus refrigerat. Omnis enim Vapor
diutius quam aër retinet fuam temperiem; fi Hyems
itaque fæviat, vel fi tempeftas anni fit frigida, vapor
hic aquofus corpori admotus neceffariò id afficit
algore. Nam calida quædam atmofphæra femper
nos circumambit, quæ aërem tepefacit antequam corpora noftra attingat. Hæc autem humiditas non
tam citò incalefcit, et quum perpetuó et æqualiter
applicatur, atque iterum iterumque renovatur, minime mirandum, eft fi corpus graviffimo frigore vi
ejus perculfum fit.

De Cœlo Chemice Sicco.

Aër poteft aridus exiftimari, quando parvam aquæ
quantitatem continet. Eurus ob hanc caufam, tem-

arefacti uncias duas; injiciantur quam ficciffimæ in ampullam magnam vitream, datam quantitatem Aëris communis continentem; et
ftatim poft falis immiffionem fit vas arctiffimè obturatum. Aqua
quæ in Aëre fuit difperfa brevi tempore fal irrigabit. Omni humi-
ditate diffusâ fic abforptâ, aqua chemicè diffoluta feorfim, ni fallor,
in Aëre remanebit. Nam Aër aquæ quam falibus ipfis caufticis magis
affinis eft, uti ex hoc clarè conftat, quod fal deliquefcens Aëri ficco
expofitum, fuam perdit humiditatem, et formam folidam affumit.
His omnibus rite peractis, jam minuetur vis aëris folvens, ampullam
vehementi frigoris gradui exponendo; et fi aquam ullam contineret,
neceffe eft ut ftatim præcipitetur fub forma guttularum per latera
vafis depluentium.

pore hyemali, ventus eft in hac regione infigniter ficcus. Flante enim per frigidos montes Tèrrafque Europæ continentis nive opertas, tota diffufa, magna itemque pars diffolutæ ejus aquæ præcipitatur. In hoc ftatu noftris corporibus adhibitus, humidam iftam atmofphæram, nobis circumfufam et à perfpiratione ortam, extemplò diffolvit. Hæc folutio frigus haud afpernendum gignit, et quoniam perficitur quamdiu emanat Perfpiratio et Ventus perflat; algor per fingula temporis punƈta fenfim augetur, ufque dum omnes ferè capillares arteriæ per fuperficiem corporis errantes contrahantur. Liquor vero Thermometri in aëre hoc arido minimè fubfidit pro ratione noftri frigoris fenfus. Homines Valetudinarii, quamvis in cubiculo et ante focum fedentes, tamen vento ab orientè excitato fenfibiliter afficiuntur; neque ullo modo poteft aƈtio ejus omnino præcaveri.

Aër ficcus in Pulmones infpiratus, Vapores aquofos Bronchiorum ftatim diffolvit, ibique etiam idem frigus ac in fuperficie corporis concitat. Ex hac caufa oritur Tuffis, et inflammatio membranæ mucofæ internè Pulmones inveftientis. Infpiratio aridi hujus aëris, alio quoque modo Pulmones inflammatione afficere poteft; nempe mucum exficcando, et inde membranam teneram Bronchiorum Frigori ftimulanti exponendo. Homines qui ereƈtâ et concitatâ voce diu publicè concionantur, fimili ftriƈtioni et iuflammationi obnoxii funt.

DE AERE PER ANGUSTAS RIMAS IN CORPUS AGENTE.

Totum corpus minori periculo quam fingulæ ejus partes aëri frigido objici poteſt. Nam fyſtema univerfum æquabiliter conſtringetur, fenſibilitas et irritabilitas minuentur, et hoc modo Frigus ipſum contra vim fuam aliquatenus præmunit, remediumque quod‑ dam fecum adfert. Sed ubi pars tantum Corporis Frigori exponitur omnes arteriæ minimæ, fympathiâ quadam, conſtrictionem patientur; dum fenſibilitas et irritibilitas in eodem ſtatu fine aliqua diminutione reſtant. Ill. VAN SWIETENUS hac de caufa benè obfervavit, aërem frigidum in corpus nudatum actum per anguſtas rimas omnium maximè nocere.*

DE POTIONE FRIGIDÆ CORPORE LABORE SUDANTE.

Plurima et triſtia obfervata in Hiſtoria Medicinæ nobis demonſtrant, multos lethales morbos, immo mortem fubitam ipfam fecutam fuiſſe, dum corpore æſtuante gelidam biberent homines.† Caufa autem tanti periculi à frigidæ potione fatis clarè patebit, fi

* Vid. VAN SWIET. Comm. vol. iii. §. 881.

† Vid. VAN SWIET. Comment. vol. ii. p. 214. Celfus de Medic. lib. i. cap. 3, &c.

imprimis confideretur quod Afpera Arteria, Pulmones, Septum Medium, aliæ quoque partes ipfi Gulæ
vicinæ, dum liquor tranfit per Œfophagum, algore
magnoperè afficiantur. Deinde quum in Ventriculum
defertur, fuam actionem per totum corpus extendit.
Vifcus enim hoc maxima præditum eft irritabilitate;
adeo ut nullam ferè impreffionem fentiat, quæ non
extemplò propagetur, miro quodam confenfu, ad
partes etiam totius fyftematis maximè remotas.

Sed Ventriculus et fuperficies corporis fympathiâ
peculiari et præ ceteris validiore inter fe videntur
effe nexi. Initio ipfo omnium fermè Febrium, Hor-
ripilatio femper adeft; eodemque tempore ftomachus
naufea et vomitione concitatur. SYDENHAMUS,
HIPPOCRATES nofter Anglicanus, hanc fympathiam
notavit in Pefte præcipuè pollere. Ægroti violentis
continuifque Vomitibus vexabantur, quos nec potio-
nes foporiferæ, nec ulla alia Medicamenta potuerunt
fedare. Nil fuit levaminis nifi ægrum ponendo in
calido lecto, et eo modo fanguinis circuitum ad
corporis exteriora determinando. Si frigida itaque
hauriatur, corpore calefcente, ventriculus gelido
liquore diftentus, non folum adjacenti Diaphragmati,
Hepati, Lieni, &c. fubitum et infolitum frigus com-
municabit, fed impreffionem ad omnes fere partes
corporis, præcipue ad ejus fuperficiem propagabit.
Quam vero periculofi, quam lethales effectus fequi
poffint, multis triftiffimisque exemplis fatis planè
demonftratur.

SECTIO QUARTA.

1. ARTERIÆ capillares in corporis superficie frigore contrahuntur; et hinc si causæ prædisponentes adsint, multi et diversi morbi nascuntur.

2. Frigus, in debilibus saltem, prohibet Perspirationem: Hicce autem effectus per se spectatus, causa morborum minimè æstimandus est. Medici quidem de natura putrida Perspirabilis materiæ, et de vitiis fluidorum ab ejus retentione natis fusissimè scripserunt. Sed hic, ni fallor, in errore magno versantur. Materiê enim transpirationis satis benè notâ, quærere vellem quænam pars ejus sanitatem corporis tantopere lædere possit? Aër, Aqua, Oleum Essentiale, et forsitan parva portio Lymphæ, Sanctorianæ exhalationis elementa propria sunt. Si aliquid etiam Volatile, corpori extraneum, viribusque nostris non subigendum, in sanguinem recipitur, sicut Alkali Volatile, Alcohol, Olea Essentialia Vegetabilium, &c. per transpirationem auferetur. Sed neque hæc extranea, nec propria perspirabilis materiæ elementa, putrida sunt æstimanda. Minimè autem nego, Perspirationem in Aëre aprico brevi tempore corrumpi; perinde ac omnes fere Vapores qui Mucilaginem continent. At nequaquam ex hoc licet

nobis deducere tranſpirationem noſtram eſſe putridam cùm primum à corpore difflatur. Gummi Arabici ſolutio dicitur Vaporem corruptioni valde ob‑noxium emittere.

Exhalationes à locis paluſtribus et uliginoſis, primâ licet elevatione minimè ſint putridæ, tamen ex copia mucilaginis vegetabilium quam continent, citò in aëre calido corrumpuntur.* Perſpiratio igitur in corpore ſano ſuppreſſa nequaquam ut ſep‑ticum humorum fermentum putanda eſt. Nec multum infert periculi, meâ quidem ſententiâ, diminutio hujus exhalationis ſi aliæ morbi cauſæ abſint : facillimè enim per Alvum, per Urinam, vel alia Organa excre‑toria poſſit exire. Gradus Perſpirationis in homi‑nibus etiam ſaniſſimis quotidie penè variatur ; adeo ut nunc ad duplicem triplicemve minuatur partem, ſine ulla ſanitatis injuria ; deinde pro eadem ratione, nullâ factâ ad meliorem valetudinem acceſſionê, au‑getur.† Tempore hyberno exhalatio per cutem magnoperè decreſcit ; nullo alio effectu interim co‑mitante niſi auctâ per renes ſecretio.‡ Quibus Per‑ſpiratio Sanctoriana maxima ex parte ſupprimitur, ii hac tamen de cauſa in Febres Intermittentes vix fiunt procliviores.‖ Perſpiratio autem et Urina, ab

* Vid. Duhamel, Phyſ. des Arbr. T. I. p. 144.

† Vid. Exp. Stat. D. Home, G. Rye, Lining, Robinson, Keil, &c.

‡ Vid. Senac de Febre Intermittente.

‖ Vid. Van Swiet. Comment. §. 586; et Diſſert. Med. Inaug. Cl. Juv. Ant. Iothergill.

experimentis Cl. B. Robinson, plane apparent inter
se respondere, adeo ut unius augmentûm alterius
diminutionem fere semper compenset. Senes ex
cute dura et copia parva vaforum exhalantium,
pauxillulum perspirant; sed nequaquam ea de causa
obferyantur in morbos incidere. Inter antiquos
maximé valuit mos, et hodie etiam valet inter multas
Africæ Gentes, oblinendi totum corpus oleo. Hæc
autem consuetudo neque olim inferebat, neque nunc
infert ullum corpori incommodum; quamvis *Africani*
tam universè se ipsos perungant, ut ne unum Vasis
osculum liberum ad exhalandum superfit.* Majores
nostri, antiqui Britanni, nullâ cum noxâ variis pig-
mentis nuda sua corpora inficiebant. Et Ill. Fran.
Baconus, patriæ suæ decus et ornamentum, à
diminutione Perspirationis vitæ productionem spe-
ravit. Hallerus affirmat Perspirabile suppreffum
non fibi ipfi fignum effe morbi. Plane apparet, à
Diariis Perspirationis, Gravedines et Catarrhos sæpe
homines invafiffe, dum hæc excretio integra remanfit;
et è contrario diminutionem Perspirationis non semper
hos morbos afferre.†

Contractio‡ autem minimarum arteriarum à frigore
orta, multos et diversos Morbos procul dubio excitat.

* Vid. Halleri Elem. Phyf. vol. v. p. 83.

† Vid. Arbuthnot on Air, p. 167.

‡ Confitendum autem eft, argumentis fupra allatis minimè ob-
ftantibus, quod omnes excretiones naturales neceffariæ fint perfectæ
fanitati; quia aliquid per unamquamque è corpore ejicitur, quod non
poteft tam commodè ullo alio modo difflari. Et in multis infuper

At non nobis licet ob brevitatem hujus Differtationis unumquemque fingulatim inveftigare.   In quatuor igitur morbis demonftrandis, qui præcipuè vi Frigoris concitantur, hoc opus infumetur.   Hi funt Febris Intermittens, Catarrhus, Diarrhœa, et Rheumatifmus.

Febris Intermittens.

Variæ Hypothefes de caufa proxima Febris Intermittentis fictæ fuerunt; et hodie etiam quæftio inter medicos vehementer agitatur.   Symptomata autem primi ftadii Morbi, plane, ut mihi videtur, indicant Arterias Capillares per totum corpus effe conftrictas. Æger expallet, ungues ejus fæpiffimè funt lividi, et cutis arida rugofaque apparet.   Pulfus eft debilis, parvus, celer et contractus, et fi vena fecatur, fanguis tardè et guttatim effluit;* quia minor copia fanguinis tunc temporis per fuperficiem corporis circumfertur. Ægrotus etiam fiti laborat, Lingua et Fauces funt aridæ, Urina lurida eft, vel fine ullo colore,† et fi

morbis Perfpiratio non folum fupprimitur, fed eodem quoque tempore minima vafa renum fæpe contrahuntur; adeo ut partes fanguinis redundantes non poffint urinâ abduci, et ab hac plenitudine corpus certiffime malè fe habebit.   Nihilominus autem minimè concedimus perfpirationis fuppreffionem feorfim fpectatam, caufam effe proximam morborum.

* Vid. Bryan Robinson on the Operation of Med. p. 97.

† Durante primo ftadio morbi, urina fit magis magifque pellucida; fecundo autem accedente, gradatim affumit rubellum colorem.   Tandem vero cum tertium incipit ftadium, deponit fedimentum lateritium.

Ulcera in ejus Corpore fint, ficca et pallida fiunt:
Refpiratio difficillima eft, et anxietas circa præcordia,
cum fenfu ponderis cujufdam, à diftenfione Vaforum
magnorum prope cor oriente, fere femper percipitur.*
Omnia hæc enumerata fymptomata contractionem
arteriarum minimarum planè indicant. Eft autem
confitendum quod in primo morbi ftadio alia fint
fymptomata, quæ caufam proximam Febris Intermittentis demonftrant non folum à fpafmo pendere.
Nam ofcitatio, languor, dolor dorfi, et fenfatio
quædam, haud verbis defcribenda, in digitorum ex-
tremitatibus, à turbata actione, ni fallor, Virium
Vitalium, originem manifeftè ducunt. Omnino itaque
verifimile videtur, quamdam generis Nervofi affectionem, fpafmodicæ Capillarium conftrictioni junctam,
caufam hujus Morbi proximam conftituere. Nimia
corporis Mobilitas, vel ab acuta magis fenfibilitate,
vel debilitate, vel epidemica anni conftitutione, vel
alio quocunque modo orta, caufa agnofcitur prædif-
ponens. *Frigus,* miafma, contagium animique affectus funt caufæ remotæ. Hic autem morbus,
multò frequentius à *Frigore,* quam ab ulla alia
origine nafcitur. Nam in locis humidis et uliginofis,
ficut in Hollandia, Flandria, Paludibus Lincolnien-
fibus, endemicè graffari confuevit. Sæpiffimè etiam

* In Febre Intermittente femper adeft fenfatio Frigoris; hæc
etiam à conftrictione capillarium arteriarum verifimillimè oritur.
Nam omnia quæ vafa fubcutanea contrahunt, uti frigus externum,
cibus quem abhorret noftra natura vel ejus Idea, hanc excitant
fenfationem.——Vid. HOME, Princ. Med. p. 72.

à Frigore fubito corpori applicato, à Ventis humidis et frigidis, Aëre aquofis particulis repleto, vel Veftitu humido excitatur.

CATARRHUS.

Hic morbus ab inflammatione membranæ mucofæ, Nares, Fauces, Afperam Arteriam, et Pulmones inveftientis provenit; et frigus cuique corporis parti, Faciei præcipuæ Colloque admotum, caufa ejus remota fere femper habetur. Frigus autem, ex vi ejus aucta vel imminuta Corporifque fenfibilitate et irritabilitate, vel Catarrhum, vel Diarrhœam, vel Febrem denique concitabit. Incolæ Regionum Auftralium, qui nimia Corporis mobilitate plerumque funt præditi, parvi levique Frigoris acceffione Febre corripiuntur: e contrario autem in Terris Septentrionalibus, Catarrhi multo fæpius invadunt.

Hic morbus in corporibus robuftis, ab inflammatione membranæ mucofæ incipit; et copiofa muci excretione ut plurimum terminatur. Sed in hominibus laxis et debilibus, excretio primum augetur et paulo poft, à ftimulo muci acris, inflammatio oritur. Infarctio Pulmonum Nariumque, et humoris tenuis et aquofi deftillatio, à circuitu fanguinis in his partibus adaucto, fat benè explicentur; neque ad acrimoniam fictam à fuppreffa perfpiratione ortam, confugere opus eft.

Diarrhœa.

Materies putrida vel Aciditates Primas Vias infes-
tantes, Medicamenta purgantia nimis. frequenter
aſſumpta, vel alia quæcumque res Inteſtina ad fre-
quentes ſtimulans dejectiones, Diarrhœam concitabit. Hæ autem cauſæ brevi tempore evaneſcunt,
et morbus fere ſemper ceſſat, ſtimulo evacuato ex
quo originem traxit. At quum Diarrhœa à Frigore
naſcitur, diuturnior eſt utplurimum, et ſymptomata
etiam graviora fiunt, adeo ut non raro in *Dyſenteriam*
abeat. Diſtenſio vaſorum minimorum membranæ
Inteſtinorum internæ, atque aucta ab arteriis ex-
halantibus excretio, hujus morbi cauſa videtur eſſe
proxima. Spaſmodica capillarium conſtrictio in corporis ſuperficie, evacuationes magnæ, putrida materies primas vias occupans, triſtes animi affectiones,
&c. cauſæ ſunt prædiſponentes; et frigus cauſa
remota ut plurimum agnoſcitur.

Hæ vero cauſæ in firma corporis conſtitutione
concurrentes, præſertim ſi bruma vel primum ver
adeſt, dyſenteriam confeſtim inducent. Sanguine
enim, aucta copiâ, in vaſa minima inteſtinorum vali-
diſſimè impulſo, vaſiſque ſummis viribus contra
renitentibus, dolor vehemens, eamque ob cauſam
inflammatio quoque naſcitur. Sin autem Ægri ha-
bitus ſit debilis et laxus, vel ſi tempus autumnale
adeſt, vaſorum renixus omnino imbecillus erit, et
copioſa muci excretio extemplò ſequitur. Sed ab

hac etiam excretione, diutius permanente, inflammatio certiffime orietur.   Ex defectu enim ftagnationis
in fuis folliculis, mucus nimis fit acris et liquidus,
adeoque ipfam membranam irritat, quam ab aliis
ftimulis defendere debet.

Rheumatismus.

Frigus, procatarcticam Rheumatifmi caufam effe,
nem ' ferè ignorat; de proxima autem caufa varias
opiniones Medici amplectuntur.   A contractione
Vaforum partis affectæ minutorum, ut mihi videtur,
oriri verifimillimum eft.   Omnia morbi fymptomata
ex hac hypothefi explicatu facilia funt.   Pallor et
contractio partis dolentis vafa folito minus plena effe
oftendunt.   Dolor, nixum quendam ad diftenfionem
indicat, qui calore et exercitatione augetur propterea
quod eo modo Arteriæ magnæ impetu agunt majori,
quo impetu fanguis in Capillaria conftricta fortius
impellitur.   Mufculorum rigiditas, torporque in
Membro Rheumatico, fpafmodici affectus quoque
figna funt. Circulatio enim obftructa vim minuit mus-
cularem, ut in operatione, Aneurifmatis caufa infti-
tuta, quum Bracchii Arteria circumligatur, cernere
eft.   Primo enim Mufculi magna ex parte agere
ceffant, ufquedum fanguis meatum novum invenerit.
Dolor etiam ex una ad alteram partem corporis tran-
fiens fpafmodicam fyftematis vafcularis affectionem
demonftrat.   Omnino manifeftum eft hanc non poffe

deduci ex metaſtaſi acris illius ſeri, aut materiæ ſalinæ
quam nonnulli proximam Rheumatiſmi cauſam eſſe
autumant; quoniam ſi carpus uterque viciſſim afficiatur, alterius dolor non ſemper ceſſat Rheumatiſmo
alterum adoriente. Præterea quum hæc acrimonia
via ſolummodo circulationis deferri poſſit; eam per
totum corpus diffuſam, peculiarem quandam partem
occupare maxime mirandum foret. Hoc etiam neceſſariò tardum eſſet, ſi modò fieri poſſet, qod expe-
rientiæ repugnat; nam dolores rheumatici ſedes ſuas
citiſſime ut plurimum mutant. Verùm de Rheumatiſmi Theoria plus ſatis diſputatum; mihi tantum
incumbit, Frigus inter præcipuas morbi eſſe cauſas
argumentis probare; et hoc HOFFMANNUS, SYDEN-
HAMUS, PRINGLE, clariſſimique Scriptores Medici
fatentur. Experientia quoque demonſtrat dolores
Rheumaticos, tempore verno vel autumnali imprimis
graſſari cum cœlum maximè mutabile eſt, vel cum
Venti contrarii ſibi invicem ſubitò ſuccedunt.

SECTIO QUINTA.

VI Frigoris in Morbis inducendis fic breviter
tractatâ, exempla pauca medicinalis ejus ufus
ad fanitatem reftituendam commemorabimus.

GANGRÆNA.

In frigidiffimis plagis frequenter evenit, ut ii quorum corpora per longum tempus gelu glacieique
expofita fuerunt, omni fenfibilitate et movendi facultate priventur. Gangræna primum incipit in partibus extremis, et inde ad cor fenfim progreditur; et
nifi remedium maturè adhibeatur, miferum cito con-
ficiet, etiam priufquam Mortificatio fiat.* Incolæ

---

* Poëta infignis THOMSON hoc infortunium patheticè defcripfit.

" As thus the fnows arife; and foul, and fierce,
" All Winter drives along the darken'd air;
" In his own loofe-revolving fields the fwain
" Difafter'd ftands; fees other hills afcend,
" Of unknown joylefs brow; and other fcenes,
" Of horrid profpect, fhag the tracklefs plain:
" Nor finds the river, nor the foreft, hid
" Beneath the formlefs wild; but wanders on
" From hill to dale, ftill more and more aftray.
         —— " Down he finks
" Beneath the fhelter of the fhapelefs drift
" Thinking o'er all the bitternefs of death,

quoque harum regionum experientia docti, huic
Gangrænæ, adhibitâ nive, vel aquâ adeo frigidâ ut
ad congelationem prope accedat, feliciſſimè occurri
reperierunt. Hoc enim modo pars morbida ad eum
caloris gradum qui vitæ neceſſarius eſt ſenſim ſenſim-
que reſtituitur ; et poſtea frictione, fomentis et
medicamentis cardiacis internè ingeſtis ſenſibilitas
movendique facultas priſtinas vires recipere· poſſunt.
Ad exiſtentiam particularum frigorificarum confugere
hic non opus eſt ; neque conjectare aquam ſpicula
ſalina, quæ cauſa Gangrænæ fuerunt, attrahere.
Efficacia Frigidæ Aquæ hinc certe oritur, quod
paucis gradibus calorem ſuperet partis cui admovetur,
unde paulatim reſtituit quantum vitæ ſufficit facultates in males calorem generantes excitare, et hæ,
aliis methodis ſupra memoratis adjutæ, curationem
perficiunt. E contrariò autem ſi aqua calida applicetur, rarefactio ſubita inde orta, Vaſa tenera partis
affectæ corrumpet et mortificatio citò ſequetur;
quemadmodum Pomum gelidum inſipidum, pul-
poſum, et putridum fit ſi ſubitò regeletur. Particulæ
glaciales in aqua poſt immerſum membrum frigore

> " Mix'd with the tender anguiſh Nature ſhoots
> " Through the wrung boſom of the dying man,
> " His wife, his children, and his friends unſeen.
> —— " On every nerve
> " The deadly Winter ſeizes; ſhuts up ſenſe;
> " And o'er his inmoſt vitals creeping cold,
> " Lays him along the ſnows a ſtiffen'd corſe !
> " Stretch'd out, and bleaching in the northern blaſt."
> Poem on the Winter, line 276.

gangrænatum fluitantes, à communibus congelationis principiis deduci poſſint; quippe quod aqua ad punctum gelationis reducta illicò congelatur.

FEBRES.

Aquæ frigidæ uſus Antiquis ipſis innotuit. GALENUS ejus potationem ad ſatietatem uſque ſuaſit. Ab HIPPOCRATE, CELSO, et RHAZE commendata fuit. CELSUS in Procemio ſuo exemplum Medici adducit qui frigidam aquam Febricitanti exhibuit, eoque modo ſitim levavit, ſomnum altum induxit, tandemque ſudore morbum expulſit. HOFFMANNUS Heroicum et magnæ efficaciæ remedium hoc in morbo nominat. Nec tamen temerè, omni tempore aut in omnibus morbi ſtatibus adminiſtranda eſt. " Bibiturus itaque frigidam aquam, non ante " id facere poteſt, quam ipſa Febris, concocto " humore evacuationeque idonea, ad ſtatum ac- " ceſſerit ſuum: jamque ipſe homo maximis af- " fectus caloribus, ſummaque ſiti, die judicatorio, " ſummum Febricitationis impetum experitur."* HOFFMANNUS dicit: " Heic igitur monuiſſe ſufficiat, " nunquam ſimul et ſemel magnis hauſtibus præ- " bendum eſſe frigidum potum, ſed ſucceſſivè et " crebro; nunquam in principio morbi, ſed elapſis " jam aliquot diebus; nunquam tempore acceſſionis

---

* Vid. LOMMII de Curand. Febrib. cap. iii. ſect. 2, p. 206.

" vel exacerbationis vel etiam fub rigore et pulfu
" parvo aut intermittente; nunquam nifi plethora
" prius foluta.   Sed quando extrema calida, pulfus
" equalis, celer et magnus."* Aqua frigida his
cautelis adminiftrata, maxima fæpè commoda affert.
Spafmum enim vaforum Capillarium folvit, fudorem
mitem ægroto commovet, Febremque omnino tollit.

Balneum Frigidum.

Inter leges œconomiæ animalis hæc una præcipua
effe vi ʲetur, quod toto fyftemate vel quavis ejus
parte irritatione aut dolore affecto motrices facultates
concitari debeant, ut nocivæ caufæ refiftant fimulque
eam repellant.   Sic Cauftico teneræ cuivis corporis
parti admoto, dolor à ftimulo ejus ortus, violenti-
orem iftius partis vaforum actionem ftatim parit, quo
tantus humorum fluxus eo deducitur, ut acrimoniam
Cauftici diluat, ejufque vim aut minuat aut omnino
auferat.   Pulvis aut quidvis aliud Oculo illatus, eam
lachrymarum fecretionem motumque convulfivum
Palpebræ concitat, quæ caufam nocivam exprimere
valeat.   Itidem Corpore in aquam frigidam fubitò
immerfo, Cutis fenfibilis ingrato more afficitur,
Capillaria omnia per ejus fuperficiem fparfa contrahuntur, fanguifque in Cor et Vafa majora violenter
impellitur.   Verum poft immerfionem (fi breviffimæ

* Hoffman Med. Rar. Syft. vol. iv. p. 356.

tantum durationis fuerit) Facultates motrices ad
conftrictionem amovendam cientur, Cor et Arteriæ
adauctis viribus contrahuntur, fanguifque ad corporis
fuperficiem rejicitur. Sin autem æger nimis diu in
gelida unda perluitur, tum vitæ vires debilitantur,
fpafmufque vel capillarium contractio continuata fuc-
cedit. Ex obfervatis fupra dictis felices Balnei
Frigidi effectus funt explicandi. Vim nervofam per
omnes corporis partes magnopere auget, fibras motrices exercet roboratque, unde Functiones omnes
animales rectiffime perficiuntur. Innumera funt tes-
timonia quæ ex fcriptoribus antiquis æque ac hodier-
nis in laudem Balnei Frigidi adduci poffint. ANTO-
NIUS MUSA, Imperatoris AUGUSTI Medicus, ufum
ejus adeo commendavit, ut hoc remedium omnibus
fere Romanis familiare effet. Et HORATIUS ait,

—— " Sane Myrteta relinqui
" Dictaque ceffantem Nervis elidere Morbum
" Sulfura contemni, Vicus gemit; invidus Ægris
" Qui Caput et Stomachum fupponere fontibus audent,
" Clufinis, Gabiofque petunt, et Frigida Rura."

HOR. Ep. xv. ad VALAM.

In Ventriculo, primifque viis infirmis ufus ejus ab
HOFFMANNO* maxime laudatur; CELSUSque in
Paralyticis, Hypochondriacis, et Hyftericis Morbis
ad Frigidum Balneum confugere monet.† · Nufquam
vero quam in Rheumatifmo chronici generis utilius
eft, quia fyftema firmat, irritabilitatem imminuit, et

* Vid. Opufc. Med. Pract. p. 204.

† CELSUS, lib. iv. cap. 5.

vaforum minutorum conftrictionem recludit. In
multis morbis quibus obnoxii funt Parvuli, in Rachi-
tide præcipue, valde infignes funt ejus effectus.
Debilitas univerfa Solidorum Vivorum in hoc morbo
imbecillitas, Perioftei et Cartilaginum vafa Materiei
Offeæ deponendæ inepta reddunt. Corpore igitur
roborato, vafifque ad debitum tonum Balnei frigidi
ope reftitutis, morbi caufa omnino tolletur. Lavatio
in *Aqua marina* noftros apud medicos admodum
celebratur. Et quum aquæ Oceani multo fale amaro
Glauberi imprægnentur, quod vim habet, exterius
adhibitum valide aftrictoriam, corpus fine dubio
robuftius reddunt. Æger etiam in marina lavatione
frigori minus obnoxius eft; 1°. Quia aqua falfa cutis
fenfibilitatem paululum hebetat. 2°. Non tamen cito
ex fuperficie corporis evaporatur quam aqua dulcis
et infulfa. 3°. Salium ftimulus, quendam forfan
calorem in cute poffit excitare. Aqua vero fontana
frigiditate falfam utplurimum excedit, quapropter ubi
actio frigoris Medicinalis folummodo requiritur,
femper eft anteponenda.

Tandem L. B. munus ACADEMIÆ hujus legibus
mihi præfcriptum abfolvi, tuæque indulgentiæ co-
namen hoc primum trado, omni illâ folicitudinê atque
diffidentiâ quæ fcriptorem juvenem in tali re circum-
fiftere folet. Si ftudia in quibus per multos annos
verfatus fui, me magis vacare fiviffent, Differtatio hæc
forfan lectu dignior fuiffet: Mihi autem perfuafum
eft, nullum neque tempus neque limæ meæ laborem
hoc effecturum fuiffe, ut mihi omninò arridere poffet.

Argumentum quod fufcepi tautam habet amplitu‑
dinem totqué partes complectitur, ut opus meum
Epitome potius quam Tractatus Philofophicus auᵗ
Medicus videatur. Thefes autem Academicæ intra
limites tam arctos coërcentur, ut carptim breviterque
fingula perftringere coactus fim. Curriculo ftudi‑
orum expleto, quum maturior ætas ingenium magis
excoluerit, erit mihi et majus otium et facultas de
hoc argumento differendi. Interea fpero, Lectorem
candidum, Errores vel fermonis vel judicii qui in hoc
Tentamine obfervari poffint, benevolè condonaturum
effe.

" Sunt delicta tamen, quibus ignoviffe velimus:
" Nam neque chorda fonum reddit quem vult manus ac mens;
" Nec femper fieret quodcunque minabitur arcus.
· · · · · · · · " Non ego paucis
" Offendar maculis, quas aut incuria fudit,
" Aut humana parum cavit natura."

HOR. Ars Poët.

MEDICAL ETHICS;

OR, A CODE OF

Institutes and Precepts,

ADAPTED TO THE

PROFESSIONAL CONDUCT

OF

PHYSICIANS AND SURGEONS:

I. In Hospital Practice.
II. In Private or General Practice.
III. In relation to Apothecaries.

IV. In Cases which may require a
Knowledge of Law.

To which is added,

𝔄𝔫 𝔄𝔭𝔭𝔢𝔫𝔡𝔦𝔵;

CONTAINING A

DISCOURSE ON HOSPITAL DUTIES;

ALSO,

NOTES AND ILLUSTRATIONS.

BY

THOMAS PERCIVAL, M.D.

F.R'S. AND A.S. LOND. F.R.S. AND R.M.S. EDINB. &C. &C.

Nulla enim. vitæ pars, neque publicis, neque privatis, neque forensibus, neque domesticis in rebus, neque si tecum agas quid, neque si cum altero contrahas, vacare officio potest: In eoque colendo sita vitæ est honestas omnis, et in negligendo turpitudo.

Cic. de Off. Lib. I. Cap. II.

TO

SIR GEORGE BAKER, BART.

PHYSICIAN TO THEIR MAJESTIES;

FELLOW OF THE ROYAL SOCIETY;

AND

LATE PRESIDENT OF THE COLLEGE OF PHYSICIANS;

&c. &c.

THIS CODE OF

PROFESSIONAL ETHICS;

WHICH HE HAS

HONOURED WITH HIS SANCTION,

AND IMPROVED BY HIS COMMUNICATIONS,

IS GRATEFULLY AND RESPECTFULLY

INSCRIBED,

BY HIS

OBLIGED AND AFFECTIONATE FRIEND,

THE AUTHOR.

E. C. PERCIVAL.

PERMIT me, my dear fon, to offer to your
acceptance this little Manual of MEDICAL
ETHICS. In the compofition of it, my thoughts
were directed towards your late excellent Brother,
with the tendereft impulfe of paternal love : and not
a fingle moral rule was framed without a fecret view
to his defignation; and an anxious wifh that it might
influence his future conduct.

To you, who poffefs, in no inferior degree, my
efteem and attachment; who are profecuting the
fame ftudies, and with the fame object; my folici-
tudes are naturally transferred. And I am perfuaded,
thefe united confiderations will powerfully and permanently operate upon your ingenuous mind.

It is the characteriftic of a wife man to act on
determinate principles ; and of a good man to, be
affured that they are conformable to rectitude and
virtue. The relations in which a phyfician ftands to
his patients, to his brethren, and to the public, are
complicated and multifarious ; involving much knowledge of human nature, and extenfive moral duties.
The ftudy of profeffional Ethics, therefore, cannot

fail to invigorate and enlarge the underſtanding; whilſt the obſervance of the duties which they enjoin, will ſoften your manners, expand your affections, and form you to that propriety and dignity of conduct, which are eſſential to the character of a GENTLEMAN. The academical advantages you have enjoyed at Cambridge, and thoſe you now poſſeſs in Edinburgh, will qualify you, I truſt, for an ample and honourable ſphere of action. And I devoutly pray, that the bleſſing of GOD may attend all your purſuits ; rendering them at once ſubſervient to your own felicity, and the good of your fellow-creatures.

Senſible that I begin to experience the preſſure of advancing years, I regard the preſent publication as the concluſion, in this way, of my profeſſional labours. I may, therefore, without impropriety, claim the privilege of conſecrating them to you, as a paternal legacy. And I feel cordial ſatisfaction in the occaſion, of thus teſtifying the eſteem and tenderneſs with which, whilſt life ſubſiſts, I ſhall remain,

Your affectionate friend,

THOMAS PERCIVAL.

Mancheſter, Feb. 20, 1803.

CONTENTS.

CHAP. II. *Of Profeffional Conduct in private, or general Practice.*

PREFACE.

----◄◄◇►►----

THE firſt chapter of the following work was compoſed in the ſpring of 1792, at the requeſt of the phyſicians and ſurgeons of the Mancheſter Infirmary : and the ſubſtance of it conſtitutes the code of laws, by which the practice of that compre‑henſive inſtitut on is now governed.* The author was afterwards induced, by an earneſt deſire to pro‑mote the honour and advancement of his profeſſion, to enlarge the plan of his undertaking, and to frame a general ſyſtem of MEDICAL ETHICS; that the official conduct and mutual intercourſe of the faculty might be regulated by preciſe and acknowledged principles of urbanity and rectitude. Printed copies of the ſcheme were, therefore, diſtributed amongſt his numerous correſpondents ; by moſt of whom it was warmly encouraged ; and by many of them was honoured with valuable ſuggeſtions for its improve‑ment.†

* See Notes and Illuſtrations, No. I.
† See Notes and Illuſtrations, No. II.

Whilft the author was thus extending his views, and carrying on his work with ardour, he loft the ftrongeft incentive to its profecution, by the death of a beloved fon, who had nearly completed the courfe of his academical education; and whofe talents, acquirements, and virtues, promifed to render him an ornament to the healing art. This melancholy event was followed, not many years afterwards, by a fecond family lofs, equally afflictive; and the defign has ever fince been wholly fufpended. The author now refumes it, animated by the hope that it may prove beneficial to another fon, who has lately exchanged the purfuits of general fcience at Cambridge, for the ftudy of medicine at Edinburgh. He feels at the fame time impreffed with the conviction, that the langour of forrow becomes culpable, when it obftructs the offices of an active vocation. " I hold every man," fays Lord Bacon, in the preface to his Elements of the Common Laws of England, " a debtor to his profeffion ; from the which as " men of courfe do feek to receive countenance and " profit, fo ought they of duty to endeavour them- " felves, by way of amends, to be a help and orna- " ment thereunto. This is performed, in fome " degree, by the honeft and liberal practice of a " profeffion ; when men fhall carry a refpect not to " defcend into any courfe that is corrupt and unwor- " thy thereof, and preferve themfelves free from the " abufes wherewith the fame profeffion is noted to " be infected : but much more is this performed, if

" a man be able to vifit and ftrengthen the roots and
" foundation of the fcience itfelf; thereby not only
" gracing it in reputation and dignity, but alfo
" amplifying it in profeffion and fubftance."

It was the author's original intention to have
treated of the POWERS, PRIVILEGES, HONOURS, and
EMOLUMENTS of the FACULTY; but he now conceives, that this would lead him into a field of inves-
tigation too wide and digreffive ; and therefore
choofes to confine himfelf to what more ftrictly
belongs to Medical Ethics.

To thefe inftitutes he has annexed an Anniverfary
Difcourfe, delivered by the late Rev. Thomas Bafs-
nett Percival, LL. B. before the prefident and
governors of the Infirmary at Liverpool. As it is
an addrefs to the gentlemen of the faculty, the officers, the clergy, and the truftees of the charity, on
their refpective hofpital duties, by one competent to
the fubject from his early ftudies, it cannot but be
deemed fufficiently appropriate to the prefent work,
exclufively of a father's claim to the privilege of its
infertion.

The aphoristic form of this code of Medical
Ethics, though adapted to fuch an undertaking, forbids, in a great meafure, all digreffion ; and even precludes the difcuffion of many interefting points,
nearly connected with the fubject. SUPPLEMEN-
TARY NOTES AND ILLUSTRATIONS, therefore, are
neceffary to the completion of the author's plan :
and he trufts the candid reader will grant him the

liberty of thus ſtating his opinions more at large;
of rectifying miſconceptions, to which the brevity
eſſential to the work may give riſe ; and of correcting whatever ſubſequent reflection, or the judicious
obſervations of his friends, may diſcover to be
erroneous.

A conſiderable portion of theſe ſheets was communicated to the Rev. THOMAS GISBORNE, M. A.
whilſt engaged in the compoſition of his ENQUIRY
into the DUTIES of MEN ; a work that reflects the
higheſt honour on the abilities and philanthropy of
the author ; and which may be juſtly regarded as the
moſt complete ſyſtem extant of PRACTICAL ETHICS.
The chapter concerning phyſicians contains a reference to theſe inſtitutes, expreſſed in the moſt gratifying terms of friendſhip ; and it treats ſo largely of
the duties of the faculty, as to ſeem, at firſt view, to
ſuperſede the uſe of the preſent manual.   But the
two publications differ not only in their plan, but
in many of their leading objects ; and it may be
hoped they will rather illuſtrate than interfere with
each other   The ſame remarks may be applied to
the excellent lectures of Dr. Gregory.   Even the
STATUTA MORALIA of the college of phyſicians,
whatever merit or authority they poſſeſs, are not
ſufficiently comprehenſive for the exiſting ſphere of
medical and chirurgical duty ; and by the few regulations which they eſtabliſh, they tacitly ſanction the
recommendation of a fuller and more adequate code
of profeſſional offices.

Copies of the former unfinished impreffion of this work have been tranfmitted to the libraries of feveral Infirmaries, in different parts of the kingdom; and the author has reafon to hope, that they have contributed to excite attention to the fubject of hofpital police. Amongft other pleafing proofs of this truth, he refers with peculiar fatisfaction to the late publications of his friends, Sir G. O. Paul, bart. and Dr. Clark, of Newcaftle-upon-Tyne.

This work was originally entitled, " MEDICAL JURISPRUDENCE;" but fome correfpondents of refpectable judgment having objected to the term Jurisprudence, it has been changed to ETHICS. According to the definition of Juftinian, however, Jurifprudence may be underftood to include moral injunctions as well as pofitive ordinances. *Juris præcepta funt hæc—honeftè vivere, alterum non lædere, fuum cuique tribuere.*—INST. JUSTIN. lib. i. p. 3.

Manchefter, Feb. 15, 1803.

—— QUICQUID DIGNUM SAPIENTE BONOQUE EST.

HOR. Lib. I. Ep. IV.

MEDICAL ETHICS;

OR,

A CODE OF INSTITUTES AND PRECEPTS,

ADAPTED TO THE

PROFESSIONAL CONDUCT

OF

PHYSICIANS AND SURGEONS.

CHAPTER I.

OF PROFESSIONAL CONDUCT, RELATIVE TO HOS-
PITALS, OR OTHER MEDICAL CHARITIES.

I. HOSPITAL Physicians and Surgeons
should minister to the sick, with due impres-
sions of the importance of their office; reflecting, that
the ease, the health, and the lives of those committed
to their charge depend on their skill, attention, and
fidelity. They should study, also, in their deportment so to unite *tenderness* with *steadiness*, and
condescension with *authority*, as to inspire the minds of
their patients with gratitude, respect, and confidence.

II. The *choice* of a *phyſician*, or *ſurgeon*, cannot be allowed to hospital patients, consistently with the regular and eſtabliſhed ſucceſſion of medical attendance. Yet perſonal confidence is not leſs important to the comfort and relief of the ſick poor, than of the rich under ſimilar circumſtances: and it would be equally juſt and humane, to enquire into and to indulge their part'alities, by occaſionally calling into conſultation the favourite practitioner. The rectitude and wisdom of this conduct will be still more apparent, when it is recollected that patients in hoſpitals not unfrequently request their diſcharge, on a deceitful plea of having received relief; and afterwards procure another recommendation, that they may be admitted under the phyſician or ſurgeon of their choice. Such practices involve in them a degree of falſehood; produce unneceſſary trouble; and may be the occaſion of irreparable loſs of time in the treatment of diseases.

III. The *feelings* and *emotions* of the patients, under critical circumſtances, require to be known and to be attended to, no leſs than the ſymptoms of their diſeaſes. Thus extreme *timidity* with reſpect to venæ ection contra-indicates its uſe in certain caſes and conſtitutions. Even the *prejudices* of the ſick are not to be contemned, or oppoſed with harſhneſs : for though ſilenced by authority, they will operate ſecretly and forcibly on the mind, creating fear, anxiety. and watchfulneſs.

IV. As miſapprehenſion may magnify real evils, or create imaginary ones, no *diſcuſſion* concerning the nature of the cafe fhould be entered into before the patients, either with the houfe furgeon, the pupils of the hofpitals, or any medical vifitor.

V. In the large wards of an Infirmary, the patients should be interrogated concerning their complaints in a *tone* of *voice* which cannot be *overheard.* Se= crecy, alfo, when required by peculiar circumstances, fhould be striêtly obferved. And females fhould always be treated with the moft fcrupulous *delicacy*. To negleêt or to fport with their feelings is cruelty; and every wound thus infl êted tends to produce a calloufnefs of mind, a contempt of decorum, and an infenfibility to modefty and virtue. Let thefe confi- derations be forcibly and repeatedly urged on the hofpital pupils.

VI. The *moral* and *religious influence* of ficknefs is fo favourable to the beft interefts of men and of fo- ciety, that it is juftly regarded as an important objeêt in the eftablifhment of every hofpital. The *inftitu=* tions for promoting it fhould, therefore, be encouraged by the phyficians and furgeons, whenever feafonable opportunities occur: and by pointing out thefe to the officiating clergyman, the facred offices will be performed with propriety, difcrimination, and greater certainty of fuccefs. The charaêter of a phyfician is ufually remote either from fuperftition or enthufiafm: and the aid which he is now exhorted to give, will tend to their exclufion from the fick wards of the hos- pital, where their effeêts have often been known to be not only baneful, but even fatal.

VII. It is one of the circumſtances which ſoftens
the lot of the poor, that they are exempt from the ſolicitudes attendant on the diſpoſal of property. Yet
there are exceptions to this obſervation : and it may
be neceſſary that an hoſp:tal patient, on the bed of
ſickneſs and death, ſhould be reminded, by ſome
friendly monitor, of the importance of a *laſt will* and
teſtament to h:s w:fe, children, or relatives, who,
otherwiſe, might be deprived of his effects, of his
expected prize money, or of ſome future reſiduary
legacy.   This kind office will be beſt performed by
the houſe ſurgeon, whoſe frequent attendance on the
sick diminiſhes their reſerve, and entitles him to their
familiar confidence.   And he will doubtleſs regard
the performance of it as a duty: for whatever is right
to be done, and cannot·by another be ſo well done,
has the full force of moral and perſonal obligation.
    VIII.   The phyſicians and ſurgeons ſhould not
ſuffer themſelves to be reſtrained, by parſimonious
conſiderations, from preſcribing *wine*, and *drugs* even
of *high price*, when required in diſeaſes of extraordinary malign:ty and danger.   The efficacy of every
medicine is proportionate to its purity and goodneſs;
and on the degree of theſe properties, *cæteris paribus*,
both the cure of the ſick, and the ſpeedineſs of its
accompl:ſhment, muſt depend.   But when drugs of
inferior quality are employed, it is requiſite to admi-
niſter them in larger doſes, and to continue the uſe of
them a longer period of time; circumſtances, which,
probably, more than counterbalance any ſavings in

their original price. If the cafe, however, were far otherwife, no œconomy, of a fatal tendency, ought to be admitted into institutions, founded on principles of the pureft beneficence, and which, in this age and country, when well conducted, can never want contributions adequate to their liberal fupport.

IX. The medical gentlemen of every charitable inftitution are, in fome degree, refponfible for, and the guardians of, the honour of eacn other. No phyfician or furgeon,t herefore, fhould *reveal* occurrences in the hofpital, which may injure the reputation of any one of his colleagues; except under the reftriction contained in the fucceeding article.

X. No *profeſſional charge* fhould be made by a phyfician or furgeon, either publicly or privately, against any affociate, without previoufly laying the complaint before the gentlemen of the faculty belonging to the inftitution, that they may judge concerning the reafonablenefs of its grounds, aud the meafures to be adopted.

XI. A proper *difcrimination* being eftablifhed in all hofpitals between the *medical* and *chirurgical cafes*, it fhould be faithfully adhered to by the phyficians and furgeons, on the admiffion of patients.

XII. Whenever cafes occur, attended with circumftances not heretofore obferved, or in which the ordinary modes of practice have been attempted without fuccefs, it is for the public good, and in an especial degree advantageous to the poor, (who, being the moft numerous clafs of fociety, are the greateft

beneficiaries of the healing art,) that *new remedies*
and *new methods* of *chirurgical treatment* should be devifed. But in the accomplifhment of this falutary purpofe, the gentlemen of the faculty fhould be fcrupu-
loufly and confcientioufly governed by found reafon,
juft analogy, or well-authenticated facts. And no
fuch trials fhould be inftituted, without a previous
confultation of the phyficians or furgeons, according
to the nature of the cafe.

XIII. To advance profeffional improvement, a
friendly and unreferved *intercourse* fhould fubfift
between the gentlemen of the faculty, with a free
communication of whatever is extraordinary or interefting in the courfe of their hofpital practice; and an
account of every *cafe* or *operation*, which is rare, curious,
or inftructive, fhould be drawn up by the phyfician
or furgeon, to whofe charge it devolves, and entered
in a regifter kept for the purpofe, but open only to
the phyficians and furgeons of the charity.

XIV. *Hofpital regifters* ufually contain only a
fimple report of the number of patients admitted and
difcharged. By adopting a more comprehenfive
plan, they might be rendered fubfervient to medical
fcience, and beneficial to mankind. The following
fketch is offered, with deference, to the gentlemen of
the faculty. Let the regifter confift of three tables;
the firft fpecifying the number of patients admitted,
cured, relieved, difcharged, or dead; the fecond, the
feveral difeafes of the patients, with their events;
the third, the fexes, ages, and occupations of the apa-

tients. The ages fhould be reduced into claffes; and the tables adapted to the four divifions of the year. By fuch an inftitution, the increafe or decreafe of ficknefs; the attack, progrefs, and ceffation of epidemicks; the comparative healthinefs of different fituations, climates, and feafons; the influence of particular trades and manufactures on health and life; with many other curious circumftances, not more interefting to phyficians than to the community; would be afcertained with fufficient precifion.

XV. By the adoption of the *regifter*, recommended in the foregoing article, phyficians and furgeons would obtain a clearer infight into the comparative fuccefs of their hofpital and private practice, and would be incited to a diligent inveftigation of the caufes of fuch difference. In particular difeafes it will be found to fubfift in a very remarkable degree: and the difcretionary power of the phyfician or furgeon, in the admiffion of patients, could not be exerted with more juftice or humanity, than in refufing to confign to lingering fuffering, and almoft certain death, a numerous clafs of patients, inadvertently recommended as objects of thefe charitable inftitutions. " In judging of difeafes with regard to the " propriety of their reception into hofpitals," fays " an excellent writer, " the following general cir- " cumftances are to be confidered :—

" Whether they be capable of fpeedy relief; be- " caufe, as it is the intention of charity to relieve as " great a number as poffible, a quick change of ob-

" jects is to be wished; and also because the inbred
" disease of hospitals will almost inevitably creep, in
" some degree, upon one who continues a long time
" in them, but will rarely attack one, whose stay is
" short.

" Whether they require in a particular manner
" the superintendance of skilful persons, either on ac-
" count of their acute and dangerous nature, or any
" singularity or intricacy attending them, or erro-
" neous opinions prevailing among the common
" people concerning their treatment.

" Whether they be contagious, or subject in a pe-
" culiar degree to taint the air, and generate pesti-
" lential diseases.

" Whether a fresh and pure air be peculiarly re-
" quisite for their cure, and they be remarkably in-
" jured by any vitiation of it."*

XVI. But no precautions relative to the reception
of patients, who labour under maladies incapable of
relief, contagious in their nature, or liable to be aggravated by confinement in an impure atmosphere, can
obviate the evils arising from *close wards*, and the
false œconomy of crowding a number of persons into
the least possible space. There are inbred diseases
which it is the duty of the physician or surgeon to
pervent, as far as lies in his power, by a strict and
persevering attention to the whole medical polity of
the hospital. This comprehends the discrimination

* See Dr. Aikin's Thoughts on Hospitals, p. 21.

of cafes admiffible, air, diet, cleanlinefs, and drugs; each of which articles fhould be fubjeted to a rigid fcrutiny, at ftated periods of time.†

XVII. The eftabli'hment of a *committee* of the *gentlemen* of the *faculty*, to be held monthly, would tend to facilitate this interefting inveftigation, and to accomplifh the moft important objeds of it. By the free communication of remarks, various improvements would be fuggefted; by the regular difcuffion of them, they would be reduced to a definite and confiftent form; and by the authority of united fuffrages, they would have full influence over the governors of the charity. The exertions of individuals, however be-nevolent or judicious, often give rife to jealoufy; are oppofed by thofe who have not been confulted; and prove inefficient, by wanting the colledive energy of numbers.

XVIII. The harmonious intercourfe which has been recommended to the gentlemen of the faculty, will naturally produce *frequent confultations*, viz. of the phyficians on medical cafes, of the furgeons on chirurgical cafes, and of both united in cafes of a com-pound nature, which, falling under the department of each, may admit of elucidation by the reciprocal aid of the two profeffions.

XIX. In confultations on medical cafes, the junior phyfician prefent fhould *deliver* his *opinion* firft, and the others in the progreffive order of their feniority. The fame order fhould be obferved in chirurgical

† See Notes and Illuftrations, No. III.

cafes; and a majority fhould be decifive in both: but if the numbers be equal, the decifion fhould reft with the phyfician or furgeon, under whofe care the patient is placed. No decifion, however, fhould reftrain the acting practitioner from makiug fuch variations in the mode of treatment, as future contingences may require, or a farther infight into the nature of the diforder may fhew to be expedient.

XX. In confultations on mixed cafes, the junior furgeon fhould *deliver* his *opinion* firft, and his brethren afterwards in fucceffion, according to progreffive feniority. The junior phyfician prefent fhould deliver his opinion after the fenior furgeon; and the other phyficians in the order above prefcribed.

XXI. In every confultation, the cafe to be confidered fhould be *concifely ftated* by the phyfician or furgeon, who requefts the aid of his brethren. The opinions relative to it fhould be delivered with brevity, agreeably to the preceding arrangement, and the decifions collected in the fame order. The order of feniority, among the phyficians and furgeons, may be regulated by the dates of their refpective appointments in the hofpital.

XXII. Due *notice* fhould be given of a confultation, and no perfon admitted to it, except the phyficians and furgeons of the hofpital, and the houfe-furgeon, without the unanimous confent of the gentlemen prefent. If an examination of the patient be previoufly neceffary, the particular circumftances of danger or difficulty fhould be carefully concealed from him, and every juft precaution ufed to guard him from anxiety or alarm.

XXIII. No important *operation* fhould be determined upon, without a confultation of the phyficians and furgeons, and the acquiefcence of a majority of them. Twenty-four hours notice fhould be given of the propofed operation, except in dangerous accidents, or when peculiar circumftances occur, which may render delay hazardous. The prefence of a *fpectator* fhould not be allowed during an operation, without the exprefs permiffion of the operator. All extra-official interference in the management of it fhould be forbidden. A decorous *filence* ought to be obferved. It may be humane and falutary, however, for one of the attending phyficians or furgeons to fpeak occafionally to the patient; to comfort him under his fufferings; and to give him affurance, if confiftent with truth, that the operation goes on well, and promifes a fpeedy and fuccefsful termination.*

As a hofpital is the beft fchool for practical furgery, it would be liberal and beneficial to invite, in rotation, two furgeons of the town, who do not belong to the inftitution, to be prefent at each operation.

XXIV. Hofpital confultations ought not to be held on Sundays, except in cafes of urgent neceffity ;

---

* The fubftance of the five preceding articles (xix. xx. xxi. xxii. xxiii.) was fuggefted by Dr. Ferriar and Mr. Simmons, at the time when I was defired, by them and my other colleagues, to frame a code of rules for the Manchefter Infirmary. The additions now made are intended to adapt them to general ufe.

and on fuch occafions an hour fhould be appointed,
which does not interfere with attendance on public
worfhip.

XXV. It is an eftablifhed ufage, in fome hofpitals,
to have a *ftated day* in the week for the performance
of operations. But this may occafion improper delay,
or equally unjuftifiable anticipation. When feveral
operations are to take place in fucceffion, one patient
fhould not have his mind agitated by the knowledge
of the fufferings of another. The furgeon fhould
change his apron, when befmeared; and the table or
inftruments fhould be freed from all marks of blood,
and every thing that may excite terror.

XXVI. Dispensaries afford the wideft fphere
for the treatment of difeafes, comprehending not only
fuch as ordinarily occur, but thofe which are fo infectious, malignant, and fatal, as to be excluded from
admiffion into Infirmaries. Happily, alfo, they neither tend to counteract that fpirit of independence,
which fhould be feduloufly foftered in the poor, nor
to preclude the practical exercife of thofe relative
duties, " the charities of father, fon, and brother,"
which conftitute the ftrongeft moral bonds of fociety.
Being inftitutions lefs fplendid and expenfive than
hofpitals, they are well adapted to towns of moderate fize; and might even be eftablifhed, without
difficulty, in populous country diftricts. Phyficians
and furgeons, in fuch fituations, have generally great
influence; and it would be truly honourable to exert

it in a caufe fubfervient to the interefts of medical
fcience, of commerce, and of philanthropy.*

The duties which devolve on gentlemen of the
faculty, engaged in the conduct of Difpenfaries, are fo
nearly fimilar to thofe of hofpital phyficians and furgeons, as to be comprehended under the fame profeffional and moral rules. But greater *authority* and
greater *condefcenfion* will be found requifite in domeftic attendance on the poor. And human nature
muft be intimately ftudied, to acquire that full afcendancy over the prejudices, the caprices, and the paffions of the fick, and of their relatives, which is
effential to medical fuccefs.

XXVII. Hofpitals, appropriated to particular
maladies, are eftablifhed in different places, and
claim both the patronage and the aid of the gentlemen of the faculty. To an ASYLUM for FEMALE
PATIENTS, labouring under SYPHILIS, it is to be
lamented that difcouragements have been too often
and fuccefsfully oppofed. Yet whoever reflects on
the variety of difeafes to which the human body is
incident, will find, that a confiderable part of them
are derived from immoderate paffions, and vicious
indulgences. Sloth, intemperance, and irregular
defires, are the great fources of thofe evils, which
contract the duration, and embitter the enjoyment, of
life. But humanity, whilft fhe bewails the vices of
mankind, incites us to alleviate the miferies which
flow from them. And it may be proved that a

* See Notes and Illuftrations, No. IV.

Lock Hospital is an inftitution founded on the moft benevolent principles, confonant to found policy, and favourable to reformation and to virtue. It provides relief for a painful and loathfome diftemper, which contaminates, in its progrefs, the innocent as well as the guilty, and extends its baneful influence to future generations. It reftores to virtue and to religion thofe votaries whom pleafure has feduced, or villainy has betrayed; and who now feel, by fad experience, that ruin, mifery, and difgrace, *are the wages of fin.* Over fuch objects pity fheds the generous tear; aufterity foftens into forgivenefs; aud benevolence expands at the united pleas of frailty, penitence, and wretchednefs.*

No *peculiar rules* of conduct are requifite in the medical attendance on Lock Hospitals. But as thefe inftitutions muft, from the nature of their object, be in a great meafure fhut from the infpection of the public, it will behove the faculty to confider themfelves as refponfible, in an extraordinary degree, for their right government; that the moral, no lefs than the medical, purpofes of fuch eftablifhments may be fully anfwered. The ftricteft decorum fhould be obferved in the conduct towards the female patients; no young pupils fhould be admitted into the houfe; every miniftering office fhould be performed by nurfes pro-

---

* See two Reports, intended to promote the eftablifhment of a Lock Hofpital at Manchefter, in the year 1774, inferted in the Author's Effays Medical, Philofophical, and Experimental. Vol. ii. p. 263, 4th edit.

perly inftructed; and books adapted to the moral improvement of the patients fhould be put into their hands, and given them on their difcharge. To provide againft the danger of urgent want, a fmall fum of money, and decent clothes, fhould at this time be difpenfed to them; and when practicable, fome mode fhould be pointed out of obtaining a reputable livelihood.

XXVIII. Asylums for Insanity poffefs accommodations and advantages, of which the poor muft, in all circumftances, be deftitute; and which no private family, however opulent, can provide. Of thefe fchemes of benevolence all claffes of men may have equal occafion to participate the benefits; for human nature itfelf becomes the mournful object of fuch inftitutions. Other difeafes leave man a rational and moral agent, and fometimes improve both the faculties of the head, and the affections of the heart. But lunacy fubverts the whole rational and moral character; extinguifhes every tender charity; and excludes the degraded fufferer from all the enjoyments and advantages of focial intercourfe. Painful is the office of a phyfician, when he is called upon to minifter to fuch humiliating objects of diftrefs: yet great muft be his felicity, when he can render himfelf inftrumental, under Providence, in the reftoration of reafon, and in the renewal of the loft image of God. Let no one, however, promife himfelf this divine privilege, if he be not deeply fkilled in the philofophy of human nature. For though cafual fuccefs may fometimes be the refult of empirical practice, the *medicina mentis* can only be adminiftered with fteady efficacy by him, who, to a knowledge of the animal œconomy, and of the phyfical caufes which regulate or difturb its movements, unites an intimate acquaintance with the laws of affociation ; the controul of fancy over judgment; the force of habit; the direction and comparative ftrength of oppofite paffions; and the reciprocal dependences and relations of the moral and intellectual powers of man.

XXIX. Even thus qualified with the pre-requifite attainments, the phyfician will find that he has a new region of medical fcience to explore. For it is a circumftance to be regretted, both by the faculty and the public, that the various difeafes which are claffed under the title of infanity, remain lefs underftood than any others with which mankind are vifited. Hofpital inftitutions furnifh the beft means of acquiring more accurate knowledge of their caufes, nature, and cure. But this information cannot be attained, to any fatisfactory extent, by the ordinary attention to fingle and unconnected cafes. The fynthetic plan fhould be adopted ; and a regular *journal* fhould be kept of every fpecies of the malady which occurs, arranged under proper heads, with a full detail of its rife, progrefs, and termination ; of the remedies adminiftered, and of their effects in its feveral ftages. The age, fex, occupation, mode of life, and (if poffible) hereditary conftitution of each patient fhould be noted; and when the event proves fatal, the brain, and other organs affe[?]ed, fhould be carefully examined, and the appearances on diffection minutely inferted in the journal. A regifter like this, in the courfe of a few years, would afford the moft interefting and authentic documents; the want of which, on a late melancholy occafion, was felt and regretted by the whole kingdom.

XXX. Lunatics are, in a great meafure, fecluded from the obfervation of thofe who are interefted in their good treatment; and their complaints of ill-ufage are fo often falfe or fanciful, as to obtain little credit or attention, even when well founded. The phyfician, therefore, muft feel himfelf under the ftrifteft obligation of honour, as well as of humanity, to fecure to thefe unhappy fufferers all the *tendernefs* and *indulgence*, compatible with fteady and effectual government.

XXXI. Certain cafes of *mania* feem to require a *boldnefs of practice*, which a young phyfician of fenfibility may feel a reluctance to adopt. On fuch occafions he muft not yield to timidity, but fortify his mind by the councils of his more experienced brethren of the faculty. Yet, with this aid, it is more confonant to probity to err on the fide of caution than of temerity.*

Hofpitals for the fmall-pox, for inoculation, for cancers, &c. &c. are eftablifhed in different places; but require no profeffional duties, which are not included under, or deducible from, the precepts already delivered.

* See Notes and Illuftrations, No. V.

CHAPTER II.

I. THE *moral rules of conduct*, prefcribed towards hofpital patients, fhould be fully adopted in private or general practice. Every cafe, committed to the charge of a phyfician or furgeon, fhould be treated with attention, fteadinefs, and humanity: reafonable indulgence fhould be granted to the mental imbecility and caprices of the fick: fecrecy, and delicacy when required by peculiar circumftances, fhould be ftrictly obferved. And the familiar and confidential inter-courfe, to which the faculty are admitted in their profeffional vifits, fhould be ufed with difcretion, and with the moft fcrupulous regard to fidelity and honour.

II. The ftricteft *temperance* fhould be deemed in-cumbent on the faculty; as the practice both of phyfic and furgery at all times requires the exercife of a clear and vigorous underftanding: and on emergencies, for which no profeffional man fhould be unprepared, a fteady hand, an acute eye, and an unclouded head, may be effential to the well-being, and even to the life, of a fellow-creature. Philip of Macedon repofed with entire fecurity on the vigilance and attention of his general Parmenio. In his hours of mirth and conviviality he was wont to fay, " Let us drink, my " friends; we may do it with fafety, for Parmenio " never drinks!" The moral of this ftory is fuffi-ciently obvious when applied to the faculty; but it fhould certainly be conftrued with great limitation by their patients.*

III. A phyfician fhould not be forward to make gloomy prognoftications; becaufe they favour of empiricifm, by magnifying the importance of his fer-vices in the treatment or cure of the difeafe. But he fhould not fail, on proper occafions, to give to the friends of the patient timely notice of danger, when it really occurs, and even to the patient himfelf, if abfolutely neceffary. This office, however, is fo pe-culiarly alarming, when executed by him, that it ought to be declined, whenever it can be affigned to any other perfon of fufficient judgment and delicacy. For the phyfician fhould be the minifter of hope and comfort to the fick; that by fuch cordials to the drooping fpirit, he may fmooth the bed of death, revive expiring life, and counteract the depreffing in-fluence of thofe maladies, which rob the philofopher of fortitude, and the Chriftian of confolation.†

IV. *Officious interference*, in a cafe under the charge of another, fhould be carefully avoided. No med-

* See Notes and Illuftrations, No. VI.
† See Notes and Illuftrations, No. VII.

dling inquiries fhould be made concerning the patient;
no unneceffary hints given, relative to the nature or
treatment of his diforder; nor any felfifh conduct
purfued, that may directly or indirectly tend to diminifh the truft repofed in the phyfician or furgeon
employed. Yet though the character of a profeffional
bufy-body, whether from thoughtleffnefs or craft, is
highly reprehenfible, there are occafions which not
only juftify but require a fpirited interpofition. When
artful ignorance grofsly impofes on credulity; when
neglect puts to hazard an important life; or rafhnefs
threatens it with ftill more imminent danger; a medical neighbour, friend, or relative, apprized of fuch
facts, will juftly regard his interference as a duty.
But he ought to be careful, that the information, on
which he acts, is well founded; that his motives are
pure and honourable; and that his judgment of the
meafures purfued is built on experience and practical
knowledge, not on fpeculative or theoretical differences of opinion. The particular circumftances of
the cafe will fuggeft the moft proper mode of conduct.
In general, however, a perfonal and confidential application to the gentlemen of the faculty concerned
fhould be the firft ftep taken; and afterwards, if
neceffary, the tranfaction may be communicated to
the patient or to his family.

V. When a phyfician or furgeon is called to a
patient, who has been before under the care of another gentleman of the faculty, a confultation with
him fhould be propofed, even though he may have

difcontinued his vifits : his practice, alfo, fhould be
treated with candour, and juftified, fo far as probity
and truth will permit. For the want of fuccefs in
the primary treatment of a cafe is no impeachment
of profeffional fkill or knowledge ; and it often ferves
to throw light on the nature of a difeafe, and to fuggeft to the fubfequent practitioner more appropriate
means of relief.*

VI. In large and opulent towns, the *diſtinction*
between the *provinces* of *phyſic* and *ſurgery* fhould
be fteadily maintained. This diftinction is fanctioned
both by reafon and experience. It is founded on the
nature and objects of the two profeffions ; on the
education and acquirements requifite for their moft
beneficial and honourable exercife ; and tends to
promote the complete cultivation and advancement
of each. For the divifion of fkill and labour is no
lefs advantageous in the liberal than in the mechanic
arts : and both phyfic and furgery are fo comprehenfive, and yet fo far from perfection, as feparately
to give full fcope to the induftry and genius of their
refpective profeffors. Experience has fully evinced
the benefits of the difcrimination recommended, which
is eftablifhed in every well-regulated hofpital, and is
thus exprefsly authorized by the faculty themfelves,
and by thofe who have the beft opportunities of
judging of the proper application of the healing art.
No phyfician or furgeon, therefore, fhould adopt

---

* See Notes and Illuftrations, No. VIII.

more than one denomination, or affume any rank or privileges different from thofe of his order.

VII. *Confultations* fhould be *promoted*, in difficult or protracted cafes, as they give rife to confidence, energy, and more enlarged views in practice. On fuch occafions no rivalfhip or jealoufy fhould be indulged: candour, probity, and all due refpect fhould be exercifed towards the phyfician or furgeon firft engaged: and as he may be prefumed to be beft acquainted with the patient and with his family, he fhould deliver all the medical directions agreed upon, though he may not have precedency in feniority or rank. It fhould be the province, however, of the fenior phyfician, firft to propofe the neceffary queftions to the fick, but without excluding his affociate from the privilege of making farther enquiries, to fatisfy himfelf, or to elucidate the cafe.

VIII. As circumftances fometimes occur to render a *fpecial confultation* defirable, when the continued attendance of another phyfician or furgeon might be objectionable to the patient, the gentleman of the faculty, whofe affiftance is required, in fuch cafes, fhould pay only two or three vifits; and feduloufly guard againft all future unfolicited interference. For this confultation a double gratuity may reafonably be expected from the patient, as it will be found to require an extraordinary portion both of time and attention.

In medical practice, it is not an unfrequent occurrence, that a phyfician is haftily fummoned, through the anxiety of the family, or the folicitation of friends, to vifit a patient, who is under the regular direction of another phyfician, to whom notice of this call has not been given. Under fuch circumftances, no change in the treatment of the fick perfon fhould be made, till a previous confultation with the ftated phyfician has taken place, unlefs the latenefs of the hour precludes meeting, or the fymptoms of the cafe are too prefling to admit of delay.

IX. *Theoretical difcuffions* fhould be avoided in confultations, as occafioning perplexity and lofs of time. For there may be much diverfity of opinion, concerning fpeculative points, with perfect agreement in thofe modes of practice, which are founded not on hypothefis, but on experience and obfervation.*

X. The rules prefcribed for hofpital confultations may be adopted in private or general practice :† and the *feniority* of a phyfician may be determined by the period of his public and acknowledged practice as a phyfician, and that of a furgeon by the period of his practice as a furgeon, in the place where each refides. This arrangement, being clear and obvious, is adapted to remove all grounds of difpute amongft medical gentlemen, and it fecures the regular continuance of the order of precedency, eftablifhed in every town, which might otherwife be liable to troublefome interruptions by new fettlers, perhaps not long ftationnary.

* See Notes and Illuftrations, No. IX.
† See Articles xix. xx. xxi. chap. i.

XI. A regular *academical education* furnishes the
only prefumptive evidence of profeffional ability, and
is fo honourable and beneficial, that it gives a juft
claim to pre-eminence among phyficians, in proportion
to the degree in which it has been enjoyed and improved: yet as it is not indifpenfably neceffary to the
attainment of knowledge, fkill, and experience, they
who have really acquired, in a competent meafure,
fuch qualifications, without its advantages, fhould
not be faftidioufly excluded from the privileges of
fellowfhip. In confultations, efpecially, as the good
of the patient is the fole object in view, and is often
dependent on perfonal confidence, the aid of an intelligent practitioner ought to be received with candour
and politenefs, and his advice adopted, if agreeable
to found judgment and truth.*

XII. *Punctuality* fhould be obferved in the vifits
of the faculty, when they are to hold confultation
together. But as this may not always be practicable,
the phyfician or furgeon, who firft arrives at the place
of appointment, fhould wait five minutes for his
affociate, before his introduction to the patient, that
the unneceffary repetition of queftions may be avoided:
no vifits fhould be made but in concert, or by mutual
agreement: no ftatement or difcuffion of the cafe
fhould take place before the patient or his friends,
except in the prefence of each of the attending gentlemen of the faculty, and by common confent: and

* See Notes and Illuftrations, No. X.

no *prognostications* should be delivered, which are not the result of previous deliberation and concurrence.

XIII. *Visits* to the sick should not be *unseasonably repeated;* because, when too frequent, they tend to diminish the authority of the physician, to produce instability in his practice, and to give rise to such occasional indulgences, as are subversive of all medical regimen.

Sir William Temple has asserted, that " an honest " physician is excused for leaving his patient, when " he finds the disease growing desperate, and can, " by his attendance, expect only to receive his fees, " without any hopes or appearance of deserving " them." But this allegation is not well founded: for the offices of a physician may continue to be highly useful to the patient, and comforting to the relatives around him, even in the last period of a fatal malady; by obviating despair, by alleviating pain, and by soothing mental anguish. To decline attendance, under such circumstances, would be sacrificing, to fanciful delicacy and mistaken liberality, that moral duty which is independent of, and far superior to, all pecuniary appreciation.

XIV. Whenever a physician or surgeon *officiates* for another, who is sick or absent, during any considerable length of time, he should receive the fees accruing from such additional practice: but if this fraternal act be of short duration, it should be gratuitously performed; with an observance always of the utmost delicacy towards the interest and character of the profeſſional gentleman previouſly connected with the family.

XV. Some general rules ſhould be adopted by the faculty, in every town, relative to the *pecuniary acknowledgments* of their patients; and it ſhould be deemed a point of honour to adhere to this rule, with as much ſteadineſs as varying circumſtances will admit. For it is obvious that an average fee, as ſuited to the general rank of patients, muſt be an inadequate gratuity from the rich, who often require attendance not abſolutely neceſſary; and yet too large to be expected from that claſs of citizens, who would feel a reluctance in calling for aſſiſtance, without making ſome decent and ſatisfactory retribution.

But in the conſideration of fees, let it ever be remembered, that though mean ones from the affluent are both unjuſt and degrading, yet the characteriſtical beneficence of the profeſſion is inconſiſtent with ſordid views, and avaricious rapacity. To a young phyſician, it is of great importance to have clear and definite ideas of the ends of his profeſſion; of the means for their attainment; and of the comparative value and dignity of each. Wealth, rank, and independence, with all the benefits reſulting from them, are the ends which he holds in view; and they are intereſting, wiſe, and laudable. But knowledge, benevolence, and active virtue, the means to be adopted in their acquiſition, are of ſtill higher eſtimation. And he has the privilege and felicity of practiſing an art, even more intrinſically excellent in its mediate than in its ultimate objects. The former, therefore, have a claim to uniform pre-eminence.*

XVI. All members of the profeffion, including apothecaries as well as phyficians and furgeons, together with their wives and children, fhould be attended *gratuitoufly* by any one or more of the faculty, refiding near them, whofe affiftance may be required. For as folicitude obfcures the judgment, and is accompanied with timidity and irrefolution, medical men, under the preffure of ficknefs, either as affecting themfelves or their families, are peculiarly dependent upon each other. But vifits fhonld not be obtruded officioufly; as fuch unafked civility may give rife to embarraffment, or interfere with that choice, on which confidence depends. Diftant members of the faculty, when they requeft attendance, fhould be expected to defray the charges of travelling. And if their circumftances be affluent, a pecuniary acknowledgment fhould not be declined: for no obligation ought to be impofed, which the party would rather compenfate than contract.

XVII. When a phyfician attends the wife or child of a member of the faculty, or any perfon very nearly connected with him, he fhould manifeft peculiar attention to his opinions, and tendernefs even to his prejudices. For the dear and important interefts which the one has at ftake, fuperfede every confideration of rank or feniority in the other; fince the mind

* See Notes and Illuftrations, No. XI.

of a hufband, a father, or a friend, may receive a
deep and lafting wound, if the difeafe terminate fatally, from the adoption of means he could not approve, or the rejection of thofe he wifhed to be tried.
Under fuch delicate circumftances, however, a confcientious phyfician will not lightly facrifice his judgment; but will urge, with proper confidence, the
meafures he deems to be expedient, before he leaves
the final decifion concerning them to his more refponfible coadjutor.

XVIII. Clergymen who experience the *res angufta
domi*, fhould be vifited gratuitoufly by the faculty:
and this exemption fhould be an acknowledged
general rule, that the feeling of individual obligation
may be rendered lefs oppreffive. But fuch of the
clergy as are qualified, either from their ftipends or
fortunes, to make a reafonable remuneration for medical attendance, are not more privileged than any
other order of patients. Military or naval fubaltern
officers, in narrow circumftances, are alfo proper objects of profeffional liberality.

XIX. As the firft *confultation* by *letter* impofes
much more trouble and attention than a perfonal
vifit, it is reafonable, on fuch an occafion, to expect
a gratuity of double the ufual amount: and this
has long been the eftablifhed practice of many refpectable phyficians. But a fubfequent epiftolary
correfpondence, on the further treatment of the fame
diforder, may juftly be regarded in the light of ordinary attendance, and may be compenfated as fuch,

according to the circumſtances of the caſe, or of the patient.

XX. Phyſicians and ſurgeons are occaſionally re-queſted to furniſh certificates, juſtifying the abſence of perſons who hold ſituations of honour and truſt in the army, the navy, or the civil departments of government. Theſe teſtimonials, unleſs under par-ticular circumſtances, ſhould be conſidered as acts due to the public, and therefore not to be compenſated by any gratuity. But they ſhould never be given without an accurate and faithful ſcrutiny into the caſe; that truth and probity may not be violated, nor the good of the community injured, by the unjuſt pre-tences of its ſervants. The ſame conduct is to be obſerved by medical practitioners, when they are ſo-licited to furniſh apologies for non-attendance on juries; or to ſtate the valetudinary incapacity of perſons appointed to execute the buſineſs of conſtables, churchwardens, or overſeers of the poor. No fear of giving umbrage, no view to preſent or future emolument, nor any motives of friendſhip, ſhould incite to a falſe, or even dubious declaration. For the general weal requires that every individual, who is properly qualified, ſhould deem himſelf obliged to execute, when legally called upon, the juridical and municipal employments of the body politic. And to be acceſſary, by untruth or prevarication, to the evaſion of this duty, is at once a high miſdemeanour againſt ſocial order, and a breach of moral and pro-feſſional honour.

XXI. The ufe of *quack medicines* fhould be difcouraged by the faculty, as difgraceful to the profeffion,
injurious to health, and often deftructive even of life.
Patients, however, under lingering diforders, are fome.
times obftinately bent on having recourfe to fuch as
they fee advertifed, or hear recommended, with a
boldnefs and confidence, which no intelligent phyfician dares to adopt, with refpect to the means that
he prefcribes. In thefe cafes, fome indulgence feems
to be required to a credulity that is infurmountable:
and the patient fhould neither incur the difpleafure of
the phyfician, nor be entirely deferted by him. He
may be apprized of the fallacy of his expectations,
whilft affured, at the fame time, that diligent attention
fhould be paid to the procefs of the experiment he is
fo unadvifedly making on himfelf, and the confequent
mifchiefs, if any, obviated as timely as poffible. Certain active preparations, the nature, compofition, and
effects of which are well known, ought not to be
profcribed as quack medicines.

XXII. No phyfician or furgeon fhould difpenfe a
fecret *noftrum*, whether it be his invention, or exclufive property. For if it be of real efficacy, the concealment of it is inconfiftent with beneficence and
profeffional liberality : and if myftery alone give it
value and importance, fuch craft implies either difgraceful ignorance, or fraudulent avarice.

XXIII. The *Efprit du Corps* is a principle of
action founded in human nature, and when duly
regulated, is both rational and laudable. Every man

who enters into a fraternity, engages, by a tacit compact, not only to submit to the laws, but to promote the honour and interest of the-association, so far as they are confistent with morality, and the general good of mankind. A physician, therefore, should cautiously guard against whatever may injure the general respectability of his profession; and should avoid all contumelious representations of the faculty at large; all general charges against their selfishness or improbity; and the indulgence of an affected or jocular scepticism, concerning the efficacy and utility of the healing art.

XXIV. As diversity of opinion and opposition of interest may, in the medical, as in other professions, sometimes occasion *controversy*, and even *contention*; whenever such cases unfortunately occur, and cannot be immediately terminated, they should be referred to the arbitration of a sufficient number of physicians or of surgeons, according to the nature of the dispute; or to the two orders collectively, if belonging both to medicine and surgery. But neither the subject matter of such references, nor the adjudication, should be communicated to the public; as they may be personally injurious to the individuals concerned, and can hardly fail to hurt the general credit of the faculty.

XXV. A wealthy physician should not give advice *gratis* to the affluent; because it is an injury to his professional brethren. The office of physician can never be supported but as a lucrative one; and it

is defrauding, in fome degree, the common funds for
its fupport, when fees are difpenfed with, which
might juftly be claimed.

XXVI. It frequently happens that a phyfician,
in his incidental communications with the patients of
other phyficians, or with their friends, may have
their cafes ftated to him in fo direct a manner, as not
to admit of his declining to pay attention to them.
Under fuch circumftances, his obfervations fhould be
delivered with the moft delicate propriety and referve.
He fhould not interfere in the curative plans purfued;
and fhould even recommend a fteady adherence to
them, if they appear to merit approbation.

XXVII. A phyfician, when vifiting a fick perfon
in the country, may be defired to fee a neighbouring
patient, who is under the regular direction of another
phyfician, in confequence of fome fudden change or
aggravation of fymptoms. The conduct to be purfued on fuch an occafion is to give advice adapted to
prefent circumftances; to interfere no farther than is
abfolutely neceffary with the general plan of treatment; to affume no future direction, unlefs it be
exprefsly defired; and, in this cafe, to requeft an
immediate confultation with the practitioner antecedently employed.

XXVIII. At the clofe of every interefting and
important cafe, efpecially when it hath terminated
fatally, a phyfician fhould trace back, in calm reflection, all the fteps which he had taken in the
treatment of it. This review of the origin, progrefs,

and conclusion of the malady; of the whole curative
plan pursued; and of the particular operation of the
several remedies employed, as well as of the doses and
periods of time in which they were administered; will
furnish the most authentic documents, on which individual experience can be formed. But it is in a
moral view that the practice is here recommended;
and it should be performed with the most scrupulous
impartiality. Let no self-deception be permitted in
the retrospect; and if errors, either of omission or
commission, are discovered, it behoves that they
should be brought fairly and fully to the mental
view. Regrets may follow, but criminality will thus
be obviated. For good intentions, and the imperfection of human skill, which cannot anticipate the
knowledge that events alone disclose, will sufficiently
justify what is past, provided the failure be made
conscientiously subservient to future wisdom and rectitude in professional conduct.

XXIX. The opportunities which a physician not
unfrequently enjoys, of promoting and strengthening
the good resolutions of his patients, suffering under
the consequences of vicious conduct, ought never to
be neglected. And his councils, or even remon-
strances, will give satisfaction, not disgust, if they be
conducted with politeness; and evince a genuine love
of virtue, accompanied by a sincere interest in the
welfare of the person to whom they are addressed.

XXX. The observance of the sabbath is a duty
to which medical men are bound, so far as is compa-

tible with the urgency of the cafes under their charge.
Vifits may often be made with fufficient convenience
and benefit, either before the hours of going to
church, or during the intervals of public worfhip.
And in many chronic ailments, the fick, together with
their attendants, are qualified to participate in the
focial offices of religion; and fhould not be induced
to forego this important privilege, by the expectation
of a call from their phyfician or furgeon.*

XXXI. A phyfician who is advancing in years,
yet unconfcious of any decay in his faculties, may
occafionally experience fome change in the wonted
confidence of his friends. Patients, who before
trufted folely to his care and fkill, may now requeft
that he will join in confultation perhaps with a
younger coadjutor. It behoves him to admit this
change without diffatisfaction or faftidioufnefs, regarding it as no mark of difrefpect; but as the exercife
of a juft and reafonable privilege in thofe by whom
he is employed. The junior practitioner may well be
fuppofed to have more ardour than he poffeffes, in
the treatment of difeafes; to be bolder in the exhi-
bition of new medicines; and difpofed to adminifter
old ones in dofes of greater efficacy. And this union
of enterprize with caution, and of fervour with
coolnefs, may promote the fuccefsful management of
a difficult and protracted cafe. Let the medical parties, therefore, be ftudious to conduct themfelves
towards each other with candour and impartiality;

* See Notes and Illuftrations, No. XII.

co-operating, by mutual conceffions, in the benevolent difcharge of profeffional duty.*

XXXII. The commencement of that period of fenefcence, when it becomes incumbent on a phyfician to decline the offices of his profeffion, it is not eafy to afcertain; and the decifion on fo nice a point muft be left to the moral difcretion of the individual. Becaufe, one grown old in the ufeful and honourable exercife of the healing art may continue to enjoy, and juftly to enjoy, the unabated confidence of the public. And whilft exempt, in a confiderable degree, from the privations and infirmities of age, he is under indif-penfable obligations to apply his knowledge and experience, in the moft efficient way, to the benefit of mankind: for the poffeffion of powers is a clear indication of the will of our Creator, concerning their practical direction. But in the ordinary courfe of nature, the bodily and mental vigour muft be ex-pected to decay progreffively, though perhaps flowly, after the meridian of life is paft. As age advances, therefore, a phyfician fhould, from time to time, fcrutinize impartially the ftate of his faculties; that he may determine, *bona fide*, the precife degree in which he is qualified to execute the active and multi-farious offices of his profeffion. And whenever he becomes confcious that his memory prefents to him with faintnefs thofe analogies, on which medical reafoning and the treatment of difeafes are founded; that diffidence of the meafures to be purfued per-

* See Notes and Illuftrations, No. XIII.

plexes his judgment; that, from a deficiency in the
acuteness of his senses, he finds himself less able to
distinguish signs, or to prognosticate events; he should
at once resolve, though others perceive not the
changes which have taken place, to sacrifice every
consideration of fame or fortune, and to retire from
the engagements of business. To the surgeon under
similar circumstances, this rule of conduct is still more
necessary: for the energy of the understanding
often subsists much longer than the quickness of eye-
sight, delicacy of touch, and steadiness of hand,
which are essential to the skilful performance of
operations. Let both the physician and surgeon
never forget, that their professions are public trusts,
properly rendered lucrative whilst they fulfil them;
but which they are bound, by honour and probity,
to relinquish, as soon as they find themselves unequal
to their adequate and faithful execution.*

* See Notes and Illustrations, No. XIV.

CHAPTER III.

OF THE CONDUCT OF PHYSICIANS TOWARDS APOTHECARIES.

I. IN the prefent ftate of phyfic, in this country, where the profeffion is properly divided into three diftinct branches, a connection peculiarly intimate fubfifts between the phyfician and the apothecary; and various obligations neceffarily refult from it. On the knowledge, fkill, and fidelity of the apothecary, depend, in a very confiderable degree, the reputation, the fuccefs, and ufefulnefs of the phyfician. As thefe qualities, therefore, juftly claim his attention and encouragement, the poffeffor of them merits his refpect and patronage.

II. The apothecary is, in almoft every inftance, the precurfor of the phyfician; and being acquainted with the rife and progrefs of the difeafe, with the hereditary conftitution, habits, and difpofition of the patient, he may furnifh very important information. It is in general, therefore, expedient, and when health or life are at ftake, expediency becomes a moral duty, to confer with the apothecary, before any decifive plan of treatment is adopted; to hear his account of the malady, of the remedies which have been adminiftered, of the effects produced by them, and of his whole experience concerning the *juvantia* and *lædentia* in the cafe. Nor fhould the future attendance of the apothecary be fuperfeded by the phyfician: for if he be a man of honour, judgment, and propriety of behaviour, he will be a moft valuable auxiliary through the whole courfe of the diforder, by his attention to varying fymptoms; by the enforcement of medical directions; by obviating mifapprehenfions in the patient, or his family; by ftrengthening the authority of the phyfician; and by being at all times an eafy and friendly medium of communication. To fubferve thefe important purpofes, the phyfician fhould occafionally make his vifits in conjunction with the apothecary, and regulate by circumftances the frequency of fuch interviews: For if they be often repeated, little fubftantial aid can be expected from the apothecary, becaufe he will have no intelligence to offer which does not fall under the obfervation of the phyfician himfelf; nor any opportunity of executing his *peculiar* truft, without becoming burthenfome to the patient by multiplied calls, and unfeafonable affiduity.

III. This amicable *intercourfe* and *co-operation* of the phyfician and apothecary, if conducted with the *decorum* and attention to *etiquette*, which fhould always be fteadily obferved by profeffional men, will add to the authority of the one, to the refpectability of the other, and to the ufefulnefs of both. The patient will find himfelf the object of watchful and unremitting care, and will experience that he is connected with his phyfician, not only perfonally, but by a fedulous reprefentative and coadjutor. The apothecary will regard the free communication of the phyfician as a privilege and mean of improvement; he will have a deeper intereft in the fuccefs of the curative plans purfued; and h's honour and repu-tation will be directly involved in the purity and excellence of the medicines difpenfed, and in the fkill and care with which they are compounded.

IV. The duty and refponfibility of the phyfician, however, are fo intimately connected with thefe points, that no dependence on the probity of the apothecary fhould prevent the occafional infpection of the drugs which he prefcribes. In London, the law not only authorizes, but enjoins a ftated examination of the fimple and compound medicines kept in the fhops: and the policy that is juft and reafonable in the metropolis, muft be proportionably fo in every provincial town, throughout the kingdom. Nor will any refpectable apothecary object to this neceffary office, when performed with delicacy, and at feafon-able times; fince his reputation and emolument will be increafed by it, probably in the exact *ratio*, thus afcertained, of profeffional merit and integrity.

V. A phyfician called to vifit a patient in the country fhould not only be *minute* in his *directions*, but fhould *communicate* to the apothecary the *parti-cular view* which he takes of the *cafe*; that the indications of cure may be afterwards purfued with precifion and fteadinefs; and that the apothecary may

ufe the difcretionary power committed to him, with
as little deviation as poffible from the general plan
prefcribed.   To fo valuable a clafs of men as the
country apothecaries, great attention and refpeƈt
is due: and as they are the guardians of health
through large diftriƈts, no opportunities fhould be
negleƈted of promoting their improvement, or con-
tributing to their ftock of knowledge, either by the
loan of books, the direƈtion of their ftudies, or by
unreferved information on medical fubjeƈts.   When
fuch occafions prefent themfelves, the maxim of
our judicious poet is ftriƈtly true, " The worft
" avarice is that of fenfe."   For praƈtical improvements ufually originate in towns, and often remain
unknown or difregarded in fituations where gentlemen of the faculty have little intercourfe, and where
fufficient authority is wanting to fanƈtion innovation.

   VI. It has been obferved, by a political and moral
writer of great authority, that " apothecaries' profit
" is become a bye-word, denoting fomething uncom-
" monly extravagant.   This great apparent profit,
" however, is frequently no more than the reafonable
" wages of labour.   The fkill of an apothecary is a
" much nicer and more delicate matter than that of
" any artificer whatever ; and the truft which is re-
" pofed in him is of much greater importance.   He
" is the phyfician of the poor in all cafes, and of the
" rich when the diftrefs or danger is not very great.
" His reward, therefore, ought to be fuitable to his
" fkill and his truft, and it arifes generally from the

" price at which he fells his drugs. But the whole
" drugs which the beſt-employed apothecary in a
" large market town will fell in a year, may not per-
" haps coſt him above thirty or forty pounds.
" Though he ſhould fell them, therefore, for three
" or four hundred, or a thouſand per cent. profit,
" this may frequently be no more than the reaſonable
" wages of his labour charged, in the only way in
" which he can charge them, upon the price of his
" drugs."* The ſtatement here given exceeds the
emoluments of the generality of apothecaries in country diſtriċts: and a phyſician who knows the education, ſkill, and perſevering attention, as well as the
ſacrifice of eaſe, health, and ſometimes even of life,
which this profeſſion requires, ſhould regard it as a
duty not to withdraw, from thoſe who exerciſe it,
any ſources of reaſonable profit, or the honourable
means of advancement in fortune. Two praċtices
prevail in ſome places injurious to the intereſt of this
branch of the faculty, and which ought to be dis-
couraged. One conſiſts in ſuffering preſcriptions to
be ſent to the druggiſt, for the ſake of a ſmall ſaving
in expence: the other in receiving an annual ſtipend,
uſually degrading in its amount, and in the ſervices
it impoſes, for being conſulted on the ſlighter indiſ-
poſitions to which all families are incident, and which
properly fall within the province of the apothecary.

VII. Phyſicians are ſometimes requeſted to viſit
the patients of the apothecary in his abſence. Com-

---

* See Smith's Wealth of Nations, book i. ch. x.

pliance in such cases should always be refused, when
it is likely to interfere with the consultation of the
medical gentleman ordinarily employed by the sick
person, or his family. Indeed this practice is so liable
to abuse, and requires in its exercise so much caution
and delicacy, that it would be for the interest and
honour of the faculty to have it altogether interdicted.
Physicians are the only proper substitutes for physicians; surgeons for surgeons; and apothecaries for
apothecaries.

VIII. When the aid of a physician is required, the
apothecary to the family is frequently called upon to
recommend one. It will then behove him to learn
fully whether the patient or his friends have any preference or partiality; and this he ought to consult,
if it lead not to an improper choice. For the maxim
of Celsus is strictly applicable on such an occasion:
*ubi par scientia, melior est amicus medicus quam ex-
traneus.* But if the parties concerned be entirely
indifferent, the apothecary is bound to decide according to his best judgment, with a conscientious and
exclusive regard to the good of the person for whom
he is commissioned to act. It is not even sufficient
that he selects the person on whom, in sickness, he
reposes his own trust; for in this case friendship justly
gives preponderancy; because it may be supposed
to excite a degree of zeal and attention which might
overbalance superior science or abilities. Without
favour or regard to any personal, family, or professional connections, he should recommend the physician

whom he confcientioufly believes, all circumftances
confidered, to be beft qualified to accomplifh the recovery of the patient.

IX. In the county of Norfolk, and in the city of
London, benevolent inftitutions have been lately
formed, for providing funds to relieve the widows
and children of apothecaries, and occafionally alfo
members of the profeffion who become indigent.
Such fchemes merit the fanction and encouragement
of every liberal phyfician and furgeon. And were
they thus extended, their ufefulnefs would be greatly
increafed, and their permanency almoft with certainty
fecured. Medical fubfcribers, from every part of
Great-Britain, fhould be admitted, if they offer fatisfactory teftimonials of their qualifications. One comprehenfive eftablifhment feems to be more eligible
than many on a fmaller fcale. For it would be conducted with fuperior dignity, regularity, and efficiency; with fewer obftacles from intereft, prejudice,
or rivalfhip; with confiderable faving in the aggregate of time, trouble, and expence; with more accuracy in the calculations relative to its funds, and
confequently with the utmoft practicable extenfion
of its dividends.

CHAPTER IV.

OF PROFESSIONAL DUTIES, IN CERTAIN CASES WHICH REQUIRE A KNOWLEDGE OF LAW.

I. GENTLEMEN of the faculty of phyfic, by the authority of different parliamentary ftatutes, enjoy an exemption from ferving on inquefts or juries; from bearing armour; from being conftables or church-wardens; and from all burdenfome offices, whether leet or parochial. Thefe privileges are founded on reafons highly honourable to medical men; and fhould operate as incentives to that diligent and affiduous difcharge of profeffional duty, which the legiflature has generoufly prefumed to occupy the time, and to employ the talents, of phyficians and furgeons, in fome of the moft important interefts of their fellow-citizens. It is perhaps on account of their being thus excufed from many civil funftions, that Sir William Black-ftone, in his learned Commentaries, judges the ftudy of the law to be lefs effential to them than to any other clafs of men. He obferves, that " there is no " fpecial reafon why gentlemen of the faculty of " phyfic fhould apply themfelves to the ftudy of the " law, unlefs in common with other gentlemen, and " to complete the charafter of general and extenfive

" knowledge, which this profeffion, beyond others,
" has remarkably deferved."* But I apprehend it
will be found that phyficians and furgeons are often
called upon to exercife appropriate duties, which require not only a knowledge of the principles of jurisprudence, but of the forms and regulations adopted
in our courts of judicature. The truth of this obfervation will fufficiently appear from the following *brief
detail* of fome of the principal cafes in which the
fcience of law is of importance to medical practitioners. To enter at large on fo comprehenfive a
fubject, would far exceed the bounds of the prefent
undertaking.

II. When a phyfician attends upon a patient,
under circumftances of imminent danger, his counfel
may be required about the expediency of a *laft will*
and *teftament*. It behoves him, therefore, to know
whether, in cafe of inteftacy, the daughters, or
younger children, of the fick perfon would be legally
entitled to any fhare of his fortune: whether the fortune would be equally divided, when fuch equality
would be improper or unjuft: whether diverfity of
claims and expenfive litigations would enfue, without
a will, from the nature of the property in queftion:
and whether the creditors of the defunct would, by
his neglect, be defrauded of their equitable claims.†

---

* Vol. i. fect. i. Introduction.

† Sir Wm. Blackftone declares it to be effential to a phyfician to
become acquainted with the *form* in which a *will* or *devife* fhould
be drawn up and executed.

For it is a culpable deficiency in our laws, that real
eſtates are not ſubject to the payment of debts by
ſimple contract, unleſs expreſsly charged with them
by the laſt will and teſtament of the proprietor; although credit is often founded, as Dr. Paley well
obſerves, on the poſſeſſion of ſuch eſtates. This acute
moraliſt adds, " He, therefore, who neglects to make
" the neceſſary appointments for the payment of his
" debts, as far as his effects extend, ſins in his grave;
" and if he omit this on purpoſe to defeat the de-
" mands of his creditors, he dies with a deliberate
" fraud in his heart."*

Property is divided by the law into two ſpecies,
perſonal and *real*; each requiring appropriate modes
of transfer or alienation, with which a phyſician
ſhould be well acquainted. It may alſo be required
of him to deliver an opinion, and even a ſolemn judicial evidence, concerning the *capacity* of his patient
to make a *will*, a point ſometimes of difficult and
nice deciſion. For various diſorders obſcure, without
perverting, the intellectual faculties: and even in
delirium itſelf there are lucid intervals, when the memory and judgment become ſufficiently clear, accurate, and vigorous, for the valid execution of a teſtament. In ſuch caſes the will ſhould commence with
the ſignature of the teſtator, concluding with it alſo,
if his hand be not, after continued mental exertions,

* See Paley's Principles of Moral and Political Philoſophy, book
iii. part i. chap. xxiii.

too tremulous for fubfcription; and it fhould be made with all poffible concifenefs, and expedition.''*

If the patient be furprized by fudden and violent ficknefs, the law authorizes a *nuncupative will* in the difpofal of perfonalty. But to guard againft fraud, the teftamentary words muft be delivered with an explicit intention to bequeath; the will muft be made at home, or among the teftator's family and friends, unlefs by unavoidable accident; and alfo in his laft ficknefs: for if he recover, it is evident that time is given for a written will.†

The law excludes from the privilege of making a will *madmen*, *ideots*, perfons in their *dotage*, or thofe who have ftupified their underftandings by drunkennefs. But there is a high degree of hypochondriacifm, which not unfrequently falls under the cognizance of a phyfician, and on which he may be required to decide whether it amounts to mental incapacity for the execution of a laft will and teftament• To define the precife boundaries of rationality is perhaps impoffible ; if it be true, according to Shakefpeare, that " the lunatic, the lover, and the poet are of imagination all compaƈt." But a partially diftempered fancy is known to fubfift with general in-

---

* " In the conftruƈtion of the ftatute, 29 Car. II. ch. iii. it has " been adjudged, that the teftator's name, written with his own " hand, at the beginning of the will, as I John Mills do make this " my laft will and teftament; is a fufficient figning, without any " name at the bottom; though the other is the fafer way." See Blackftone's Comment. book ii. ch. xxiii.

† Id. book ii. c. xxxii.

telligence: And a man, like Mr. Simon Browne, believing the extinction of his rational foul by the judgment of GOD, may uniformly evince, in every other
inſtance, very diſtinguiſhed intellectual powers; and
be capable of directing his concerns, and diſpoſing of
his property, with ſufficient diſcretion. To preclude
one, ſo affected, from being a teſtator, ſeems inconſiſtent either with wiſdom or juſtice; eſpecially if the
will which has been made, diſcover, in its eſſential
parts, no traces of a diſturbed imagination or
unſound judgment. But whenever falſe ideas of
a *practical kind* are ſo firmly united as to be conſtantly and invariably miſtaken for truth, we properly
denominate this unnatural alliance INSANITY: and
if it give riſe to a train of ſubordinate wrong aſſociations, producing incongruity of behaviour, incapacity for the common duties of life, or unconſcious
deviations from morality and religion, MADNESS has
then its commencement.*

III. A lunatic, or *non compos mentis*, in the eye of
the law, is one who has had underſtanding, but has
loſt it by diſeaſe, grief, or other accident. The king
is the truſtee for ſuch unfortunate perſons, appointed
to protect their property, and to account to them, if
they recover, for their revenues, or, after their de-
ceaſe, to their repreſentatives. The Lord Chancellor,
therefore, grants a commiſſion to inquire into the ſtate
of mind of the inſane perſon; and if he be found *non*

---

* See the Author's Moral and Literary Diſſertations, p. 127, ſecond edit.;—alſo Notes and Illuſtrations, No. XV.

compos, by a jury, he ufually commits the care of his
perfon, with a fuitable allowance for his maintenance,
to fome friend, who is then called his committee."*
The phyfician, who has been confulted about the
cafe, will doubtlefs be called upon to deliver an opinion concerning his patient : and before he becomes
acceffary to his deprivation, as it were, of all legal exiftence, he will weigh attentively the whole circumftances of the diforder, the original caufe of it, the
degree in which it fubfifts, its duration, and probable
continuance. For if the malady be not fixed, great,
and permanent, this folemn act of law muft be deemed
inexpedient, becaufe it cannot be reverfed without
difficulty : and when infanity has been once formally declared, there may be grounds of apprehenfion,
that the party will be configned to neglect and oblivion. With regard to the wafte or alienation of property by the perfon thus afflicted, little rifque is incurred, if he be put under the ordinary reftraint of a
judicious *curator.* For whilft his mind remains in
the ftate of alienation, he is incapable of executing
any act with validity; and the next heir or other perfon interefted may fet it afide, on the plea of his incapacity. But the ufe of a guardian or committee of
a lunatic is chiefly to renew, in his right, under the
direction of the Court of Chancery, any leafe for lives
or years, and to apply the profits for the benefit of the
infane perfon, of his heirs, or executors.

* Blackftone's Comment. book i. chap. viii.

IV. The law juftifies the *beating of a lunatic, in
such manner as the circumftances may require.** But
it has been before remarked that a phyfician, who
attends an afylum for infanity, is under an obligation
of honour as well as of humanity, to fecure to the
unhappy fufferers, committed to his charge, all the
tendernefs and indulgence compatible with fteady and
effectual government :† and the ftrait waiftcoat, with
other improvements in modern practice, now preclude
the neceffity of coercion by corporal punifhment.

V. Houfes for the reception of lunatics are fubject
to ftrict regulations of law.   Thefe regulations refer
to the perfons keeping fuch houfes, to the admiffion
of patients into them, and to their infpection by vi-
fitors duly authorifed and qualified.   If any one conceal more than a fingle lunatic without a licence, he
becomes liable to a penalty of five hundred pounds.
The licences in the cities of London and Weftmin-
fter, or within feven miles of the metropolis, are
granted by the College of Phyficians ; who are empowered to elect five of their fellows to act as commiffioners for infpecting the lunatic afylums within
their jurifdiction. Houfes for the reception of lunatics
in the country are to be licenfed by the juftices of
the peace, during their quarter-feffions: and at the
time when the licence is granted, the magiftrates are
d'rected to nominate two of their own body, and alfo
one phyfician, to vifit and infpect fuch licenfed houfes.

* I. Hawkins, 130. Burn's Juftice, vol. iii. p. 117.
† Chap. i. fect. xxx.

This infpection they are empowered to make as often
as they judge it to be expedient; and an allowance
is to be granted for the expences incurred. The
keeper of every licenfed houfe is bound, under the penalty of one hundred pounds, not to admit or confine any perfon as a lunatic, without having a
certificate in writing, under the hand and feal of fome
phyfician, furgeon, or apothecary, that fuch perfon
is proper to be received into the houfe, as being
non compos mentis. And he is further required, under
the fame penalty, to give notice of this certificate to
the fecretary of the commiffioners, appointed either
by the college of phyficians, or the magiftrates
at their quarter-feffions. The act of parliament,
which eftablifhes thefe regulations, ftates this important provifo: " That in all proceedings which fhall
be had under his Majefty's writ of *Habeas Corpus,*
and in all indictments, informations, and actions, that
fhall be preferred or brought againft any perfon or
perfons for confining or ill treating any of his Majefty's fubjects, in any of the faid houfes, the parties
complained of fhall be obliged to juftify their proceedings according to the courfe of the common law, in
the fame manner as if this act had not been made."*

The legal allowance to a medical commiffioner, for
the vifitation and infpection of a lunatic afylum, is
fixed, by the ftatute, at one guinea. This gratuity,
which cannot be regarded as a juft compenfation for

* See Statutes at Large, vol. viii. 14 Geo. III. c. 49.

the time and trouble beſtowed, it may often be proper to decline. For to a phyſician, of a liberal mind, an inadequate pecuniary acknowledgment is felt as a de-gradation; but he will be amply remunerated by the conſcioufneſs of having performed an office, enjoined at once by the laws of humanity and of his country.

VI. In the caſe of *ſudden death*, the law has made proviſion for examining into the cauſe of it by the *Coroner*, an officer appointed for the purpoſe, who is empowered to ſummon ſuch evidence as is neceſſary, for the diſcharge of his inquiſitorial and judicial func-tions. On theſe occaſions, the attendance of a phy-ſician or ſurgeon may often be required, who ſhould be qualified to give teſtimony confonant to legal as well as to medical knowledge. To this end he muſt not only be acquainted with the ſigns of natural death, but alſo of thoſe which occur, when it is produced by accident or violence: and he ſhould not be a ſtranger to the ſeveral diſtinctions of homicide, eſta-bliſhed in our courts of judicature. For the diviſion of this act into *juſtifiable*, *excuſable*, and *felonious*, will aid his inveſtigation, and give preciſion to the opi-nion which he delivers.

VII. When a crime, which the law has adjudged to be capital, is attempted to be committed by force, the reſiſtance of ſuch force, even ſo as to occaſion the death of the offender, is deemed *juſtifiable homicide*. Mr. Locke, in his Eſſay on Government, carries this doctrine to a much greater extent; aſſerting, that " all manner of force without a right upon a man's

" perfon puts him in a ftate of war with the aggreffor,
" and of confequence, being in fuch a ftate of war,
" he may lawfully kill him that puts him under this
" unnatural reftraint."* But Judge Blackftone con-
fiders this conclufion as applicable only to a ftate of
uncivilized nature; and obferves, that the law of
England is too tender of the public peace, too careful
of the life of the fubject, to adopt fo contentious a
fyftem; nor will fuffer with impunity any crime to
be *prevented* by death, unlefs the fame, if committed,
would alfo be punifhed by death.†

VIII. With cafes of juftifiable homicide, however,
gentlemen of the faculty are feldom likely to be profeffionally concerned. But *excufable homicide* may
frequently fall under their cognizance, and require
their deliberate attention, and accurate inveftigation.
It is of two forts; either *per infortunium*, by mifadventure; or *se defendendo*, upon a principle of felf-
prefervation. Death may be the confequence of a
lawful act, done without any intention of hurt. Thus
if an officer, in the correction of a foldier, happen to
occafion his death, it is only mifadventure; ‡ the
punifhment being lawful. But if the correction be
unwarrantably fevere, either in the manner, the inftrument, or the duration of punifhment, and death
enfue, the offender is at leaft guilty of manflaughter,
and in fome circumftances, of murder: a furgeon,

* Effay on Government, Part ii. ch. iii.
† Blackftone's Comment. book iv. ch. xiv. ‡ Ibid.

therefore, is ufually prefent, when foldiers are chaf-
tifed with the lafh in purfuance of the fentence of a
court-martial; and on his teftimony muft depend the
juftification of the mode and degree of punifhment
inflicted.—When medicines adminiftered to a fick patient, with anhoneft defign, to produce the allevia tion
of his pain, or cure of his difeafe, occafion death,
this is mifadventure, in the view of the law; and the
phyfician or furgeon who directed them, is not liable
to punifhment criminally, though a civil action might
formally lie for neglect or ignorance.* But it hath
been holden that fuch immunity is confined to *regular*
phyficians and furgeons. Sir Matthew Hale, however, juftly queftions the legality of this determination; fince phyfic and falves were in ufe before
licenfed phyficians and furgeons. " Wherefore he
" treats the doctrine as apocryphal, andfitted only to
" qualify and flatter licenciates and doctors in phyfic;
" though it may be of ufe to make people cautious
" how they meddle too much in fo dangerous an em-
" ployment." The college of phyficians, however,
within their jurifdiction, which extends feven miles
round London, are vefted by charter with the power
of fine and imprifonment *pro mala praxi.* Yet Dr.
Groenvelt, who was cited, in the year 1693, before
the Cenfors of the College, and committed to Newgate, by a warrant from the prefident, for prefcribing
cantharides in fubftance, was acquitted on the plea

---

* Confult " Efprit des Loix," lib. xxix. ch. xiv.

that bad practice must be accompanied with a bad
intention, to render it criminal. This profecution,
whilst it ruined the doctor's reputation, and injured
his fortune, fo that he is faid to have died in want, excited general attention to the remedy, and afterwards
eftablifhed the ufe of it: though it muft be acknowledged that his dofes were too bold and hazardous.
But whatever be the indulgence of the law towards
medical practitioners, they are bound by a higher authority than that of the moft folemn ftatute, not to
exercife the healing art without due knowledge, tendernefs, and difcretion : And every rafh experiment,
every miftake originating from grofs inattention, or
from that ignorance which neceffarily refults from defective education, is, in the eye of confcience, a crime
both againft GOD and man.

It muft frequently devolve on the faculty to decide concerning the nature and effects of blows,
ftrokes, or wounds inflicted; and how far the death
of the fufferer is to be afcribed to them, or to fome
antecedent or fubfequent difeafe. In homicide, alfo,
se defendendo, the manner and time of the defence
are to be confidered. For if the perfon affaulted fall
upon the aggreffor, when the fray is over and he is
running away, this is revenge and not defence: and
though no witnefs were prefent, the fituation of the
wound or of the blow would afford, if in the back of
the affailant, prefumptive evidence of *felonious homicide*.

IX. This crime, which in atrocity exceeds every other, is confidered by the law under the three heads of *fuicide*, *manflaughter*, and *murder*; concerning each of which the faculty are occafionally obliged to give profeffional evidence. A *felo de se* is one who has deliberately put an end to his exiftence, or committed any unlawful malicious act, the immediate confequence of which proved death to himfelf. To conftitute this act a crime, the party muft have been of years of difcretion, and in the poffeffion of reafon. A phyfician, therefore, may be called upon, by the coroner, to ftate his opinion of the mental capacity of the defunct: and the law will not authorife the plea, that every melancholic or hypochrondriac fit deprives a man of the power of difcerning right from wrong. Even if a lunatic kill himfelf in a lucid in-terval, Sir M. Hale affirms that he is a *felo de se:* And the phyfician who has attended him, is beft qualified to judge of the degree, the duration, or periodical feafons of fuch returns of fanity. But there are cafes of temporary diftraction, when death may be rufhed upon apparently with defign, but really from the influence of terror, or the want of that prefence of mind, which is neceffary to the exercife of judgment, and the difcrimination of actual from imaginary evil. Of this kind the reader will find an affecting inftance, related by Dr. Hunter, in the Medical Obfervations and Inquiries publifhed by a Society of Phyficians, in London."*

* Vol. vi. p. 279.

X. *Manflaughter* is defined "the unlawful killing " of another, without malice, exprefs or implied; " which may be either *voluntarily*, upon a fudden " heat; or *involuntarily*, but in the commiffion of " fome unlawful act." Yet though this definition is delivered from Sir Matthew Hale, by the excellent commentator on the laws of England fo often quoted, it is not fufficiently precife and comprehenfive. For when a perfon does an act lawful in itfelf, but which proves fatal to a fellow-citizen, becaufe done without due circumfpection, it may, according to circumftances, be either mifadventure, manflaughter, or murder. Thus when a workman kills any one, by flinging down a ftone or piece of timber into the ftreet, if the accident be in a country village, where there are few paffengers, and if he give warning by calling out to them, it is only mifadventure : But if it be in London, or any other populous town, where perfons are continually paffing, it is manflaughter, though warning be loudly given: And it is murder, if he know of their paffing, and yet gives no warning ; for this is malice againft all mankind.*

On the like grounds we may reafon concerning the cafes of death, occafioned by drugs defigned to produce abortion. This purpofe is not always unlawful: for the configuration of the *pelvis* in fome females is fuch as to render the birth of a full-grown child impoffible, or inevitably fatal. But even in

---

* Blackftone's Comment. book. iv. ch. xiv.

such instances the guilt of manslaughter may be incurred by ignorance of the drastic quality of the medicine prescribed, or want of due caution in the dose administered: and when no moral or salutary end is in view, the simple act itself, if fatal in the issue, falls under the denomination of murder.† "If a "woman be quick with child, and, by a potion or "otherwise, killeth it in her womb, this is a great "misprision, yet no murder : but if the child be born "alive, and dieth of the potion or other cause, this "is murder."‡ The procuring of abortions was common amongst the Romans; and it is said, was liable to no penalty before the reigns of Severus and Antoninus. Even those princes made it criminal only in the case of a married woman practising it to defraud her husband of the comforts of children, from motives of resentment. For the *foetus* being regarded as a portion of the womb of the mother, she was supposed to have an equal and full right over both. This false opinion may have its influence in modern, as well as in ancient times; and false it must be deemed, since no female can be privileged to injure her own bowels, much less the *foetus*, which is now well known to constitute no part of them. To extinguish the first spark of life is a crime of the same nature, both against our Maker and society, as to destroy an infant, a child, or a man; these regular and successive stages of existence being the ordinances of

† See Burn's Justice of Peace, vol. i. page 216.
‡ Id. vol. ii. p. 110.

God, fubject alone to his divine will, and appointed by fovereign wifdom and goodnefs as the exclufive means of preferving the race, and multiplying the enjoyments, of mankind. Hence the father of phyfic, in the oath enjoined on his pupils, which fome univerfities now impofe on the candidates for medical degrees, obliged them folemnly to abjure the practice of adminiftering the τεσσος φθοριος. But in weighing the charge againft any perfon of having procured abortion, the methods employed fhould be attentively confidered by the faculty; as this effect has often been afcribed to caufes inadequate to its production. Even the peffary, fo fanctimonioufly forbidden by Hippocrates, has little of that activity and power, which fuperftition affigned to it.

XI. The law of England guards, with affiduous care, the lives of infants, when endangered by motives which counteract, and too often overbalance, the ftrong operation of maternal love. In cafes of *baftardy*, therefore, it is declared, by a ftatute paffed in the reign of James I. that " If any woman be de-
" livered of any iffue of her body, male or female,
" which being born alive, fhould by the laws of this
" realm be a baftard, and fhe endeavour privately,
" either by drowning, or fecret burying thereof, or
" any other way, either by herfelf, or the procuring
" of others, fo to conceal the death thereof, as that
" it may not come to light whether it was born alive
" or not, but be concealed, fhe fhall fuffer death, as
" in cafe of murder; except fhe can prove, by one

" witnefs at leaft, that the child was born dead."*
This law, though humane in its principle, is much
too fevere in its conftruction.   To give certainty to
punifhment, by facilitating conviction, is doubtlefs an
effential object of jurifprudence: and it has been
well obferved, that the ftatute, which made the poffeffion of the implements of coining a capital offence,
by conftituting fuch poffeffion complete evidence of
guilt, has proved the moft effectual mean of enforcing
the denunciation of law againft this dangerous and
tempting crime.†   But the analogy, which the able
moralift has drawn between this ordinance and that
relating to baftardy, is not fully conclufive.   For
poffeffion, in the former cafe, clearly implies a fpecific
purpofe, for which the legiflature, with fufficient
wifdom and juftice, has provided a fpecific punifhment:
whereas fecrecy in the mother, concerning the death
of her illegitimate offspring, hardly amounts to the
loweft degree of prefumptive evidence of felonious
homicide.   Gentlemen of the faculty have often melancholy experience of the diftraction and mifery,
which females fuffer under thefe unhappy circumftances: and when it becomes their painful office to deliver evidence on fuch occafions, juftice and humanity
require, that they fhould fcrutinize the whole truth,
and *nothing extenuate, nor fet down aught in malice.*
" What is commonly underftood to be the murder of
" a baftard child by the mother," fays Dr. Hunter,

* Burn's Juftice, vol. i. p. 216.
† See Paley's Moral and Political Philofophy, 4to. p. 350.

"if the real circumftances were fully known, would
"be allowed to be a very different crime in different
"circumftances. In fome (it is to be hoped *rare*)
"inftances, it is a crime of the very deepeft dye." . . .
"But, as well as I can judge, the greateft number of
"what are called murders of baftard children, are of a
"very different kind. The mother has an uncon-
"querable fenfe of fhame, and pants after the pre-
"fervation of character: fo far fhe is virtuous and
"amiable. She has not the refolution to meet and
"avow infamy. In proportion as fhe lofes the hope
"either of having been miftaken with regard to
"pregnancy, or of being relieved from her terrors by
"a fortunate mifcarriage, fhe every day fees her dan-
"ger greater and nearer, and her mind overwhelmed
"with terror and defpair. In this fituation many
"of thefe women, who are afterwards accufed of
"murder, would deftroy themfelves, if they did not
"know that fuch an action would infallibly lead to
"an inquiry, which would proclaim what they are
"fo anxious to conceal. In this perplexity, and
"meaning nothing lefs than the murder of the in-
"fant, they are meditating different fchemes for con-
"cealing the death of the child; but are wavering
"between difficulties on all fides, putting the evil
"hour off, and trufting too much to chance and for-
"tune. In that ftate often they are overtaken be-
"fore they expect it; their fchemes are fruftrated;
"their diftrefs of body and mind deprives them of
"all judgment and rational conduct; they are deli-

" vered by themfelves wherever they happen to retire
" in their fright or confufion; fometimes dying in the
" agonies of child-birth; and fometimes being quite
" exhaufted, they faint away, and become infenfible
" of what is paffing; and when they recover a little
" ftrength, find that the child, whether ftill-born or
" not, is completely lifelefs.   In fuch a cafe, is it to
" be expected, when it would anfwer no purpofe,
" that a woman fhould divulge the fecret?   Will not
" the beft difpofitions of mind urge her to preferve
" her character?   She will therefore hide every ap-
" pearance of what has happened as well as fhe can,
" though, if the difcovery be made, that conduct will
" be fet down as a proof of her guilt." . . . " Here
" let us fuppofe a cafe, which every body will
" allow to be very poffible:—An unmarried wo-
" man becoming pregnant is ftriving to conceal her
" fhame, and laying the beft fcheme that fhe can
" devife, for faving her own life and that of the child,
" and at the fame time concealing the fecret; but her
" plan is at once difconcerted by her being taken ill
" by herfelf, and delivered of a dead child.   If the
" law punifh fuch a woman with death for con-
" cealing her fhame, does it not require more from
" human nature, than weak human nature can bear ?
" In a cafe fo circumftanced, furely the only crime is
" the having been pregnant, which the law does not
" mean to punifh with death; and the attempt to
" conceal it by fair means fhould not be punifhable

" with death, as that attempt feems to arife from a
" principle of virtuous fhame."*

The obfervations here quoted have a juft claim to
attention, from the extenfive experience which the
author poffeffed, and ftill more from his intimate
knowledge of the female chara&ter. Yet to the
moral and political philofopher, Dr. Hunter may
appear to have exalted the fenfe of fhame into the
principle of virtue; and to have miftaken the great
end of penal law, which is not vengeance, but the
prevention of crimes. The ftatute, indeed, which
makes the concealment of the birth of a baftard child
full proof of murder, confounds all diftin&tions of innocence and guilt; as fuch concealment, whenever
pra&ticable, would be the wifh and a&t of all mothers,
amiable or vicious, under the fame unhappy predicament. Law, however, which is the guardian and
bulwark of the public weal, muft maintain a fteady
and even rigid watch over the general tendencies of
human a&tions: and when thefe are not only clearly
underftood, but interpreted according to the rules of
wifdom and re&titude, that may juftly be conftituted a
civil crime, which, if permitted, might give occafion
to atrocious guilt, though in its own nature innocent.
The meafure of punifhment, however, fhould be
proportionate, as nearly as poffible, to the temptation
to offend, and to the kind and degree of evil produced by the offence. If inadequate to the former,
it will be nugatory; and if too fevere for the latter,

* Med. Obf. and Inq. vol. vi. p. 271, et feq.

it will defeat itfelf, by furnifhing a juft plea for fuper-feding its execution.* A revifion of our fanguinary ftatutes is much wanted ; and it would be happy if means could be devifed of fuppreffing the punifhment, by obviating the crime, when it is merely pofitive or municipal. This we have feen accomplifhed with refpect to the coinage of money, by the fimple intro-duction of a ftandard weight in the payment of gold: and a fagacious legiflator might doubtlefs difcover and adopt fimilar improvements in other branches of penal jurifprudence.

Much obfervation is required to difcriminate be-tween a child ftill-born, and one that has lived after birth only a fhort fpace of time. Various appear-ances, alfo, both internal and external, may be miftaken for marks of violent death. Even the fwimming of the lungs in water, a teft on which fo much reliance is placed, will, on many occafions, be found fallacious. But thefe are points of profeffional fcience, which do not ftrictly fall under the fubject of this fection; and the reader is particularly referred to the paper already quoted, and alfo to the *Elementa Medicinæ Forenfis Joh. Fred. Fafelii;* or to a valuable epitome of the fame work in Englifh by Dr. Farr.†

---

* " L' atrocité des lois en empêche l'exécution.
" Lorfque la peine eft fans mefure, on eft fouvent obligé
    de lui préférer l'impunité."——MONTESQUIEU.

† Elements of Medical Jurifprudence; or a fuccinct and compen-dious Defcription of fuch Tokens in the Human Body, as are requi-fite to determine the Judgment of a Coroner, and of Courts of Law, in Cafes of Divorce, Rape, Murder, &c. London, Becket, 1788.

XII. *Duelling* is another fpecies of felony, even though the confequences of it fhould not prove fatal: and gentlemen of the faculty are peculiarly interefted in the knowledge of the laws relating to it; becaufe they are not only liable to be fummoned on the trial of the parties, if either or both of them be wounded, but are frequently profeffional attendants on them in the field of combat. It is aftonifhing that a practice, which originated in ages of Gothic ignorance, fuperftition, and barbarifm, fhould be continued in the prefent enlightened period, though condemned by the ordinances of every ftate, and repugnant to the fpirit and precepts of Chriftianity. Sir Francis Bacon, when attorney-general, in the reign of James I. delivered a charge, before the court of Star-Chamber, touching duels, which gives a clear and animated view of the light in which they were then regarded. " The firft " motive," he fays, " is a falfe and erroneous ima-" gination of honour and credit; and therefore the " king, in his proclamation, doth moft aptly call them " *bewitching duels*. For if one judge of it truly, it is " no better than a forcery, that enchanteth the fpi-" rits of young men; and a kind of fatanical illufion " and apparition of honour againft religion, againft " law, and againft moral virtue. Hereunto may be " added, that men have almoft loft the true notion " and underftanding of fortitude and valour. For " fortitude diftinguifheth of the grounds of quarrels, " whether they be juft; and not only fo, but whether " they be worthy; and fetteth a better price upon

" men's lives than to beſtow them idly. Nay, it is
" weakneſs and diſeſteem of a man's ſelf, to put a
" man's life upon ſuch liedger performances : a man's
" life is not to be trifled away ; it is to be offered up
" and ſacrificed to honourable ſervices, public merits,
" good cauſes, and noble adventures. It is in expence
" of blood, as it is in expence of money ; it is no
" liberality to make a profuſion of money upon every
" vain occaſion ; nor no more is it fortitude to make
" effuſion of blood, except the cauſe be of worth."*

The decree of the Star-Chamber againſt Prieſt and
Wright, the objeƈts of Sir Francis Bacon's charge,
was, that they ſhould both be committed to priſon ;
that the former ſhould be fined 500l. and the latter
500 marks ; and that at the next aſſizes they ſhould
publickly acknowledge their high contempt of and
offence againſt GOD, the king's majeſty, and his
laws, ſhewing themſelves penitent for the ſame.—
Though this judgment appears to have been founded
in wiſdom and equity, yet, happily for our country,
the court, which paſſed the ſentence, has been long
ſuppreſſed ; and we are now governed not by arbitrary will, but by known and fixed laws. Thoſe
which ſubſiſt againſt duelling, I ſhall quote on the
authorities of Foſter, Blackſtone, Hawkins, and Burn.
" Deliberate duelling, if death enſueth, is, in the
" eye of the law, murder ; for duels are generally
" founded in deep revenge ; and though a perſon
" ſhould be drawn into a duel, not upon a motive ſo

* Bacon's Works, 4to. Birch's edit. vol. ii. p. 565.

" fo criminal, but merely upon the punctilip of what
" the fwordfmen falfely call honour, that will not
" excufe; for he that deliberately feeketh the blood
" of another upon a private quarrel, acteth in defi-
" ance of all laws human and divine."* " Exprefs
" malice is when one, with a fedate deliberate mind
" and formed defign, doth kill another. This takes
" in the cafe of deliberate duelling, where both par-
" ties meet avowedly, with any intent to murder;
" thinking it their duty as gentlemen, and claiming it
" as their right, to wanton with their own lives, and
" thofe of their fellow-creatures, without any war-
" rant or authority from any power either human or
" divine, but in direct contradiction to the laws both of
" GOD and man. And therefore, the law has juftly
" fixed the crime and punifhment of murder on them,
" and on their feconds alfo."†—" The law fo abhors
" all duelling in cold blood, that not only the prin-
" cipal who actually kills the other, but alfo his
" feconds, are guilty of murder, whether they fought
" or not: and it is holden that the feconds of the
" party flain are alfo guilty as acceffaries."‡ From
variations in the moral and intellectual character of
man, it is impoffible to afcertain the precife period,
when the paffions may be fuppofed to become cool,
after having been violently agitated. Judgment,

---

* Sir Michael Fofter's Reports, 8vo. p. 297.

† Blackftone's Comment. book iv. ch. xiv.

‡ I. Hawkins, 82; and Burn's Juftice, vol. ii. p. 509.

therefore, muſt be founded on the circumſtances of deliberation, which are delivered in the courſe of evidence. In many caſes, it has been determined that death, in conſequence of an appointment and meeting, a few hours ſubſequent to the provocation, is murder.*

XIII. Before a ſurgeon engage profeſſionally to *attend* a *duelliſt* to the *field* of *combat*, it behoves him to conſider well, not only how far he is about to countenance a deliberate violation of the duties of morality and religion; but whether, in the conſtruction of law, he may not be deemed an aider and abettor of a crime, which involves in it ſuch turpitude, that death is alike denounced againſt the principal and the acceſſary. Does he not voluntarily put himſelf into a predicament ſimilar, in many eſſential points, to that of the *ſecond*, who is expreſsly condemned by the legiſlature of this country? Both are apprized of the purpoſe to commit an act of felony ; both take an intereſt in the circumſtances attendant upon it; and both are preſent during the execution; the one to regulate its antecedents, the other to alleviate its conſequences. But I ſuggeſt theſe conſiderations with much diffidence; and though I obſerve ſome paſſages in Sir Michael Foſter's Diſcourſe concerning Accomplices, which ſeem to confirm them; yet it may be proper to quote the following, apparently adverſe, opinion of this excellent judge. " In

* See Legg's ca. Kelyng, 27 ; Eden's Principles of Penal Law, p. 224.

" order to render a perfon an accomplice and a prin-
" cipal in felony, he muft be aiding and abetting at
" the fact, or ready to afford affiftance, if neceffary.
" And therefore, if A happeneth to be prefent at a
" murder, for inftance, and taketh no part in it, nor
" endeavoureth to prevent it, nor apprehendeth the
" murderer, nor levieth hue and cry after him ; this
" ftrange behaviour of his, though highly criminal,
" will not of itfelf render him either principal or
" acceffary."*

But whatever be the objections againft the attendance of a furgeon in the field of combat, they cannot
be conftrued to extend to the affording of all poffible
affiftance to any unfortunate fufferer in an affair of
honour; provided fuch affiftance be not preconcerted,
but required as in ordinary accidents or emergencies.
For in the offices of the healing art, no difcrimination
can be made, either of occafions or of characters :
and it muft be acknowledged, that many of the vic-
tims of duelling have been men, from their talents
and virtues, poffeffing the jufteft claim to affiduous
and tender attention. That lives of fuch ineftimable
value to their friends, to their families, and to the
public, fhould be at the mercy of any profligate rake,
who wantonly gives affronts, or idly fancies he receives them, is a great aggravation of the folly, as
well as of the guilt of duelling. This reflection feems
to fhew the propriety of a change in the penal code,

* Fofter's Crown Law, 8vo. p. 350.

refpecting it; and that the punifhment inflicted fhould
be confined to the aggreffor; ftrict inquifition into
the circumftances of the cafe being previoufly made
by the coroner, or fome magiftrate authorized and
bound to exercife this important truft. And he may,
with reafon, be regarded as the aggreffor, who either
violates the rules of decorum, by any unprovoked
rudenefs or infult; or who converts into an offence
what was intended only as convivial pleafantry.*

XIV. A phyfician has no fpecial intereft in an acquaintance with the ftatutes relative to duelling. But
as he poffeffes the rank of a gentleman, both by his
liberal education and profeffion, the *law of honour*, if
that may be termed a law which is indefinite and
arbitrary, has a claim to his ferious ftudy and attention : as a philofopher, alfo, it becomes him to trace
its origin, and to inveftigate the principles on which
it is founded: and as a moralift, duty calls upon him
to counteract its baneful influence and afcendancy.
For, in principle, it is diftinct from virtue ; and, as a
practical rule, it extends only to certain formalities
and decorums, of little importance in the tranfactions
of life, and which are fpontaneoufly obferved by thofe,
who are actuated with the true fenfe of propriety and
rectitude. Genuine honour, in its full extent, may
be defined a quick perception and ftrong feeling of
moral obligation, in conjunction with an acute fenfibility to fhame, reproach, or infamy. In different

* See Notes and Illuftrations, No. XVI.

characters, thefe conftituent parts of the principle are found to exift in proportions fo diverfified, as fometimes to appear almoft fingle and detached. The former always *aids and ftrengthens virtue*; the latter may occafionally *imitate her actions*,* when fafhion happily countenances, or high example prompts to rectitude. But being connected, for the moft part, with a jealous pride and capricious irritability, it will be more fhocked with the *imputation*, than with the *commiffion* of what is wrong. And thus it will conftitute that fpurious honour, which, by a perverfion of the laws of affociation, *puts evil for good, and good for evil;* and, under the fanction of a name, perpetrates crimes without remorfe, and even without ignominy.†

XV. *Homicide* by *poifon* is another very important object of medical jurifprudence. When it is the effect of inadvertency, or the want of adequate caution, in the ufe of fubftances dangerous to health and life, the law regards it as a mifdemeanour: When it is the confequence of rafhnefs, of wanton experiment, or of motives unjuft, though not malicious,‡ it be-

---

* Addifon's Cato.

† See the Author's Mor. and Lit. Diff. p. 295, 2d edit.

‡ " If an action unlawful itfelf be done deliberately, and *with
" intention of mifchief*, or great bodily harm to particulars, or of
" mifchief indifcriminately, fall it where it may, and death enfue
" againft or befide the original intention of the party, it will be
" murder. But if fuch *mifchievous intention* doth not appear, which
" is matter of fact, and *to be collected from circumftances*, and the
" act was done heedlefsly and incautioufly, it will be manflaughter;
" not accidental death, becaufe the act which enfued was unlawful."
Fofter, p. 261.

comes manflaughter: And when the exprefs purpofe
is to kill, by means of fome deleterious drug, it conftitutes a moft atrocious fpecies of murder.   In cafes
of this nature, the faculty are called upon to give evidence concerning the nature of the poifon, the fymptoms produced by it, and the actual fatality of its
operation.   The period of this fatal operation is extended, as in the infliction of blows and wounds, to
a year and a day.   But if it be, the moft nice and
accurate inveftigation of the progreffive advances of
difeafe and death will be incumbent on the phyfician
or furgeon, who is confulted on the occafion.   No
fubject has given rife to more mifconception and fuperftition, than the action of poifons.   Numberlefs
fubftances have been claffed as fuch, which, if not
inert, are at leaft innoxious ; and powers have been
afcribed to others, far exceeding their real energy.
Even Lord Verulam, the great luminary of fcience,
in his charge againft the Earl of Somerfet, for the
murder of Sir Thomas Overbury, in the Tower of
London, feems to give credit to the ftory of Livia,
who is faid to have poifoned the figs upon the tree,
which her hufband was wont to gather with his own
hands.   And he ferioufly ftates, that " Wefton
" chafed the poor prifoner with poifon after poifon;
" poifoning falts, poifoning meats, poifoning fweet-
" meats, poifoning medicines and vomits, until at laft
" his body was almoft come, by the ufe of poifons,
" to the ftate that Mithridates's body was by the
" ufe of treacle and prefervatives, that the force of

" the poifons was blunted upon him: Wefton con-
" feffing, when he was tried for not difpatching him,
" that he had given enough to poifon twenty men."*
In this criminal tranfaction the truth probably was,
what has been judicioufly fuggefted by Rapin, that
the lieutenant of the tower, refufing to be concerned
in the crime, yet not daring to difcover it, from the
fear of the Vifcount Rochefter's refentment, feized
the victuals fent from time to time for the prifoner,
and threw them into the houfe of office. Sir Thomas
Overbury, however, fell a victim at laft to an em-
poifoned glyfter.

When the particular drug, or other mean employed,
can be accurately afcertained, its deleterious qualities
fhould be fully inveftigated; and thefe fhould be
cautioufly compared with the effects afcribed to it, in
the cafe under confideration. It may often be expedient, alfo, to examine the body of the fufferer by
diffection; and this fhould be accomplifhed as expe-
ditioufly as poffible; that the changes imputed to
death may not be confounded with thofe which are
imputed to poifon. But on fuch points reference can
alone be made to the knowledge and experience of
the practitioner, and to the lights which he may acquire by confulting Fafelius, and other works of a
fimilar nature. I fhall, therefore, clofe this article
with a few paffages of the charge of Mr. Juftice
Buller to the grand jury, relative to the trial of

* Bacon's Works, vol. ii. p. 614.

Capt. Donellan, for the murder of Sir Theodofius Boughton, at the Warwick affizes, in March 1781. " In this cafe, gentlemen," he fays, " you will have " two objects to confider; firft, whether the deceafed " did die of *poifon?* fecondly, whether·the perfon " fufpected did affift in *adminiftering* the poifon? " With refpect to the firft of thefe confiderations, " you will, no doubt, *hear the fentiments of thofe who* " *are fkilled in the nature and effects of poifon,* which " is of various forts, and moft fubtile in its operation. " From the *information* of fuch perfons you will be " able to form an opinion of the effects which *different* " *poifons* have on *different perfons;* and alfo the effects " the *fame poifons* have on perfons of *different habits* " *and conftitutions.* If you find he did get his death " by poifon ; the next cafe is, to confider who gave " him that poifon? Where poifon is knowingly given, " and death enfues, it is wilful murder; and if one " *who knows what is intended,* be prefent, when " poifon is given by another, he is not an acceffary, " but a principal."*

XVI. In all civilized countries, the honour and chaftity of the female fex are guarded from violence, by the fevereft fanctions of law. And this protection is at once humane, juft, and neceffary to focial morality. It is confonant to humanity that weaknefs fhould be fecure againft the attacks of brutal ftrength: it is juft that the moft facred of all perfonal property

* Hift. Sketches of Civil Liberty, p. 209.

fhould be preferved from invafion:—and it is effential
to morality that licentious paffion fhould be reftrained;
that modefty fhould not be wounded; nor the mind
contaminated, in fome inftances, before it is capable
of forming adequate conceptions of right and wrong.
The crime of *rape*, therefore, fubjefts the perpetrator
to condign punifhment by every code of jurifprudence,
ancient or modern.*   Amongft the Jews death was
inflifted, if the damfel were betrothed to another
man: and if not betrothed, a fine, amounting to fifty
fhekels of filver, was to be paid to her father by him
who had *laid hold of the virgin*, and fhe was to become his wife: and becaufe *he had humbled her*, *he*
might not put her away all his days :† for the privilege of divorce was authorized by the Jewifh inftitutions.   The Romans made this offence capital,
fuperadding the confifcation of goods.   Even the
carrying-off a woman from her parents or guardians,
and cohabiting with her, whether accomplifhed by
force, or with her full confent, were made equally
penal with a rape, by an imperial edift.   For the
Roman law feems to have fuppofed, that women
never deviate from virtue, without being feduced by
the arts of the other fex: and, therefore, by impofing a powerful reftraint on the folicitations of men,
they aimed at a more effeftual fecurity of the chaftity
of women.   *Nifi etenim eam folicitaverit, nifi odiofis*

* See Notes and Illuftrations, No. XVII.
† Deuteronomy xxii. 28, 29.

artibus circumvenerit, non faciet eam velle in tantum dedecus sese prodere. But the Englifh law, as Judge Blackftone has obferved, does not entertain fuch fub-lime ideas of the honour of either fex, as to lay the blame of a mutual fault on one only of the trans-greffors: and it is, therefore, effential to the crime of rape, that the woman's will is violated by the execution. But, by a ftatute of·Queen Elizabeth, if the crime be perpetrated on a female child under the age of *ten* years, the confent or non-confent is immaterial, as fhe is fuppofed to be of infufficient judgment. Sir Matthew Hale is even of opinion, that fuch profligacy committed on an infant under *twelve* years, the age of female difcretion by common law, either with or without confent, amounts to a rape and felony. But the decifions of the courts have, generally, been founded on the ftatute above-mentioned.

A male infant, under the age of fourteen years, is deemed, by the law, incapable of committing, and therefore cannot be found guilty of a rape, from a prefumed imbecility both of body and mind. This deteftable crime being executed in fecrecy, and the knowledge of it being confined to the party injured, it is juft that her fingle teftimony fhould be adducible in proof of the fact. Yet the excellent obfervation of Sir Matthew Hale merits peculiar attention: " It " is an accufation," fays he, " eafy to be made, and " harder to be proved; but harder to be defended " by the party accufed, though innocent." He then

relates two extraordinary cafes of malicious profecution for this crime, which had fallen under his own
cognizance; and concludes, "I mention thefe in-
"ftances, that we may be more cautious upon trials
"of offences of this nature, wherein the court and
"jury may, with fo much eafe, be impofed upon,
"without great care and vigilance; the heinoufnefs of
"the offence many times tranfporting the judge and
"jury with fo much indignation, that they are over-
"haftily carried to the conviction of the perfon ac-
"cufed thereof, by the confident teftimony of fome-
"times falfe and malicious witneffes." Collateral
and concurrent circumftances of time and place;*
appearances of violence on examination, &c. are,
therefore, neceffary to be added to the mere affirmative evidence of the profecutor. And the infpeftion
of a furgeon is often required, to afcertain the reality
of the alleged violence. On fuch occafions, his tes-
timony fhould be given with all poffible delicacy, as
well as with the utmoft caution. Even external figns
of injury may originate from difeafe, of which the
following examples, which have occurred in Manchefter, are adduced on very refpeftable authorities.

A girl, about four years of age, was admitted into
the Manchefter Infirmary, on account of a mortification in the female organs, attended with great fore-
nefs and general depreffion of ftrength. She had

* Thefe circumftances are particularly adverted to in the Mofaic
Law. See Deut. xxii. 25, 26, 27.

been in bed with a boy, fourteen years old; and there was reafon to fufpeft, that he had taken criminal liberties with her. The mortification increafed, and the child died. The boy, therefore, was apprehended, and tried at the Lancafter affizes; but was acquitted on fufficient evidence, that feveral inftances of a fimilar difeafe had appeared, near the fame period of time, in which there was no poffibility of injury or guilt. In one of thefe cafes the body was opened after death. The diforder had been a *typhus* fever, accompanied with the mortification of the *pudenda*. There was no evident caufe of this extraordinary fymptom difcoverable on infpeftion. The lumbar glands were of a dark colour; but all the *vifcera* were found.*

XVII. Concerning *nuifances*, the inveftigation and teftimony of the faculty may be required, whenever they are of a nature offenfive by the vapours which they emit, and injurious to the health of individuals, or of the community. The law defines any thing that worketh hurt, inconvenience, or damage, to be a nuifance.† Thus if a perfon keep hogs, or other noifome animals, fo near the houfe of another, that the ftench incommodes him, and renders the air unwholefome, this is a nuifance; becaufe it deprives him of the enjoyments and benefits of his habitation. A fmelting-houfe for lead, the fmoke of which kills

* See Notes and Illuftrations, No. XVIII.
† See Blackftone's Comment. book iii. ch. xiii.;and book iv. ch. xiii.

the grafs and corn, and injures the cattle of a neighbouring proprietor of land, is deemed a nuifance.
Dye-houfes, tanning-yards, &c. are nuifances, if erected fo near a water-courfe, as to corrupt the ftream.
But a chandler's factory, even when fituated in a
crowded town, is faid to be privileged from action
or indictment, becaufe candles are regarded as neceffaries of life. Hawkins, however, queftions the authority of this opinion, fince the making of candles
may be carried on in the country without annoyance.† But this is fcarcely practicable in a populous
neighbourhood: and as Lord Mansfield has adjudged, that, in fuch cafes, what makes the enjoyment of being and property uncomfortable is, in the
view of the law, a nuifance;* various works and
trades, effential to the happinefs and intereft of the
community, may fall under this conftruction. But
chemiftry, mechanics, and other arts and fciences,
furnifh methods of diminifhing or obviating almoft
every fpecies of noifome vapour: and there can
be no doubt that vitriol works, aquafortis works,
marine acid bleaching-works, the fingeing of velvets,
&c. may be carried on with very little inconvenience
to a neighbourhood, by means neither difficult nor
expenfive. The fame obfervation may be applied to
the bufinefs of the dyer, the fell-monger, the tanner,
the butcher, and the chandler: and as thefe, with
many other difguftful trades are, in fome degree,
neceffary in large towns, juftice and policy require,

† 1 Hawk. 199. Burn's Juftice, vol. iii. p. 239.
* Burron. Mansfield, 333. Burn U. S.

that they fhould only be profecuted as nuifances, when
not conducted in the leaft offenfive mode poffible. To
guard againft arbitrary powers in municipal government, and to render the decifion and inveftigation of
fuch points perfectly confiftent with the liberty of the
fubject, the reference fhould be made to a jury; or
at leaft, any individual fhould be allowed an appeal
to one, if he think himfelf aggrieved.

The frequency of fires, in large manufacturing
towns, makes it expedient that magiftrates, or commiffioners, fhould be authorized to fcrutinize rigidly
into the caufes of them, when they occur; to punifh
neglect or careleffnefs, as well as malicious intention;
and to enforce fuitable meafures of prevention. The
plans propofed for this laft very important purpofe
by Mr. Hartley and Lord Stanhope have been proved
to be effectual, and are not expenfive. The adoption
of them, therefore, or of other means which may
hereafter be difcovered, fhould be required, under a
heavy penalty, in cafes deemed by infurers *doubly
hazardous.*

XVIII. It is a complaint made by coroners, magiftrates, and judges, that medical gentlemen are
often reluctant in the performance of the offices required from them as citizens qualified, by profeffional
knowledge, to aid the execution of public juftice.
Thefe offices, it muft be confeffed, are generally painful, always inconvenient, and occafion an interruption
to bufinefs, of a nature not to be eafily appreciated or
compenfated. But as they admit of no fubftitution,

they are to be regarded as appropriate debts to the community, which neither equity nor patriotifm will allow to be cancelled.

When a phyfician or furgeon is called to give evidence, he fhould avoid, as much as poffible, all obfcure and technical terms, and the unneceffary difplay of medical erudition. He fhould deliver, alfo, what he advances, in the pureft aud moft delicate language, confiftent with the nature of the fubject in queftion.—When two or more gentlemen of the faculty are to offer their opinions or teftimony, it would fometimes tend to obviate contrariety, if they were to confer freely with each other before their public examination. Intelligent and honeft men, fully acquainted with their refpective means of information, are much lefs likely to differ, than when no communication has previoufly taken place. Several years ago, a trial of confiderable confequence occurred, relative to a large copper work ; and two phyficians of eminence were fummoned to the affizes, to bear testimony concerning the falubrity or infalubrity of the fmoke iffuing from the furnaces. The evidence they offered was entirely contradictory. One grounded his teftimony on the general prefumption that the ores of copper contain arfenic; and confequently that the effluvia, proceeding from the roafting of them, muft be poifonous becaufe arfenical. The other had made actual experiments on the ore employed in the works under profecution, and on the vapours which it yielded : he was thus furnifhed with full proof that no arfenic was difcoverable in either. But the affirmative prevailed over the negative teftimony, from the authority of the phyfician who delivered it; an authority which he probably would not have mis-applied, if he had been antecedently acquainted with the decifive trials made by his opponent.*

XIX. It is the injunction of the law, fanctioned by the folemnity of an oath, that in judicial teftimony, *the truth, the whole truth*, and *nothing but the truth* fhall be delivered. A witnefs, therefore, is under a facred obligation to ufe his beft endeavours that his mind be clear and collected, unawed by fear, and un-influenced by favour or enmity. But in criminal pro-fecutions, which affect the life of the perfon accufed, fcruples will be apt to arife in one who, by the ad-vantages of a liberal education, has been accuftomed to ferious reflection, yet has paid no particular atten-tion to the principles of political ethics. It is incum-bent, therefore, on gentlemen of the faculty, to fettle their opinions concerning the right of the civil ma-giftrate to inflict capital punifhment ; the moral and focial ends of fuch punifhment ; the limits prefcribed to the exercife of the right ; and the duty of a citizen to give full efficiency to the laws.

The magiftrate's *right* to inflict punifhment, and the ends of fuch punifhment, though intimately connected, are in their nature diftinct. The right is clearly a fubftitution or transfer of that which be-

* See Notes and Illuftrations, No. XIX.

longs to every individual, by the law of nature, viz. inſtant ſelf-defence, and ſecurity from future violence or wrong. The ends are more comprehenſive, ex‑ tending not only to complete ſecurity againſt offence, but to the correction and improvement of the offen‑ der himſelf, and to counteract in others the diſpoſition to offend. Penal laws are to be regulated by this ſtandard; and the lenity or ſeverity, with which they are executed, ſhould, if poſſible, be exactly propor‑ tionate to it. In different circumſtances, either per‑ ſonal or public conſiderations may preponderate: and in caſes of great moral atrocity, or when the common wea is eſſentially injured, all regard to the reformation of a criminal is ſuperſeded; and his life is juſtly for‑ feited to the good of ſociety. In the participation of the benefits of the ſocial union, he has virtually ac‑ ceded to its conditions, and the violation of its fun‑ damental articles renders him a rebel and an enemy, to be expelled or deſtroyed, both for the ſake of ſe‑ curity, and as an awful warning to others. When capital puniſhments are viewed in this light, the moſt humane and ſcrupulous witneſs may conſider himſelf as ſacrificing private emotions to public juſ‑ tice and ſocial order; and that he is performing an act at once beneficial to his country and to mankind. For political and moral economy can ſubſiſt in no community, without the ſteady execu‑ tion of wiſe and ſalutary laws: and every atrocious act, perpetrated with impunity, operates as a terror to the innocent, a ſnare to the unwary, and an incentive to the flagitious. The criminal, alfo, who evades the fentence of juftice, like one infected with the peftilence, contaminates all whom he approaches. He, therefore, who, from falfe tendernefs, or mifguided confcience, has prevented conviction, by withholding the neceffary proofs,* is an acceffary to all the evils which enfue. The maxim, that *it is better ten villains fhould be difcharged than a fingle perfon fuffer by a wrong adjudication*, is one of thofe partial truths which are generally mifapplied, becaufe not accurately underftood. It is certainly eligible that the rules and the forms of law fhould be fo precife and immutable, as not to involve the innocent in any decifion obtained by corruption, or dictated by paffion and prejudice; though this fhould fometimes furnifh an outlet for the efcape of actual offenders. The plea, alfo, may have fome validity, in crimes of a nature chiefly political, (with which, however, the faculty can profeffionally have no concern,) fuch as coining and forgery, or in cafes wherein the punifh-ment much exceeds the evil or turpitude of the offence. For Lord Bacon has well obferved, that " over-great penalties, befides their acerbity, deaden " the execution of the law."† And when they are

* " The oath adminiftered to the witnefs is not only that " what he depofes fhall be true, but that he fhall alfo depofe the " whole truth: *So that he is not to conceal any part of what he* " *knows, whether interrogated particularly to that point or not.*"— Blackftone, book iii. ch. xxiii.

† See propofal for amending the Laws of England.—Bacon's Works, 4to. vol. ii. p. 542.

difcovered to be unjuftly inflicted, its authority is impaired, its fanctity difhonoured, and veneration gives place to difguft and abhorrence.

But the dread of *innocent blood being brought upon us*, by explicit and honeft teftimony, is one of thofe fuperftitions which the nurfe has taught, and which a liberal education ought to purge from the mind: and if, in the performance of our duty, innocence fhould unfortunately be involved in the punifhment of guilt, we fhall affuredly ftand acquitted before God and our own confciences. The convict himfelf, lamentable as his fate muft be regarded, may derive confolation from the reflection, that, though his fentence be unjuft, " he falls for his country, whilft he " fuffers under the operation of thofe rules, by the " general effect and tendency of which the welfare of " the community is maintained and upheld."*

XX. When profeffional teftimony is required, in cafes of fuch peculiar malignity as to excite general horror and indignation, a virtuous mind, even though fcrupulous and timid, is liable to be influenced by too violent impreffions; and to transfer to the accufed that dread and averfion, which, before conviction, fhould be confined to the crime, and as much as poffible withheld from the fuppofed offender. If the charge, for inftance, be that of parricide, accomplifhed by poifon, and accompanied with deliberate malice, ingratitude, and cruelty; the inveftigation fhould be made with calm and unbiaffed precifion, and

---

* Paley's Moral and Political Phil. b. vi. ch. ix. p. 553, 4to.

the teſtimony delivered with no colouring of paſſion, nor with any deviation from the *ſimplicity of truth*. When *circumſtantial proofs* are adduced, they ſhould be arranged in the moſt lucid order, that they may be contraſted and compared, in all their various relations, with facility and accuracy; and that their weight may be ſeparately and collectively determined in the balance of juſtice. For, in ſuch evidence, there ſubſiſts a regular gradation from the ſlighteſt preſumption to complete moral certainty: and if the witneſs poſſeſs ſufficient information in this branch of philoſophical and juridical ſcience, he will always be competent to ſecure himſelf, and on many occaſions the court alſo, from fallacy and error. The Marquis de Beccaria has laid down the following excellent theorems, concerning judicial evidence:—

" When the proofs of a crime are dependent on each
" other, that is, when the evidence of each witneſs,
" taken ſeparately, proves nothing; or when all the
" proofs are dependent upon one, the number of
" proofs neither increaſes nor diminiſhes the proba-
" bility of the fact; for the force of the whole is no
" greater than the force of thoſe on which they de-
" pend; and if this fail, they all fall to the ground.
" When the proofs are independent of each other,
" the probability of the fact increaſes in proportion to
" the number of proofs; for the falſehood of one
" does not diminiſh the veracity of another. . . . .
" The proofs of a crime may be divided into two
" claſſes, perfect and imperfect. I call thoſe perfect,

" which exclude the poffibility of innocence; imper-
" fect, thofe which do not exclude this poffibility.
" Of the firft, one only is fufficient for condemnation;
" of the fecond, as many are required as form a per-
" fect proof; that is to fay, each of thefe, feparately
" taken, does not exclude the poffibility of innocence;
" it is neverthelefs excluded by their union."*

* Beccaria's Effay on Crimes and Punifhments, ch. xiv.

AN

APPENDIX:

CONTAINING,

I. *A DISCOURSE,*

ADDRESSED TO

THE GENTLEMEN OF THE FACULTY, THE OFFICERS, THE
CLERGY, AND THE TRUSTEES OF THE INFIRMARY
AT LIVERPOOL,

ON THEIR RESPECTIVE HOSPITAL DUTIES.

BY THE

Rev. THOMAS BASSNETT PERCIVAL, LL. B.

Of St. John's-College, Cambridge; Chaplain to the Marquis of Waterford; and to the
Company of British Merchants at St. Petersburgh.

II. *NOTES AND ILLUSTRATIONS.*

. . . . " Lo! a goodly Hofpital afcends,
" In which they bade each lenient aid be nigh,
" That could the fick bed fmooth of that fad company.
" It was a worthy edifying fight,
" And gives to human kind peculiar grace,
" To fee kind hands attending day and night,
" With tender miniftry, from place to place:
" Some prop the head; fome, from the pallid face
" Wipe off the faint cold dews weak nature fheds;
" Some reach the healing draught; the whilft to chafe
" The fear fupreme, around their foften'd beds,
" Some holy man by prayer all opening heaven difpreds."

THOMSON's Caftle of Indolence; Canto ii.

A

DISCOURSE

ON

HOSPITAL DUTIES:

BEING AN

ANNIVERSARY SERMON,

PREACHED IN MAY 1791;

FOR THE BENEFIT OF THE INFIRMARY AT LIVERPOOL.*

———

*" Let us not be weary in well doing, for in due season we shall
" reap, if we faint not."*—GALAT. vi. 9.

IF we confider the circumftances of man, as placed
in this great theatre of action; as connected with
his fellow-creatures by various ties and relations;
and with GOD himfelf, his creator and judge: if we
confider the powers and faculties with which he is
endowed, and that thefe are talents committed to his
truft, capable of indefinite degrees of improvement,
and which the LORD, at his coming, will demand
with ufury; we fhall fee the fulleft reafon for the
apoftolical injunction, *be not weary in well doing,* and

* See Notes and Illuftrations, No. XX.

rejoice in the affurance, that *in due feafon we fhall reap, if we faint not.* The fphere of human duty has no limits to its extent. Every advance in knowledge widens its boundaries; every increafe of power and wealth multiplies and diverfifies the objects of it; and length of years evinces their unceafing fucceffion. Therefore, *whatfoever thy hand findeth to do, do it with all thy might.* Vigour and perfeverance are effential to every noble purfuit; and no virtuous effort is in vain. To be difcouraged by oppofition; to be alarmed by danger; or overcome by difficulty, is a ftate of mind unfitted for the Chriftian warfare.

But the prefent interefting occafion calls for a fpecific application of the precept contained in our text. What is juft and true, concerning the whole duty of man, muft be equally juft and true of every individual branch of moral and religious obligation: and it can require no deep refearch, no abftrufe inveftigation, to work conviction on our minds, that the higher is the object we have in view, the more active and inceffant fhould be our exertions in the attainment of it. The inftitution, which now claims your moft ferious attention, is founded on the *wifeft policy;* adapted to the nobleft purpofes of *humanity;* and capable of being rendered fubfervient to the *everlafting welfare* of mankind.

The *wifdom* of fuch charitable foundations can admit of no difpute. On the lower claffes of our fellow-citizens alone, we depend for food, for raiment, for the habitations in which we dwell, and for all the conveniences and comforts of life. But health is effential to their capacity for labour; and in this labour, I fear, it is too often facrificed. An additional obligation, therefore, to afford relief, fprings from fo affecting a confideration. He who at once toils and fuffers for our benefit, has a multiplied claim to our fupport; and to withhold it, would be equally chargeable with folly, ingratitude, and injuftice.

But *humanity* prompts, when the ftill voice of wifdom is not heard. Sicknefs, complicated with poverty, has pleas, that to a feeling mind are irre-fiftible. *To weep with thofe that weep*, was the cha-racter of our Divine Mafter; and, to the honour of our nature, we are capable of the fame generous fympathy. Vain and idle, however, are the fofteft emotions of the mind, when they lead not to corres-pondent actions : and he who views the naked, without clothing them, and thofe who are fick, with-out miniftering unto them, incurs the dreadful de-nunciation, *Depart from me, ye curfed, into everlafting fire, prepared for the devil and his angels. For in-afmuch as ye did it not to one of the leaft of thofe my brethren, ye did it not unto me.*

It were an eafy and pleafing tafk to enlarge on thefe general topics. But they come not fufficiently " home to men's bufinefs and bofoms:" and honour-ed as I am, by being thus called to the privilege of addreffing you, I feel it incumbent on me to be more appropiate, by fuggefting to your candid attention the diftinct and relative duties attached to the feveral orders, which compofe this moft excellent community. Permit me therefore to claim your indulgence, whilft I offer, with all deference and refpeft, but with the plainnefs and freedom of gofpel fincerity, a few words of exhortation :

I. To the Faculty;
II. To the Officers and Superintendants;
III. To the Clergy;·

And laftly, To the general Body of Trus-tees and Contributors.

I. To the Faculty. As man is placed by Divine Providence in a fituation which involves a variety of interefts and duties, often complicated and mixed to-gether, the motives which influence human aftions muft neceffarily be mixed and complicated. Wifdom and virtue confift in the feleftion of thofe which are fit and good, and in the arrangement of all by a juft appreciation of their comparative dignity and import-ance. In the acceptance of your profeffional offices, in this Infirmary, it is prefumed that you have been governed by the *love of reputation;* by the *defire of acquiring knowledge and experience;* and by that *fpirit of philanthropy,* which delights in and is never weary of well-doing. Let us briefly confider each of thefe principles of aftion, and how they ought to be regulated.

If we analize the *love of reputation,* as it exifts in liberal and well-informed minds, it will be found to fpring from the love of moral and intelleftual excel-lence. For of what value is praife, when not founded

on defert? But the confcioufnefs of defert, by the
conftitution of our nature, is ever attended with felf-
approbation: and this delightful emotion, which is
at once the concomitant, and the reward of virtue,
widely expands its operation, and by a focial fympathy, encircles all who are the witneffes or judges of
our generous deeds. From the fame principle, piety
itfelf derives its origin. For how fhall he who loveth
not, or is regardlefs of the approbation of his brother,
whom he hath feen, love or regard the favour of
GOD, whom he hath not feen!

But let us remember not to fubftitute for the
legitimate and magnanimous love of fame, that fpurious and fordid paffion which feeks applaufe by
gratifying the caprices, by indulging the prejudices,
and by impofing on the follies of mankind. To court
the public favour by adulation, or empirical arts, is
meannefs and hypocrify; to claim it by high and
affumed pretenfions, is arrogance and pride; and to
exalt our own character by the depreciation of that
of our competitor, is to convert honourable emulation
into profeffional enmity and injuftice.

You have been elevated by the fuffrages of your
fellow-citizens: you have been honoured by their
favour and confidence. rejoice in the diftinction conferred upon you; fulfil with affiduity and zeal the
truft repofed in you; and by being unwearied in well-
doing, rife to higher and higher degrees of public
favour and celebrity!

The *acquisition of knowledge and experience* is a farther incentive to your generous exertions in this receptacle of disease and misery. It is one important design of the institution itself; which affords peculiar advantages for ascertaining the operation of remedies, and the comparative merit of different modes of medical and chirurgical treatment. For the strict rules which are enjoined; the steadiness with which their observance is enforced; and the unremitting attendance of those who are qualified to make accurate observations, and to note every symptom, whether regular or anomalous, in the diseases under cure; are circumstances incompatible with the ordinary domestic care of the sick. To avail yourselves of them, therefore, is agreeable to sound policy, and consonant to the purest justice and humanity. For every improvement in the healing art is a public good, beneficial to the poor as well as to the rich, and to the former in a proportionably greater degree, as they are more numerous, and consequently more frequently the objects of it. On this point, however, peculiar delicacy is required; and as the discretionary power with which you are entrusted, is almost without controul, it should be exercised with the nicest honour and probity. When novelties in practice are introduced, be careful that they are conformable to reason and analogy; that no sacrifice be made to fanciful hypothesis, or experimental curiosity; that the infliction of pain or suffering be, as much as possible, avoided; and that the end in view fully warrant the means for its attainment.

But your nobleſt call to duty and exertion ariſes from the exalted *ſpirit of philanthropy:* and on this occaſion I may addreſs you individually, in the language of the firſt of orators to the ſovereign of imperial Rome: *Nihil habet fortuna tua majus quam ut poſſis, nec natura melius quam ut velis, ſervare quam plurimos.* It is your honour and felicity to be engaged in an occupation which leads you, like our bleſſed LORD, during his abode on earth, to go about doing good; healing the ſick, and curing all manner of diſeaſes. To you learning has opened her ſtores, that they may be applied to the ſublimeſt purpoſes; to alleviate pain; to raiſe the drooping head; to renew the roſes of the cheek, and the ſparkling of the eye; and thus to gladden, whilſt you lengthen life. Let this hoſpital be the theatre on which you diſplay, with aſſiduous and perſevering care, your ſcience, ſkill, and humanity: and let the manner correſpond with, and even heighten, the meaſure of your benevolence. With patience hear the tale of ſymptoms; ſilence not harſhly the murmurs of a troubled mind; and by the kindneſs of your looks and words, evince that Chriſtian condeſcenſion may be compatible with profeſſional ſteadineſs and dignity.

It is, I truſt, an ill-founded opinion, that compaſſion is not the virtue of a ſurgeon. This branch of the profeſſion has been charged with hardneſs of heart:

and some of its members have formerly juftified the
ftigma, by ridiculing all foftnefs of manners; by af-
fuming the contrary deportment; and by ftudioufly
banifhing from their minds that fympathy, which they
falfely fuppofed would be unfuitable to their character,
and unfavourable to the practical exercife of their
art. But different fentiments now prevail. And a
diftinction fhould ever be made between true compaffion, and that unmanly pity which enfeebles the
mind; which fhrinks from the fight of woe; which
infpires timidity; and deprives him, who is under its
influence, of all capacity to give relief. Genuine
compaffion roufes the attention of the foul; gives
energy to all its powers; fuggefts expedients in danger; incites to vigorous action and difficulty; and
ftrengthens the hand to execute, with promptitude,
the purpofes of the head. The pity which you fhould
reprefs, is a turbulent emotion. The commiferation
which you fhould cultivate, is a calm principle. It
is benevolence itfelf directed forcibly to a fpecific object. And the frequency of fuch objects diminifhes
not, but augments its energy: for it produces a tone
or conftitution of mind, conftantly in unifon with
fuffering; and prepared, on every call, to afford the
full meafure of relief. Appear, therefore, to your
patients to be actuated by that fellow-feeling, which
nature, education, and Chriftianity require. Make
their cafes, in a reafonable degree, your own; *and
whatfoever ye would that men fhould do unto you, do
ye even fo unto them.*

II. To you, the OFFICERS and SUPERINTEN-
DANTS of this hofpital, we may juftly afcribe views
the moft pure and public-fpirited. But zeal in the
caufe of charity, however fincere, can only be rendered ufefully efficient by due attention to, and fteady
perfeverance in, the wifeft means for its accomplifhment. On the miftaken humanity of crowding your
wards with numerous patients, by which difeafe is
generated, and death multiplied in all its horrors; on
the fatal calculations of favings in ˎmedicines, diet,
or clothing; and on a ftrict attention to ventilation,
cleanlinefs, and all the domeftic arrangements, which
have order, utility, or comfort for their objects; I
truft it is needlefs to enlarge. But you will fuffer
me, I hope, to offer a few hints on the *moral* and
religious application of the Inftitution which you govern; a topic hitherto little noticed, though of high
importance.

The yifitation of ficknefs is a wife and kind difpenfation of Providence, intended to humble, to refine,
and to meliorate the heart: and its falutary influence extends beyond the fufferer, to thofe relatives
and friends, whofe office it is to minifter unto him;
exciting tendernefs and commiferation; drawing clofer
the bonds of affection; and roufing to exertions, virtuous in their nature, profitable to man, and well-
pleafing to GOD. A parent, foothed and fupported
under the angu fh of pain, by the loving kindnefs of
his children; a hufband nurfed with unwearied affiduity by the partner of his bed; a child experiencing

all the tenderneſs of paternal and maternal love; are ſituations which form the ground-work of domeſtic virtue, and domeſtic felicity. They leave indelible impreſſions on the mind, impreſſions which exalt the moral character, and render us better men, better citizens, and better Chriſtians. It is wiſdom, there-fore, and duty, not to fruſtrate the benevolent conſtitutions of Heaven, by diſſolving the ſalutary connections of ſickneſs, and tranſporting into a public aſylum thoſe who may, with a little aid, enjoy in their own homes, benefits and conſolations which, elſewhere, it is in the power of no one to confer.*

But numerous are the ſufferers under ſickneſs and poverty, to whom your hoſpitable doors may be opened, with the higheſt moral benefit to themſelves and to the community. When admitted within theſe walls, they form one great family, of which you are the heads, and conſequently reſponſible for all due attention to their preſent behaviour, and to the means of their future improvement. Withdrawn from the habitations of penury, ſloth, and dirtineſs; from the converſation of the looſe and the profligate; and from all their aſſociates in vice, they may here form a taſte for the ſweets of cleanlineſs; learn the power of bridling their tongues; and be induced, by this temporary abſence, to free themſelves from all farther connection with their idle and debauched companions. Let it be your ſedulous care to foſter

* See Notes and Illuſtrations, No. XXI.

thefe excellent tendencies: Encourage in the patients every attention to neatnefs: Tolerate no filth or flovenlinefs, either in their perfons or attire : Keep a ftrict guard on the decency of their behaviour: Urge them to active offices of kindnefs and compaffion to each other: Furnifh the convalefcents with bibles, and with books of plain morality, and practical piety, fuited to their capacities and circumftances; and which will neither delude the imagination, nor perplex the underftanding: Oblige them to a regular attendance on the public worfhip of the hofpital, or of their refpective churches: And, agreeably to your laws, neglect not to make provifion for the ftated and frequent adminiftration of the holy facrament. There is fomething in this office peculiarly adapted to comfort and fortify the mind, under the preffure of poverty, pain, and ficknefs.   In the contemplation of that love which CHRIST manifefted for us by his fufferings and death, all the confolation is experienced which divine fympathy can afford. *We have a high-prieft touched with the feeling of our infirmities,* and who holds forth to us this foothing invitation: *Come unto me, all ye that are weary and heavy laden, and I will give you reft.* Promote the celebration of an ordinance, adapted thus to fill the mind with gratitude, and to alleviate every woe. And let the example of our Saviour's refignation to the appointment of GOD be enforced by it, who in his agony exclaimed, *Father, if it be thy will, let this cup pafs from me; neverthelefs, not my will, but thine be done.*

III. I doubt not the cordial and entire concurrence of you, my Rev. Brethren, the Clergy who officiate in this hofpital, in the recommendation of the holy facrament, not only as a ftated, but as a frequent ordinance of the Inftitution.   With you it will reft to obviate every objeftion to the rite, and to give it the full meafure of fpiritual efficacy.   Enthufiafm and fuperftition cannot be dreaded in the offices of rational piety, condufted by thofe who are rational and pious: and you will neither betray men into falfe confidence, nor alarm them, when languifhing under ficknefs and pain, with unfeafonable terrors. *The fpirit of a man will fuftain his infirmity, but a wounded fpirit who can bear?*   Under fuch circumftances, vain will be the aid of fkill or medicine, without the fupports and comforts, which it is your facred funftion to afford.   You can

> - - - - - - " minifter to a mind difeafed ;
> " Pluck from the memory a rooted forrow,
> " Raze out the written troubles of the brain ;
> " And, with fome fweet oblivious antidote,
> " Cleanfe the full bofom of that perilous ftuff
> " Which weighs upon the heart."   Shakespeare,

Being thus the *Phyficians* of the foul, you are effential conftituents of this enlarged fyftem of philanthropy.   Apply, therefore, with diligence and zeal, the fpiritual *medicines* which it is your office to difpenfe.   Here you have a wide field *for exhortation, for correction, and for inftruction in righteoufnefs.* Convalefcence peculiarly furnifhes the *mollia tempora*

fandi, the foft feafons of impreffive counfel. The
mind is then open to ferious conviction; difpofed to
review paft offences with contrition; and to look
forward with fincere refolutions of amendment.
Many difeafes are the immediate confequences of vice:
and he who has recently experienced the fufferings
of guilt, will deeply feel its enormity; and cherifh
thofe precepts, which will fecure him from relapfe,
and convert his paft mifery into future bleffings.

IV. But this large aggregate of good, which it is
the defign of the prefent anniverfary to commemorate,
depends, for its fupport and extenfion, on the
GENERAL BODY OF CONTRIBUTORS to the charity.
How deeply interefting, then, are the claims which
your fellow-citizens have to make on your philanthropy! How important is it to the health of
thoufands, in rapid fucceffion, that you fhould per-
fevere in beneficence, and continue unwearied in well
doing! Ordinary bounty terminates almoft in the
moment when it is beftowed. The object of it being
withdrawn, folicitude and refponfibility are no more.
But in this noble Inftitution, charity exerts itfelf in
fteady and unceafing operations. It is a ftream ever
full, yet ever flowing; and through the grace of
GOD, I truft, will be inexhauftible. From your zeal,
your concord, and liberality, thefe SACRED *waters
of life* proceed. Be watchful that they are not
poifoned in their fource, nor contaminated in their
progrefs. Let your *zeal* be employed in fearching
out and recommending proper objects of relief.

Call to you, according to the injunction of our Saviour, *the halt, and the maimed, the lame, and the blind; for they cannot recompenfe you: Ye fhall be recompenfed at the refurrection of the juft.* Suffer no prejudices, either political or religious, to contract the bounds of your charity. *Pafs not by on the other fide from a fellow-creature who has fallen among thieves*, becaufe he is not of your party, of your fect, or even of your nation. But, like the good Samaritan, *have compaffion on him, and let oil and wine be poured into his wounds* in this hofpitable *Beth fda* Guard, moft feduloufly guard, againft the fpirit of diffenfion. You are united in the labours of Chriftian love; and having one common and glorious caufe, the conteft fhould be for pre-em nence in doing good, not for the gratification of pride, the indulgence of refentment, or even for the interefts of friendfhip.* To your liberality in contribution no appeal can be required, no new incitement can be urged. What your judgment approves, what experience has fanctioned, and what touches the tendereft feelings of your hearts, muft have pleas that are irrefiftible.

It only remains, then, that we cordially unite in offering our devout fupplications to the throne of grace, in behalf of all thofe *who are afflicted or diftreffed in mind, body, or eftate; that it may pleafe the God of all confolation to relieve them, according to their feveral neceffities; giving them patience under their fufferings, and a happy iffue out of all their*

* See Notes and Illuftrations, No. XXII.

affli&ions: And finally, that we may. be delivered from all hardnefs of heart ; from all covetous defires, and inordinate love of riches ; and, having been taught that all our doings, without charity, profit nothing, that this moft excellent gift, the bond of peace, and of all virtues, may be poured into us abundantly, through the merits and mediation of our blefsed Lord and Saviour.

NOTES

ILLUSTRATIONS.

———❦❦———

Note I. *Preface. Page* 367.

HOSPITAL AT MANCHESTER.

THIS inſtitution comprehends an Infirmary, Lunatic Hoſpital, and Diſpenſary; and has now connected with it a Houſe of Recovery, for the reception of patients ill of contagious fevers. It provides, alſo, for inoculation, both variolous and vaccine; and for the delivery of pregnant women at their own habitations, in caſes certified by the ordinary midwives to be attended with great difficulty and danger. From the 24th of June 1792, to the 24th of June 1802, the in-patients, admitted during the ſpace of ten years, amounted to 8083; of which number 361 died:—the out-patients amounted to 31,890; of which number 676 died:—the home-patients amounted to 24,439; of which number 1970 died. The Lunatic Hoſpital was eſtabliſhed in

the year 1766; from which time to June 24th,
1802, the patients admitted have amounted to 1575.
Of this number 627 have been cured; 212 have
been relieved; 488 have been difcharged at the
requeft of their friends; 171 have died; 8 have
been deemed incurable; and 69 remained in the
houfe on the 24th of June 1802. The Houfe of
Recovery, for the admiffion of patients ill of contagious fever, is appropriated to thofe, who, from
extreme penury, are incapable of receiving proper
aid in their own clofe and noifome habitations, or
who are liable to communicate contagion to a numerous family, and, if in a crowded neighbourhood,
even to perpetuate its virulence. It is attended by
the phyficians of the Infirmary; and is furnifhed
with wine and medicines from the funds of that
charity; but all the other expences are defrayed by
an eftablifhment, entitled the BOARD OF HEALTH,
which commenced in the fpring of 1796.

The general objects of this benevolent Inftitution
are threefold. I. To obviate the generation of difeafes. II. To prevent the fpread of them by contagion. III. To fhorten the duration of exifting
difeafes; and to mitigate their evils, by affording the
neceffary aids and comforts to thofe who labour
under them.—I. Under the firft head are comprehended—the infpection and improvement of the
general accommodations of the poor;—the prohi-
bition of fuch habitations, as are fo clofe, noifome, or
damp, as to be incapable of being rendered tolerably

falubrious:—the removal of privies placed in improper fituations;—provifion for white wafhing and cleanfing the houfes of the poor twice every year; attention to their ventilation by windows with open cafements, &c.:—the infpection of cotton-mills, or other factories, at ftated feafons; with regular returns of the condition as to health, clothing, appearance, and behaviour of the perfons employed in them; of the time allowed for their refrefhment, at breakfaft and dinner; and of the accommodations of thofe who are parochial apprentices, or who are not under the immediate direction of their parents or friends:—the limitation and regulation of lodging-houfes; on the eftablifhment of *caravanferas* for paffengers, or thofe who come to feek employment, unrecommended or unknown:—the eftabl'fhment of public warm and cold baths; provifion for particular attention to the cleaning of the ftreets, which are inhabited by the poor; and for the fpeedy removal of dunghills, and every other fpecies of filth:—the diminution, as far as is practicable, of noxious effluvia from different fources, fuch as thofe which arife from the work-houfes of the fellmonger, the yards of the tanner, and the flaughter-houfes of the butcher:— the fuperintendance of the feveral markets; with a view to prevent the fale of putrid flefh or fifh, and of unfound flour, or other vegetable productions.

Under the fecond general head are included—the fpeedy removal of thofe who are attacked with fymptoms of fever, from the cotton-mills, or factories, to the habitations of their parents or friends, or to commodious houfes which may be fet apart for the reception of the fick, in the different diftricts of Man-chefter :—the requifite attentions to preclude unne-ceffary communications with the fick, in the houfes wherein they are confined ; and to the fubfequent changing and ventilation of their chambers, bedding, and apparel :—and the allowance of a fufficient time for perfect recovery, and complete purification of their clothes, before they return again to their works, or mix with their companions in labour.   III. Under the third head are comprehended—medical atten-dance:—the care of nurfes:—and fupplies of medicine, wine, appropriate diet, fuel, and clothing.

From the opening of the Houfe of Recovery on the 31ft of May 1796, to the 31ft of May 1802, 3210 patients have been admitted; of whom 2939 have been cured; and 271 have died.

Note II. *Preface.   Page 2.*

DISTRIBUTION OF PRINTED COPIES OF THE
MEDICAL ETHICS.

When it was firft recommended to me to enlarge and publifh this code of profeffional Ethics, I felt extremely difficult in the adoption of an undertaking fo liable to the charge of prefumption, in an individual

confcious of inadequate powers, and poffeffing no claim
or authority to dictate rules to his medical brethren.
With much folicitude, therefore, I availed myfelf of
the aid and fupport of various judicious and learned
friends, in different ftations of life, by communicating
to them printed copies of the general fcheme.   And
I record not only with *gratitude*, but as the *neceffary
fanction* of my work, the names of thofe who have
honoured it with their approbation or affiftance.
John Aikin, M. D.; Sir George Baker, bart.; S. A.
Bardfley, M. D.; Thomas Butterworth Bayley, efq.;
Fofter Bower, efq; barrifter; John Crofs, efq; barrifter; James Currie, M. D.; Erafmus Darwin,
M. D.; William Falconer, M. D.; John Ferriar,
M. D.; Rev. Thomas Gifborne, M. A.; John Hay-
garth, M. D.; William Heberden, M. D.; Mr.
Thomas Henry; Samuel Heywood, efq; ferjeant at
law; Edward Holme, M. D.; George Lloyd, efq;
barrifter; Rev. Archdeacon Paley; Sir G. O. Paul,
bart.; Robert Percival, of Dublin, M. D.; Mr.
Simmons; Richard Warren, M. D.; Right Rev.
Richard Watfon, D. D. Bifhop of Landaff; Charles
White, efq; and William Withering, M. D.

If it were not from the apprehenfion of fwelling
this long lift of names, I fhould not omit the prefent
opportunity of expreffing my grateful acknowledgments to many other refpectable friends, to whom
copies of the Medical Ethics were tranfmitted, fub-
fequently to the firft circulation of the fcheme.

Note III. *Chap.* I. *Sect.* XVI.

SITUATION, CONSTRUCTION, AND GOVERNMENT
OF HOSPITALS.

" In the town of Funchal, in the ifland of Ma-
" deira, the Infirmary in particular drew our attention,
" as a model which might be adopted in other coun-
" tries with great advantage. It confifts of a long
" room, on one fide of which are the windows, and
" an altar for the convenience of adminiftering the
" facrament to the fick. The other fide is divided
" into wards, each of which is juft big enough to
" contain a bed, and neatly lined with gally-tiles.
" Behind thefe wards, and parallel to the room in
" which they ftand, there runs a long gallery, with
" which each ward communicates by a door; fo that
" the fick may be feparately fupplied with whatever
" they want, without difturbing their neighbours."
—See *Voyages round the World*, publifhed by Dr.
Hawkefworth, vol. ii. page 8.

In the year 1790, I was confulted concerning the
fituation, ftructure, and government of a large county-
hofpital, about to be erected; and I fhall here infert
the hints, which I then fuggefted.

The SITUATION muft, in fome meafure, be dependent on local circumftances: but, as far as is compatible with thefe, it fhould be dry, airy, moderately

elevated, at a commodious diftance from the town, and well fupplied with falubrious water. If fwampy grounds happen to be in the neighbourhood, particular attention fhould be paid to the winds which moft frequently prevail, that it may be as little as poffible influenced by the vapours thofe winds are likely to convey. The fame precaution is applicable to the fmoke of the town. The hofpital at Manchefter is three-fourths of the year involved in fmoke, by being erected on the eaftern fide of the town; an evil which might eafily have been avoided by the choice of an oppofite fite.

The STRUCTURE includes accommodation and ventilation: and the form beft adapted *(mutatis mutandis)* to thefe effential purpofes appears to be that of the new prifon at Manchefter, which is conftructed on the well-known plan of Mr. Howard. The building which forms the gateway, will afford a large and commodious room above, for the governors of the charity; and below, a fhop for the apothecary; and a hall for the reception of out-patients, who would thus have no communication with the Infirmary, and confequently incur no rifque either of bringing or carrying back with them febrile or other contagion. The central part of the building is well adapted for kitchens and other offices, over which the chapel might be conftructed. The four *radii*, or buildings which project from the centre, might each contain fix wards, fifteen feet fquare by thirteen high, in each ftory, with a gallery interpofed. No ward fhould

have more than two beds in it; for the contamination
of the air arises chiefly from the crowding too many
fick perfons in one chamber: and contagion not only
fpreads by this means, but the patients fuftain great
injury from the multiplied fpeĉtacles of fuffering to
which they are witneffes in the large apartments of an
hofpital.   Small chambers, alfo, have the advantage
of being quickly ventilated.   The three ftories fhould
be of the fame height; and if the roof be lined with
boards under the flates, the temperature of the higheft
ftory will be much lefs than ufually affeĉted by the
heat of fummer, or cold of winter.   In each gallery
a room fhould be fet apart for the convalefcents, and
for thofe patients who are able to quit their bed-
chambers occafionally in the day-time.

In the provifion for ventilating the wards, it fhould
be remembered, that though adequate fupplies of
FRESH AIR are effential to its purity, the *temperature*
of it, alfo, muft be regarded with a view to falubrity.
For cold is not only ungrateful to the feelings of the
fick, commonly very acute, but in many difeafes injurious by its fedative aĉtion: and it has often been
fufpeĉted of giving energy to infeĉtion.   The ventilation, too, fhould be accomplifhed without any current of wind perceptible by the patients; who, being
ignorant of the nature and effeĉts of conʌagion, have
no apprehenfion of danger from it, but entertain
ftrong prejudices againft a flow of cool air; efpecially
when in bed, or afleep.   Thefe prejudices, if they
are to be deemed fuch, claim not only tendernefs, but

indulgence. For though filenced by authority, as I have before obferved, they will operate fecretly and forcibly on the mind, creating fear, anxiety, and watchfulnefs.

The GOVERNMENT of the hofpital is an object of great importance, and will demand very mature confideration. The fyftem adopted in moft of our charitable inftitutions appears to me neither fufficiently comprehenfive nor efficient; and fome unhappy difputes in the Manchefter Infirmary induced me to draw up the following propofitions, for the confideration of the truftees:—

I. A committee, for the purpofe of mediation, fuperintendance, and improvement, fhould be chofen by ballot from among the truftees: it fhould confift of nine gentlemen of talents, refpectability, and independence, to give dignity and authority to their proceedings: it fhould be ftiled the COUNCIL of the Infirmary; or be diftinguifhed by fome other honourable and expreffive appellation: and, when regularly convened, five members fhould be competent to tranfact bufinefs.

II. No officer of the Infirmary, nor any phyfician or furgeon belonging to it, fhould be eligible into the council.

III. No member of the council fhould continue in office more than three years: three members fhould annually go out of office, and three others be chofen in their room; and the fame gentlemen may be re-elected after the expiration of one or more years.

IV. The council fhould be a board of arbitration, for adjufting whatever differences or difputes may arife between the feveral members of the Infirmary: it fhould take cognizance of every thing relative to the polity of this inftitution, and of its appendages, the Lunatic Hofpital, and Difpenfary: it fhould inquire into the progrefs and prefent ftate of the charity: it fhould fuggeft to the annual board of truftees fuch improvements as may be deemed expedient: and it fhould receive, methodize, and deliberate upon the feveral laws or regulations which may be propofed by the weekly board, or by any individual truftee, according to the prefcribed form of notice, previous to a final decifion.

V. The council fhould be convened fourteen days before each quarterly board, or oftener, if neceffary: they fhould then communicate to the phyficians and furgeons of the Infirmary whatever laws or regulations, relative to the medical or chirurgical departments, fall under their difcuffion: and they fhould attend, either perfonally or by their chairman, the fucceeding quarterly or annual board, to ftate the refult of their inveftigations, and to affift the deliberations or decifions of the general body of truftees.

VI. The phyficians and furgeons of the Infirmary fhould be requefted to form themfelves into a committee, to aid the council with their experience, knowledge, and advice; and to take into confideration whatever laws or regulations may be propofed, relative to their peculiar departments, before they be referred to the decifion of the general body of truftees.

VII. The meetings of the committee of phyficians and furgeons fhould be held the day after the affembly of the council: and they fhould deliver, in writing, by the fenior phyfician or furgeon, the refult of their deliberations, in due time before the fucceeding annual or quarterly board, to an adjourned meeting of the council.

N. B. The council may be either a permanent or a temporary inftitution, and fubfift only during the fpace of two or three years, being renewable at ftated periods of time, or whenever emergencies fhall require fuch an eftablifhment.

Note IV. Chap. I. Sect. XXVI.

HOUSE OF RECEPTION FOR PATIENTS ILL OF CONTAGIOUS FEVERS.

In Note, No. I. it has been ftated that a houfe of reception for patients ill of infectious fevers now forms part of the fyftem of the Manchefter Difpenfary. To aid the eftablifhment of fimilar inftitutions in other places, I fhall infert the regulations which form the polity of the houfe.

REGULATIONS FOR THE ADMISSION OF PATIENTS
INTO THE HOUSE OF RECOVERY.

I. The phyfician of the Infirmary fhall be authorifed to give one or two fhillings, from the funds of
the inftitution, (by a ticket to the fecretary of the Board
of Health,) to the perfon who fhall furnifh the earlieft
information of the appearance of fever in any poor
family, within the limits of their refpective diftricts.

II. As foon as the fecretary has received this ticket,
he fhall apply, or take care that application be made,
to fome truftee of the Board of Health, living within
the diftrict, and who is a fubfcriber to the Infirmary,
for an immediate recommendation of the fick perfon
as an home patient.

III. Such patients as the phyficians fhall deem
peculiar objects of recommendation, either on account
of their extreme poverty, or of the clofe and crowded
ftate of their habitations, fhall be conveyed in a fedan-
chair (provided with a moveable wafhing lining, kept
for this fole purpofe, and diftinguifhed by proper
marks) to the Houfe of Recovery.

IV. The phyficians fhall be requefted to form the
neceffary regulations, for the domeftic government of
the families of the home-patients, afflicted with fever.

V. A reward, to the amount of   fhall be
given to the heads of the family, after the ceffation
of the fever, on condition that they have faithfully

obferved the rules prefcribed for cleanlinefs, ventilation, and the prevention of infection amongft their
neighbours. This reward fhall be doubled in cafes
of extraordinary danger, and when the attentions
have been adequate and fuccefsful.

VI. After the vifitation of fever has ceafed in any
poor dwelling-houfe, the fum of   , or a fufficient fum, fhall be allowed (to be expended under the
direction of an infpector) for white-wafhing and
cleanfing the premifes, and for the purchafe of new
bed-clothes, or apparel, in lieu of fuch as it may be
deemed neceffary to deftroy, to obviate the continuance or propagation of fever.

VII. An infpector fhall be appointed in each diftrict
of the Infirmary, to aid the execution, and to enforce
the obfervance, of the foregoing regulations. And
the gentlemen of the Strangers' Friend Society fhall
be requefted to undertake this office.

INTERNAL REGULATIONS FOR THE HOUSE OF RECOVERY.

I. Every patient, on admiffion, fhall change his
infectious, for clean, linen; the face and hands are
to be wafhed clean with lukewarm water, and the
lower extremities fomented.

II. The clothes brought into the houfe by patients
fhall be properly purified and aired.

III. All linen and bed-clothes, immediately on being removed from the bodies of the patients, shall be immersed in cold water, before they are carried down stairs.

IV. All discharges from the patients shall be removed from the wards without delay.

V. The floors of the wards shall be carefully washed twice a week, and near the beds every day.

VI. Quick-lime shall be slaked in large open vessels in every ward, and renewed whenever it ceases to bubble on the affusion of water. The walls and roofs shall be frequently washed with this mixture.

VII. No relation or acquaintance shall be permitted to visit the wards, without particular orders from one of the physicians.

VIII. No strangers shall be admitted into the wards; and the nurses shall be strictly enjoined not to receive unnecessary visits.

IX. No linen or clothes shall be removed from the House of Recovery till they have been washed, aired, and freed from infection.

X. No convalescents shall be discharged from the house, without a consultation of the physicians.

XI. The nurses and servants of the house shall have no direct communication with the Infirmary; but shall receive the medicines in the room already appropriated to messengers from the home patients.

XII. The committee of the Strangers' Friend Society shall be requested to undertake the office of inspecting the House of Recovery.

XIII. A weekly report of the patients admitted and difcharged fhall be publifhed in the Manchefter newfpapers.

XIV. When a patient dies in the wards, the body fhall be removed as foon as poffible into a room appropriated to that ufe; it fhall then be wrapt in a pitched cloth, and the friends fhall be defired to proceed to the interment as early as is confiftent with propriety.

XV. All provifions and attendance for the patients in this Houfe of Recovery fhall be provided from the funds of this inftitution, without any communication with the Infirmary.

The eftablifhment of fever-wards was propofed in 1774, and a few years afterward carried into complete execution by my excellent and truly philanthropic friend Dr. Haygarth; whofe life has been actively devoted to the promotion of fcience, the improvement of his profeffion, and the general good of mankind. The reader will find in his writings views concerning the nature, caufes, and prevention of contagion, derived from philofophic principles, and confirmed by extenfive and accurate obfervation.* Thefe interefting fubjects have lately, in a peculiar degree, engaged the attention, and employed the pens, of various other diftinguifhed writers, as appears by the works of Dr. Wall, Dr. Currie, Dr. Ferriar, and Dr. Clark.†

---

* See Haygarth's Enquiry how to prevent the Small-Pox; Sketch of a Plan to exterminate the cafual Small-Pox; Letter to Dr. Percival on the Prevention of Infectious Fevers.

† See the Reports of the Society for bettering the Condition and Increafing the Comforts of the Poor; Dr. Stanger's Remarks on

Note V.   *Chap.* I.   *Sect.* XXXI.

CAUTION OR TEMERITY IN PRACTICE.

It is the obfervation of an elegant writer on the fubject of morals, and applicable to medical practice, that " the beft character is that which is not fwayed " by temper of any kind; but alternately employs " enterprize and caution, as each is ufeful to the par- " ticular purpofe intended.   Such is the excellence " which St. Evremond afcribes to Marefchal Turenne; " who difplayed every campaign, as he grew older, " more temerity in his military enterprifes; and " being now, from long experience, perfectly ac- " quainted with every incident in war, he advanced " with greater firmnefs and fecurity, in a road fo " well known to him."*   Yet it is faid of the great Duke of Marlborough, that ten years of fuch unin- terrupted and fplendid fuccefs as no other general could boaft of, never betrayed him into a fingle rafh action.†

That boldnefs in medical practice is more frequently the antecedent than the confequence of experience, is a melancholy truth; for it is generally founded

the Neceffity and Means of fuppreffing Contagious Fever; alfo Thoughts on the Means of preferving the Health of the Poor, by the Rev. Sir W. Clarke, bart.; and feveral other valuable modern works.

* Hume's Effays, vol. ii. p. 284.

† See Smith's Theory of Moral Sentiments, vol. ii. p. 158.

either on theoretical dogmas, or on pride which dis-
claims authority.   To the confideration of phyficians,
who are thus prematurely confident in their own
powers, the remark of Lord Verulam may be recommended.   " This is well to be weighed, that bold-
" nefs is ever blind; for it feeth not dangers and
" inconveniences; therefore it is ill in counfel, good
" in execution: fo that the right ufe of bold perfons
" is, that they never command in chief, but be fe-
" conds, and under the direction of others.   For in
" counfel it is good to fee dangers; and in execution
" not to fee them, except they be very great."

Note VI.   *Chap*. II.   *Sect*. II.

TEMPERANCE OF PHYSICIANS.

" Though much has been faid, and with fome
" truth, of the good effects of wine in producing
" rapidity and vivacity of thought, it has fcarcely
" ever been pretended that it favoured the exercife
" of difcrimination and judgment.   The only perfons
" in whom it has ever been fuppofed not to have the
" oppofite effects, are fome gentlemen of the faculty.
" The ignorant vulgar would think, *a priori*, that,
" *cæteris paribus*, a phyfician who was fober, would
" attend more accurately to the cafe of his patient,
" and compare and diftinguifh all circumftances
" better, and judge more foundly, and prefcribe more

" rationally, than he could do when he was drunk.
" But fome phyficians, who fhould be fuppofed to
" know themfelves beft, and who certainly muft have
" known how they acquitted themfelves in thofe
" different fituations, have boafted that they pre-
" fcribed as well drunk as fober.   In this they could
" not be miftaken; for, whether we confider the
" matter phyfically or logically, their boaft amounts
" precifely to this, that they prefcribed no better
" when they were fober than they did when they
" were drunk; which is undoubtedly a noble accom-
" plifhment; but it is not furely either wonderful
" or rare."*

Tacitus, in his admirable treatife *De Moribus
Germanorum*, has ftated, that thofe nations—*de re-
conciliandis invicem inimicis, et jungendis affinitatibus,
et adfcifcendis principibus, de pace denique ac bello,
plerumque in conviviis confultant: tamquam nullo magis
tempore aut ad fimplices cogitationes pateat animus, aut
ad magnas incalefcat.   Gens non aftuta nec callida
aperit adhuc fecreta pectoris licentiâ loci.   Ergo de-
tecta et nuda omnium mens pofterâ die retractatur; et
falva utriufque temporis ratio eft.   Deliberant dum
fingere nefciunt: conftituunt dum errare non poffunt.*†

---

* See the Introduction to Philofophical and Literary Effays, by
Dr. Gregory, of Edinburgh, p. 187.

† Taciti Opera à Lipfio. fol. 1627, p. 444.—The learned editor
obferves, in his note on this paffage, *Perfarum fimilis mos, et
Cretenfium, et Græcorum omnium veterum.*

In deliberation, it may, on fome peculiar occafions, be of importance to break off all former ftrong affociations. A fit of drunkennefs accomplifhes this fully: fleep has the fame tendency; and hence the proverb, *I will fleep upon it.* But fuch deliberation bears no analogy to what is required from a phyfician, when he is to confider the cafe of a patient.

" Univerfal temperance," fays Mr. Gifborne,
" both in eating and drinking, is particularly incum-
" bent on a phyfician in every period of his practice;
" not merely as being effentially requifite to preferve
" his faculties in that alert and unclouded ftate, which
" may render him equally able at all times to pro-
" nounce on the cafes which he called to infpect,
" but becaufe it is a virtue which he will very fre-
" quently find himfelf obliged to inculcate on his
" patients; and will inculcate on them with little
" effect, if it be not regularly exemplified in his own
" conduct."*

Note VII. *Chap.* II. *Sect.* III.

" A PHYSICIAN SHOULD BE THE MINISTER OF HOPE AND COMFORT TO THE SICK."

Mr. Gifborne, in one of his interefting letters to me on the fubject of Medical Ethics, fuggefts, that it would be advifeable to add, *as far as truth and fin-*

* Duties of Men, vol. ii. p. 139. Note.

cerity will admit. " I know very well," fays he,
" that the fentence, as it now ftands, conveys to you,
" and was meant by you to convey to others, the
" fame fentiment which it would exprefs after the
" propofed addition. But if I am not miftaken in
" my idea, that there are few profeffional temptations
" to which medical men are more liable, and fre-
" quently from the very beft principles, than that of
" unintentionally ufing language to the patient and
" his friends more encouraging than fincerity would
" vindicate on cool reflexion ; it may be right fcru-
" puloufly to guard the avenues againft fuch an error."

In the *Enquiry into the Duties of Men,* the fame
excellent moralift thus delivers his fentiments more at
large. " A profeffional writer, fpeaking, in a work
" already quoted,* refpecting the performance of
" furgical operations in hofpitals, remarks, that it
" may be a falutary as well as an humane act, in the
" attending phyfician, occafionally to affure the patient
" that every thing goes on well, *if that declaration
" can be made with truth.* This reftriction, fo pro-
" perly applied to the cafe in queftion, may with
" equal propriety be extended univerfally to the
" conduct of a phyfician, when fuperintending opera-
" tions performed, not by the hand of a furgeon, but
" by nature and medicine. Humanity, we admit,
" and the welfare of the fick man commonly require,
" that his drooping fpirits fhould be revived by every

* Percival's Medical Ethics, chap. i.

" encouragement and hope, which can honeftly be
" fuggefted to him. But truth and confcience for-
" bid the phyfician to cheer him by giving pro-
" mifes, or raifing expectations, which are known,
" or intended, to be delufive. The phyfician may
" not be bound, unlefs exprefsly called upon, inva-
" riably to divulge, at any fpecific time, his opinion
" concerning the uncertainty or danger of the cafe:
" but he is invariably bound never to reprefent the
" uncertainty or danger as lefs than he actually be-
" lieves it to be; and whenever he conveys, directly
" or indirectly, to the patient or to his family, any
" impreffion to that effect, though he may be mifled
" by miftaken tendernefs, he is guilty of pofitive
" falfehood. He is at liberty to fay little; but let
" that little be true. St. Paul's direction, *not to do*
" *evil that good may come*, is clear, pofitive, and
" univerfal."*

Whether this fubject be viewed as regarding general morality, or profeffional duty, it is of high importance; and we may juftly prefume, that it involves
confiderable difficulty and intricacy, becaufe oppofite
opinions have been advanced upon it by very diftinguifhed writers. The ANCIENTS, though fublime
in the abftract reprefentations of virtue, are feldom
precife and definite in the detail of rules for its obfervance. Yet in fome inftances they extend their
precepts to particular cafes: and Cicero, in the Third

---

* Duties of Men, vol. ii. p. 148.

Book of his Offices, exprefsly admits of limitations to the abfolute and immutable obligation of fidelity and truth.

The maxim of the poet, alfo, may be adduced as intended to be comprehenfive of the moral laws by which human conduct is to be governed:

> ———— " Sunt certi denique fines,
> " Quos ultrá citráque nequit confiftere rectum."†

The early FATHERS of the Chriftian church, Origen, Clement, Tertullian, Lactantius, Chryfoftom, and various others, till the period of St. Auguftine, were latitudinarians on this point. But the holy father laft mentioned, if I miftake not, in the warmth of his zeal, declared that he would not utter a lie, though he were affured of gaining heaven by it. In this declaration there is a fallacy, by which Auguftine probably impofed upon himfelf. For a lie is always underftood to confift in a *criminal* breach of truth, and therefore under no circumftances can be juftified. It is alleged, however, that falfehood may lofe the effence of lying, and become even praife-worthy, when the adherence to truth is incompatible with the prac-tice of fome other virtue of ftill higher obligation. This opinion almoft the whole body of CIVILIANS adopt, with full confidence of its rectitude. The fentiments of Grotius may be feen at large in the fa-

---

† Horat. Sat. lib. i. Sat. i. 106.

tisfactory detail which he has given of the controverfy relating to it.*

Puffendorff, who may be regarded as next to this
great man in fucceffion as well as authority, delivers
the following obfervations in his *Law of Nature and
Nations*, which are pointedly applicable to the prefent
fubjects, yet carried affuredly to a very reprehenfible
extent: " Since thofe we talk to may often be in
" fuch circumftances, that if we fhould tell them the
" downright truth of the matter, it would prejudice
" them, and would incapacitate us for procuring that
" lawful end we propofe to ourfelves for their good;
" we may in thefe cafes ufe a fictitious or figurative
" way of fpeech, which fhall not directly reprefent
" to our hearers our real thoughts and intentions: for
" when a man is defirous, and it is his duty, to do a
" piece of fervice, he is not bound to take meafures
" that will certainly render his attempts unfuccefs-
" ful."†—" Thofe are by no means guilty of lying,
" who, for the better information of children, or
" other perfons not capable of relifhing the naked
" truth, entertain them with fictions and ftories: nor
" thofe who invent fomething that is falfe, for the
" fake of a good end, which by the plain truth they
" could not have compaffed; as, fuppofe, for pro-
" tecting an innocent, for appeafing a man in his

---

* See the fecond, third, and fourth paragraphs of the 10th Sect.
cap. 1, lib. 3, of Grotius de Jure Bell. ac Pac.—Alfo, the 14th, 15th,
and 16th Sections of the fame chapter.

† Spavan's Puffendorff, vol. ii. cap. i. p. 6.

" paffion, for *comforting the afflicted*,, for *animatiug*
" *the timorous*, for *perfuading a naufeating patient to*
" *take his phyfic*, for overcoming an obſtinate humour,
" for making an ill defign mifcarry."*

Several modern ETHICAL WRITERS, of confiderable celebrity, have been no lefs explicit and indulgent on this queſtion. Amongſt thefe, it may fuffice to cite the teſtimony of the late Dr. Francis Hutchefon, of Glafgow; of whom it is faid by his excellent biographer, that " he abhorred the leaſt " appearance of deceit, either in word or action."†
" When in certain affairs," fays he, " it is known " that men do not conceive it an injury to be de-" ceived, there is no crime in falfe fpeech about fuch " matters.—No man cenfures a phyfician for deceiv-" ing a patient too much dejected, by expreſſing good " hopes of him; or by denying that he gives him a " proper medicine, which he is foolifhly prejudiced " againſt: the patient afterwards will not reproach " him for it.—Wife men allow this liberty to the " phyfician, in whofe fkill and fidelity they truſt: " or if they do not, there may be a juſt plea from " neceſſity."‡—" Thefe pleas of neceſſity fome would " exclude by a maxim of late received, *We muſt not* " *do evil that good may come of it.* The author of this

* Spavan's Puffendorff, vol. ii. cap. i. p. 9.

† Dr. Lechman's Biographical Preface to Hutchefon's Syſtem of Moral Philofophy, p. 26.

‡ Hutchefon's Syſtem of Moral Philofophy, vol. i. p. 32, 33.

" maxim is not well known. It feems by a paffage
" in St. Paul, that Chriftians were reviled as teaching
" that fince the mercy and veracity of God were dis-
" played by the obftinate wickednefs of the Jews,
" they fhould continue in fin, that this good might
" enfue from it. He rejeéts the imputation upon his
" doétrine; and hence fome take up the contradiétory
" propofition, as a general maxim of great importance
" in morality. Perhaps it has been a maxim
" among St. Paul's enemies, as they upbraid him with
" counteraéting it. Be the author who they pleafe,
" it is of no ufe in morals, as it is quite vague and
" undetermined. Muft one do nothing for a good
" purpofe, which would have been evil without this
" reference ? It is evil to hazard life without a view
" to fome good ; but when it is neceffary for a pub-
" lic intereft, it is very lovely and honourable.
" It is criminal to expofe a good man to danger for
" nothing; but it is juft even to force him into the
" greateft dangers for his country. It is criminal to
" occafion any pains to innocent perfons without a
" view to fome good; but for reftoring of health we
" reward chirurgeons for fcarifyings, burnings, and
" amputations. *But*, fay they, *fuch aétions, done for*
" *thefe ends, are not evil. The maxim only determines*
" *that we muft not do, for a good end, fuch aétions as*
" *are evil even when done for a good end.* But this
" propofition is identic and ufelefs ; for who will
" tell us next, what thefe aétions, fometimes evil, are,
" which may be done for a good end ? and what

" actions are so evil that they muſt not be done even
" for a good end ?   The maxim will not anſwer this
" queſtion ; and truly it amounts only to this trifle ;
" *you ought not for any good end to do what is evil,* or
" *what you ought not to do even for a good end.*"*

Dr. Johnſon, who admits of ſome exception to the
Law of Truth, ſtrenuouſly denies the right of telling
a lie to a ſick man for fear of alarming him.   " You
" have no buſineſs with conſequences," ſays he,
" you are to tell the truth. Beſides, you are not ſure,
" what effect your telling him that he is in danger
" may have.   It may bring his diſtemper to a criſis,
" and that may cure him.   Of all lying I have the
" greateſt abhorrence of this, becauſe I believe it has
" been frequently practiſed on myſelf."†

If the medical reader wiſh to inveſtigate this nice
and important ſubject of caſuiſtry, he may conſult
Grotius de Jure Bell. ac Pacis; Puffendorff; Grove's
Ethics; Balguy's Law of Truth; Cambray's Tele-
machus; Butler; Hutcheſon; Paley; and Giſborne.
Every practitioner muſt find himſelf occaſionally in
circumſtances of very delicate embarraſſment, with
reſpect to the contending obligations of veracity and
profeſſional duty: and when ſuch trials occur, it
will behove him to act on fixed principles of rectitude,
derived from previous information, and ſerious reflection.   Perhaps the following brief conſiderations,

---

* Hutchinſon's Syſtem of Mor. Phil. vol. ii. p. 132.
† See Boſwell's life of Johnſon, p. 570.

by which I have confcientioufly endeavoured to govern my own conduct, may afford fome aid to his decifion.

Moral truth, in a profeffional view, has two references; one to the party to whom it is delivered, and another to the individual by whom it is uttered. In the firft, it is a *relative duty*, conftituting a branch of juftice; and may be properly regulated by the divine rule of equity prefcribed by our Saviour, to *do unto others as we would*, all circumftances duly weighed, *they should do unto us.* In the fecond, it is a *perfonal duty*, regarding folely the fincerity, the purity, and the probity of the phyfician himfelf. To a patient, therefore, perhaps the father of a numerous family, or one whofe life is of the higheft importance to the community, who makes enquiries which, if faithfully anfwered, might prove fatal to him, it would be a grofs and unfeeling wrong to reveal the truth. His right to it is fufpended, and even annihilated; becaufe its beneficial nature being reverfed, it would be deeply injurious to himfelf, to his family, and to the public: and he has the ftrongeft claim, from the truft repofed in his phyfician, as well as from the common principles of humanity, to be guarded againft whatever would be detrimental to him. In fuch a fituation, therefore, the only point at iffue is, whether the practitioner fhall facrifice that delicate fenfe of veracity, which is fo ornamental to, and indeed forms a characteriftic excellence of, the virtuous man, to this claim of profeffional juftice and focial duty. Under such a painful conflict of obligations, a wife and good man must be governed by those which are the most imperious; and will therefore generously relinquish every consideration, referable only to himself. Let him be careful, however not to do this, but in cases of real emergency, which happily seldom occur; and to guard his mind sedulously against the injury it may sustain by such violations of the native love of truth.

I shall conclude this long note with the two following very interesting biographical facts. The husband of the celebrated Arria, Cæcinna, Pætus, was very dangerously ill. Her son was also sick at the same time, and died. He was a youth of uncommon accomplishments; and fondly beloved by his parents. Arria prepared and conducted his funeral in such a manner, that her husband remained entirely ignorant of the mournful event which occasioned that solemnity. Pætus often enquired with anxiety about his son; to whom she cheerfully replied, that he had slept well, and was better. But if her tears, too long restrained, were bursting forth, she instantly retired, to give vent to her grief; and when again composed, returned to Pætus, with dry eyes, and a placid countenance, quitting, as it were, all the tender feelings of the mother at the threshold of her husband's chamber.†

---

† Plin. Epist. 16. lib.. iii.

Lady Ruſſel's only ſon, Wriotheſley Duke of Bedford, died of the ſmall-pox in May 1711, in the 31ſt year of his age. To this affliction ſucceeded, in Nov. 1711, the loſs of her daughter, the Ducheſs of Rutland, who died in child-bed. Lady Ruſſel, after ſeeing her in the coffin, went to her other daughter, married to the Duke of Devonſhire, from whom it was neceſſary to conceal her grief, ſhe being at that time in child-bed likewiſe; therefore ſhe aſſumed a cheerful air, and with aſtoniſhing reſolution, verbally agreeable to truth, anſwered her anxious daughter's enquiries with theſe words,—" I have ſeen your ſiſter out of bed to-day."*

Note VIII. *Chap*. II. *Sect*. V.

THE PRACTICE OF A PRIOR PHYSICIAN SHOULD BE TREATED WITH CANDOUR, AND JUSTIFIED SO FAR AS TRUTH AND PROBITY WILL PERMIT.

MONTAIGNE, in one of his eſſays, treats, with great humour, of phyſic and phyſicians; and makes it a charge againſt them, that they perpetually direct variations in each other's preſcriptions. " Whoever ſaw," ſays he, " one phyſician approve of the preſcription of another, without taking ſomething away,

---

* Note to the Letters of Lady Ruſſel, 4to. Letter 149, p. 204.

or adding fomething to it ? By which they fufficiently betray their aft, and make it manifeft to us,
that they therein more confider their own reputation,
and confequently their profit, than their patient's
intereft."*

Note IX. Chap. II. Sect. IX.

THEORETICAL DISCUSSIONS SHOULD BE GENERALLY AVOIDED.

THIS rule is not only applicable to confultations;
but to any reafonings on the nature of the cafe, and
of the remedies prefcribed, either with the patient
himfelf or his friends. It is faid by my lamented
friend Mr. Seward, in his entertaining anecdotes,
that the late Lord Mansfield gave this advice to a
military gentleman, who was appointed governor of
one of our iflands in the Weft-Indies, and who expreffed his apprehenfions of not being able to dis-
charge his duty as chancellor of his province:—"When
you decide, never give reafons for your decifion. You
will in general decide well; yet may give very bad
reafons for your judgment."†

---

* Montaigne's Effays, book ii. ch. xxxvii. p. 703.—Confult alfo
the fame chapter, page 719.

   Anecdotes of diftinguifhed Perfons, vol. ii. p. 361.

Note X. *Chap.* II. *Sect.* XI.

REGULAR ACADEMICAL EDUCATION.

" IT has been the general opinion," fays Dr. Johnfon, " that Sydenham was made a phyfician by accident and neceffary; and Sir R. Blackmore reports, in the preface to his Treatife on the Small-pox, that he engaged in practice without any preparatory ftudy, or previous knowledge of the medicinal fciences; affirming, that when he was confulted by him what books he fhould read to qualify him for the faid profeffion, he recommended Don Quixote. That he recommended Don Quixote to Blackmore (continues Dr. Johnfon) we are not allowed to doubt; but the relator is hindered, by the felf-love which dazzles all mankind, from difcovering that he might intend a fatire, very different from a general cenfure of all the ancient and modern writers on medicine ; fince he might perhaps mean, either ferioufly, or in jeft, to infinuate, that Blackmore was not adapted by nature to the ftudy of phyfic ; and that whether he fhould read Cervantes or Hippocrates, he would be equally unqualified for practice, and equally unfuccefs-ful in it. Whatfoever was his meaning, nothing is more evident than that it was a tranfient fally of an imagination warmed with gaiety; or the negligent effufion of a mind intent upon fome other employment, and in hafte to difmifs a troublefome intruder." Sydenham himfelf has declared, that after he determined upon the profeffion of phyfic, he applied in earneft to it, and fpent feveral years in the Univerfity of Oxford, before he began to practife in London. He travelled afterwards to Montpelier in queft of more information; fo far was he from any contempt of academical inftitutions ; and fo far from thinking it reafonable to learn phyfic by experiments alone, which muft neceffarily be made at the hazard of life."*

But it is highly injurious to the ufefulnefs and honour of the profeffion, to fuppofe the education of a phyfician may be confined to the purfuit of medicine as an *art.*   Sir W. Blackftone, in his introduction to his Commentaries on the Laws of England, has reprobated the cuftom of placing the juridical ftudent at the defk of fome fkilful attorney, in order to initiate him early in all the depths of practice, and to render him more dexterous in the mechanical part of bufinefs.   This illiberal path to the bar is not to be fanctioned, he obferves, by a few particular inftances of perfons, who, through the force of tranfcendant genius, have been able to overcome every difadvantage: and he points out, in very forcible terms, and with found argument, how effential it is to the lawyer to form his fentiments by the perufal of the pureft claffical authors ; to learn to reafon with pre-

* See Johnfon's Life of Sydenham.

cifion by the fimple but clear rules of unfophifticated logic; to fix the attention, and fteadily to purfue truth through the moft intricate deduftions, by an acquaintance with mathematical demonftration; and to acquire enlarged conceptions of nature and of art, by a view of the feveral branches of experimental philofophy. Now if this be the *vantage ground,* to adopt the language of Lord Bacon, from which the ftudy of the law fhould commence; it ought to be deemed at leaft equally neceffary to qualify for the profecution of medicine—a fcience which has man, as a compound of matter and mind, for its fubjeft, and an infinitude of fubftances derived from the animal, vegetable, and mineral kingdoms, for its inftruments. This fentiment feems to have been early prevalent in the celebrated fchool of phyfic, eftablifhed at Salerno in Italy. For it was enafted, A. D. 1237, by the heads of colleges there, that the pupils fhould be bound to pafs three years in the acquifition of phy- lofophy, and five fubfequent years in that of medi- cine.* The like regulations were afterwards adopted

* Vide Bulæi Hift. Univers. Paris, vol. p. 158.—Henry's Hiftory of Great-Britain, vol. viii. p. 206.

Dr. Freind, in his *Hift. Medicinæ,* has given a fomewhat different account of the celebrated School of Salernum. " *Sunt in eo decem* " *Doftores, qui fibi invicem, juxta creationis ordinem, fuccedunt.* " *Candidatorum examinatio feveriffima eft, quæ fit aut in Galeni* " *Therapeuticis, aut in primo primi Canonis Avicennæ, aut in* " *Aphorifmis. Is qui Doftoratum ambit unum ac viginti annos* " *habere debet (verum hic lapsum ſubeſſe autumo, cum ſcribendum ſit* " *viginti quinque vel ſeptem) ac teſtimonia proferre, quæ per ſeptem* " *annos eum Medicinæ ſtuduiſſe doceant. Quod ſi inter Chirurgos* " *recipi cupiat, Anatomiam per anni ſpatium didiciſſe hunc oportet:*

in other Univerfities; but in various countries have
fallen into difufe.*

On the firft revival of learning in Europe, fcience
was held in the higheft eftimation; and the three faculties of law, phyfic, and divinity, affumed particular
honours and privileges.   Academical degrees were
conferred on their members; and thefe titles, with the
rank annexed to them, were admitted *ubique gentium;*
being, like the order of knighthood, of univerfal validity.   Doctors indeed contended fometimes with
knights for precedence, and the difputes were not unfrequently terminated by advancing the former to
the dignity of knighthood.   It was even afferted that
a doctor had a right to that title, without creation.†

Note XI. *Chap.* II. *Sect.* XV.

PECUNIARY ACKNOWLEDGMENTS.

THE following fact, related in Dr. Johnfon's Life
of Addifon, is applicable to the profeffional conduct

"*jurandum ei est, fidelem se ac morigerum Societati futurum,*
"*præmia a pauperibus oblata recufaturum, neque Pharmacopolarum,*
"*lucri participem fore. Tum liber in ejus manum traditur, annulus*
"*digito induitur, Caput laurea redimitur, atque ipfe ofculo dimit-*
"*titur. Multa alia Statuta sunt ad Praxeos ordinationem per-*
"*tinentia; Pharmacopolæ præfertim, ut juxta Medici præcepta*
"*componant Medicamenta, et ut ea certo pretio divendant, obligantur.*"
I. FREIND OPERA MED. p. 537.

* Efprit des Loix, liv. xxix. chap. xiv.
† Confult *Seb. Bachmeifteri Autiqitates Roftoch; Crevier Hift.
de l'Univers. de Paris;* and Dr. Robertfon's Proofs and Illuftrations,
annexed to his View of the State of Europe.—Hift. Charles V. vol. i.
p. 387, 8vo.

of phyſicians towards their friends. " When Addiſon was in office, (under the Duke of Wharton, as
Lord-Lieutenant of Ireland,) he made a law to himſelf, as Swift has ſtated, never to remit his regular
fees, in civility to his friends. " For," ſaid he, " I
may have an hundred friends, and if my fee be two
guineas, I ſhall, by relinquiſhing my right, loſe two
hundred guineas, and no friend gain more than two;
there is therefore no proportion between the good im-
parted, and the evil ſuffered."*   In recording Mr.
Addiſon's *prudential* conduct, his probity, with reſpect
to pecuniary acknowledgments, ſhould not be unno-
ticed.   In a letter, relative to the caſe of Major
Dunbar, he ſays, " And now, Sir, believe me, when
I aſſure you, I never did, nor ever will, on any pretence whatſoever, take more than the ſtated or cus-
tomary fees of my office.   I might keep the contrary
practice concealed from the world, were I capable of
it ; but I could not from myſelf; and I hope I ſhall
always fear the reproaches of my own heart, more
than thoſe of all mankind."†

At a period when empirics and empiriciſm ſeem to
have prevailed much in Rome, the exorbitant demands of medical practitioners, particularly for certain
ſecret compoſitions which they diſpenſed, induced the
Emperor Valentinian to ordain, that no individual of
the faculty ſhould make an expreſs charge for his
attendance on a patient ; nor even avail himſelf of

---

* See Johnſon's Lives of the Poets.   † Idem.

any promife of remuneration during the period of
ficknefs; but that he fhould reft fatisfied with the
donative voluntarily offered at the clofe of his minis-
tration.*   By the fame law, however, the Emperor
provided that one practitioner, at leaft, fhould be
appointed for each of the fourteen fections into which
the Roman metropolis was divided, with fpecial privileges, and a competent falary for his fervices; thus
indirectly, yet explicitly, acknowledging that a phyfician has a full claim in equity to his profeffional
emoluments.   Is it not reafonable, therefore, to
conclude, that what fubfifted as a *moral right*, ought
to have been demandable, under proper regulations,
as a *legal right?*   For it feems to be the office of
law to recognize and enforce that which natural
juftice recognizes and fanctions.

The Roman advocates were fubject to the like reftrictions, and from a fimilar caufe.   For their rapacity occafioned the revival of the Cincian ordinance,
" *quâ cavetur antiquitus, ne quis ob caufam orandam*
pecuniam donumve accipiat."   But Tacitus relates,
that when the fubject was brought into difcuffion
before Claudius Cæfar, amongft other arguments in
favour of receiving fees, it was forcibly urged, *fub-*
latis ftudiorum pretiis, etiam ftudia peritura ; and that,
in confequence, the prince " *capiendis pecuniis pofuit*
modum, ufque ad dena feftertia, quæ egreffi repetunda-
rum tenerentur."†

* Vid. Cod. Theodos. lib. x.iii. tit. iii.
† Annal. lib. xi. p. 168, edit. Lipfii.

A precife and invariable *modus*, however, would be injurious both to the barrifter and the phyfician, becaufe the fees of each ought to be meafured by the value of his time, the eminence of his character, and by his general rule of practice. This rule, with its antecedents, being well known, a *tacit compact* is eftablifhed, reftrictive on the claims of the practitioner, and binding on the probity of the patient. Law cannot properly, by its ordinances, eftablifh the cuftom, which will and ought to vary in different fituations, and under different circumftances. But a court of judicature, when formally appealed to, feems to be competent to authorize it if juft, and to correct it if unjuft. Such decifions could not wholly change the honorary nature of fees; becaufe they would continue to be increafed, at the difcretion of the affluent, according to their liberality and grateful fenfe of kind attentions; and diminifhed, at the option of the phyfician, to thofe who may, from particular circumftances, require his beneficence.

From the Roman code, the eftablifhed ufage, in different countries in Europe, relative to medical fees, has probably originated. This ufage, which conftitutes common law, feems to require confiderable modification to adapt it to the prefent ftate of the profeffion. For the general body of the faculty, efpecially in the united kingdoms of Great-Britain and Ireland, are held in very high eftimation, on account of their liberality, learning, and integrity:* and it would be difficult to affign a fatisfactory reafon why they fhould be excluded from judicial protection, when the juft remuneration of their fervices is wrongfully withheld. Indeed a medical practitioner, one efpecially who is fettled in a provincial town, or in the country, may have accumulated claims from long-protracted and often expenfive attendance; and his pecuniary acknowledgments may be refufed from prejudice, from captioufnefs, from parfimony, or from difhonefty. Under fuch circumftances, confiderations of benevolence, humanity, and gratitude, are wholly fet afide: becaufe when difputes arife, they muft be fufpended or extinguifhed; and the queftion at iffue can alone be decided on the principles of *commutative juftice.*

* Of this truth, it has been my duty and inclination to offer feveral proofs, of unqueftionable authority, in different parts of the prefent work. Two additional ones now occur to my recollection, which I fhall here infert. Mr. Pope, writing to Mr. Allen, concerning his obligations to Dr. Mead, and other phyficians, about a month before his death, fays, " There is no end of my kind treat-
" ment from the faculty. They are in general the moft amiable
" companions and the beft friends, as well as the moft learned men
" I know." The Rev. Dr. Samuel Parr, in a letter with which he honoured me in September 1794, thus expreffes himfelf: " I have
" long been in the habit of re ling on medical fubjects; and the
" great advantage I have derived from this circumftance is, that I
" have found opportunities for converfation and friendfhip with a
" clafs of men, whom, after a long and attentive furvey of literary
" characters, I hold to be the moft enlightened profeffional perfons
" in the whole circle of human arts and fciences."

Note XII. *Chap.* II. *Sect.* XXX.

PUBLIC WORSHIP, SCEPTICISM, AND
INFIDELITY.

THE neglect of focial worſhip, with which phyſicians have been too juſtly charged, may be traced, in
many inſtances, to the period of their academical education, particularly in the univerſities, where young
men are permitted to live at large, and are ſubject to
no collegiate diſcipline. Sunday, affording a receſs
from public lectures, is devoted, by thoſe who are
ardent in ſtudy, to a review of the labours of the
paſt week; to preparations for medical or ſcientific
diſcuſſions in the ſocieties of which they are members;
or to other purſuits, belonging to their profeſſion,
but unconnected with religion. The idle and the
gay, in ſuch ſituations, are eager to avail themſelves
of opportunities ſo favourable to their taſte for recre-
tation, or to their averſion to buſineſs and confinemen.
In each of theſe claſſes, though actuated by different
principles, there is much danger that devotional impreſſions will be gradually impaired, for want of
ſtated exerciſe and renewal: and a foundation will
thus be laid for habitual and permanent indifference,
in future life, to divine ſervices, whenever medical avo-
cations furniſh a *ſalvo* to the mind, and a plauſible

excufe to the world, for non-attendance on them. This coldnefs of heart, this moral infenfibility, fhould be feduloufly counteracted before it has acquired an invincible afcendancy. No apology fhould be ad-mitted for abfence from the ftated offices of piety, but that of duties to be performed of immediate and preffing neceffity. When the church is entered with Juft views, it will be found that there is a fympathy in religious homage, which at once infpires and heightens devotion: and that to hold communion with GOD in concert with our families, our friends, our neighbours, and our fellow-citizens, is the higheft privilege of human nature. But with a full con-viction of the obligation of public worfhip, as a focial inftitution, founded on common confent, and enjoined by legal authority; as a moral duty connect-ing us by the moft endearing ties with our brethren of mankind, who are joint dependants with our-felves, on the pardon, the protection, and the bounty of GOD; and as a debt of general homage to our creator, benefactor, and judge; yet there may fubfift in a devout and benevolent mind fcruples, refpecting doctrines and forms, fufficient to produce an aliena-tion from the facred offices of the temple. Such doubts, when they originate from ferious enquiry, and are not the refult of faftidioufnefs or arrogance, have a claim to tendernefs and indulgence; becaufe, to act in contradiction to them, whilft they fubfift, would be a violation of fincerity, amounting in fome cafes to the guilt of hypocrify. But in a country where private judgment is happily under no reftraint, and where fo great diverfity of fefts prevails, it will be ftrange, if a candid and well-informed man can find no Chriftian denomination, with which he might accord in fpirit and in truth. Sir Thomas Brown, in the ftatement which he has given in his *Religio Medici*, feems to have allowed himfelf on thefe points very extenfive latitude.—" We have reformed from " them, viz. the Papifts, not againft them—and there- " fore I am not fcrupulous to converfe and live with " them, to enter their churches in defeft of ours, " and either pray with them or for them. I could " never perceive that a refolved confcience may not " adore her Creator any where, efpecially in places " devoted to his fervice; where, if their devotions " offend him, mine may pleafe him; if theirs profane " it, mine may hallow it. I could never hear the *Ave* " *Maria* bell without an elevation, or think it a fuffi- " cient warrant, becaufe they erred in one circum- " ftance, for me to err in all—that is in filence and " dumb contempt: whilft therefore they direft their " devotions to the Virgin, I offer mine to God, and " reftify the errors of their prayers by rightly order- " ing my own."

But authority, much more refpeftable than that of Sir Thomas Brown, may be adduced in favour of the fpirit of Catholicifm in Chriftian communion. Mr. Locke, a fhort time before his death, received the facrament according to the rites of the Church of England, though it is evident from his writings that

he diſſented from many of her doctrines. When the
office was finiſhed, he told the miniſter, " that he was
in perfect charity with all men, and in ſincere communion with the church of CHRIST, by what name ſoever
it might be diſtinguiſhed."*—Dr. David Hartley
was originally intended for the clerical profeſſion, but
was prevented from going into holy orders by his
ſcruples concerning ſubſcription to the thirty-nine
articles. He continued, however, to the end of his
life, a well-affected member of the Eſtabliſhment, ap-
proving of its practical doctrines, and conforming to
its public worſhip. " He was a catholic chriſtian,"
ſays his ſon and biographer, " in the moſt extenſive
and literal ſenſe of the term." On the ſubject of
religious controverſy, he has left the following teſtimony of his ſentiments:—" The great differences of
" opinion and contentions, which happen on religious
" matters, are plainly owing to the violence of men's
" paſſions, more than to any other cauſe. When
" religion has had its due effect in reſtraining theſe,
" and begetting true candour, we may expect an unity
" of opinion both in religious and other matters, as
" far as is neceſſary for uſeful and practicable pur-
" poſes."

Theſe examples of the conduct of wiſe and con-
ſcientious chriſtians evince, that, in their eſtimation,
forms, ceremonies, and doctrines, are of a moment
ſubordinate to the benefits and obligations of ſocial
worſhip. But they are not adduced to ſanction an

* See Brit. Biog. vol. vii. p. 13.

indifference, either to religious rites, or religious truth. The mind will always be in the beft frame for holy exercifes, when the modes by which they are con-ducted are confonant to its fentiments of propriety and rectitude. And that church fhould be habitually reforted to, if practicable, the public fervices of which accord moft fatisfactorily with the views of the indi-vidual, concerning the attributes of GOD, and the revelation of his will and promifes to man. No perfonal friendfhip, no party connection, no profeffi-onal intereft fhould be allowed to predominate in the choice. For genuine piety, which is the joint offspring of reafon and of fentiment, admits of no fubftitutions. It confifts in a full conviction of the underftanding, accompanied with correfpondent affections of the heart; and in its exercifes calls forth their united and nobleft energies.

It will not be foreign to the fubject of this note to inveftigate briefly the imputation of fcepticifm and infidelity, which has been laid againft the medical faculty. The Rev. Dr. Samuel Parr, whofe can-dour is unqueftionable, and whofe learning and genius entitle him to the higheft refpect, has lately fanctioned it, as will appear by the following paffage from his *Remarks on the Statement of Dr. Charles Combe*, pages 82, 83.—" While I allow," fays he, " that peculiar and important advantages arife from " the appropriate ftudies of the three liberal pro- " feffions, I muft confefs, that in erudition, in fcience, " and in habits of deep and comprehenfive thinking,

" the pre-eminence, in fome degree, muft be af-
" figned to phyficians. The propenfity which fome
" of them have fhewn to fcepticifm, upon religious
" topics, is indeed to be ferioufly lamented; and it
" may be fatisfactorily explained, I think, upon me-
" taphyfical principles, which evince the ftrength
" rather than the weaknefs of the human mind, when
" contemplating, under certain circumftances, the
" multiplicity and energy of phyfical caufes. But I
" often confole myfelf with reflecting on the founder
" opinions of Sir Thomas Browne, Sydenham, Boer-
" haave, and Hartley, in the days that are paft; and
" of our own times, pofterity will remember that
" they were adorned by the virtues, as well as the
" talents, of a Gregory, a Heberden, a Falconer, &c."*

Mr. Gifborne, in his *Enquiry into the Duties of
Men, in the higher and middle Claffes of Society*,
a work to which I have already referred, as an admirable fyftem of practical and appropriate ethics,
has very explicitly and forcibly delivered his fentiments on this interefting fubject. " The charge,"
he fays, " may have been made on partial and infufficient grounds; but the exiftence of it fhould excite the efforts of every confcientious phyfician, to
refcue himfelf from the general ftigma. It fhould
ftimulate him, not to affect a fenfe of religion which
he does not entertain, but openly to avow that which

---

* " Of our own times, pofterity will remember that they were
adorned by the virtues, as well as the talents of a Gregory, a Heberden, a Falconer, *and a Percival*." Vide Remarks &c. by Dr.
Parr. (Note of the Editor.)

he actually feels. If the charge be in fome meafure true, it is of importance, to the phyfician, to afcertain the caufes from which the fact has originated, that he may be the more on his guard againft their influence. The following circumftances may not have been without their weight. They who are accustomed to deep refearches into any branch of philofophical fcience; and find themfelves able to explain, to their own fatisfaction, almoft every phænomenon, and to account, as they apprehend, for almoft every effect, by what are termed natural caufes, are apt to acquire extravagant ideas of the fufficiency of human reafon on all fubjects; and thus learning to doubt the neceffity, become prejudiced againft the belief, of divine revelation. In the next place, they who juftly difclaim the empire of authority in medical theories, may carelefsly proceed to regard religious doctrines as theories, refting on no other foundation, and deferving of no better fate. Thirdly, it is to be obferved, that men may be divided into two diftinct claffes, with refpect to the fort of teftimony on which they receive truths of any kind. They who are chiefly addicted to inveftigations and reafonings, founded on analogy, look primarily and with extreme partiality to that fpecies of evidence; and if the thing afferted appear contrary to the common courfe of nature, more efpecially if it militate againft any theory of their own, (and fuch perfons are much difpofed to theorife,) they are above meafure reluctant to admit the reality of it; and withhold their affent, until fuch a number of particular proofs, incapable of being refolved into fraud or mifconception, is produced, as would have been far more than fufficient to convince an unbiaffed judgment. Whereas other men, little ufed to analogical enquiries, look not around for fuch teftimony, either in fupport or in refutation of an extraordinary circumftance affirmed to them ; but readily give credit to the fact on its own diftinct proofs, or from confidence in the veracity and difcernment of the relator. It is evident that phyficians are to be ranked in the clafs firft defcribed, and are confequently liable to its prejudices: and it is equally evident, that thofe prejudices will render all on whom they faften particularly averfe to recognize the truth of miracles ; and will probably prevent them from examining, with impartiality, the evidence of a religion founded on miracles, and perhaps from examining it at all.   Fourthly; to the preceding circumftances muft be added the neglect of divine worfhip, too cuftomary among perfons of the medical profeffion.   This neglect feems to have contributed not only to excite and ftrengthen the opinion of their fcepticifm and infidelity; but fometimes to produce fcepticifm and infidelity itfelf.   For it is a natural progrefs, that he who habitually difregards the public duties of religion, fhould foon omit thofe which are private ; fhould fpeedily begin to wifh that religion, may not be true ; fhould then proceed to doubt its truth; and at length fhould difbelieve it."   Vol. II. p. 192, edit. 4.

The late Dr. Gregory, of Edinburgh, anxious to support the honour of a profeſſion which he loved, and of which he was a diſtinguiſhed ornament, very ſtrenuouſly repels the charge againſt it of ſcepticiſm and infidelity. Though his excellent lectures are, doubtleſs, in the hands of moſt phyſicians, yet I am tempted to make a tranſcript from them, becauſe I wiſh the preſent important ſubject to be viewed in the ſeveral lights, in which it has been preſented to the mind by different writers of acknowledged probity, information, and judgment. "I think the charge," he obſerves, "ill-founded, and will venture "to ſay, that the moſt eminent of our faculty have "been diſtinguiſhed for real piety. I ſhall only men- "tion as examples, Harvey, Sydenham, Arbuthnot, "Boerhaave, Stahl, and Hoffmann.—It is eaſy, "however, to ſee whence this calumny has ariſen. "Men whoſe minds have been enlarged by know- "ledge, who have been ac uſtomed to think and to "reaſon upon all ſubjects with a generous freedom, "are not apt to become bigots to any particular ſect "or ſyſtem. They can be ſteady to their own "principles, without thinking ill of thoſe who differ "from them; but they are impatient of the autho- "rity and controul of men, who would lord it over "their conſciences, and dictate to them what they "are to believe. This freedom of ſpirit, this mode- "ration and charity for thoſe of different ſentiments, "have frequently been aſcribed, by narrow minded "people, to ſecret infidelity, ſcepticiſm, or, at leaſt, to

" lukewarmnefs in religion; while fome who were
" fincere Chriftians, exafperated by fuch reproaches,
" have fometimes expreffed themfelves unguardedly,
" and thereby afforded their enemies a handle to
" calumniate them. This, I imagine, has been the
" real fource of that charge of infidelity, fo often and
" fo unjuftly brought againft phyficians."

" The ftudy of medicine, of all others, fhould be
" the leaft fufpected of leading to impiety. An inti-
" mate acquaintance with the works of nature raifes
" the mind to the moft fublime conceptions of the
" Supreme Being; and at the fame time dilates the
" heart with the moft pleafing views of Providence.
" The difficulties that neceffarily attend all deep en-
" quiries into a fubject fo difproportionate to the
" human faculties, fhould not be fufpected to furprize
" a phyfician, who, in his practice, is often involved
" in perplexity, even in fubjects expofed to the exa-
" mination of his fenfes."

" There are, befides, fome peculiar circumftances
" in the profeffion of a phyfician, which fhould natu-
" rally difpofe him to look beyond the prefent ftate
" of things, and engage his heart on the fide of
" religion. He has many opportunities of feeing
" people, once the gay and the happy, funk in deep
" diftrefs; fometimes devoted to a painful and lin-
" gering death; and fometimes ftruggling with the
" tortures of a diftracted mind. Such afflictive fcenes,
" one fhould imagine, might foften any heart, not
" dead to every feeling of humanity; and make it

" reverence that religion, which alone can fupport the
" foul in the moft complicated diftreffes; that reli-
" gion, which teaches to enjoy life with cheerfulnefs,
" and to refign it with dignity."

The judicious and animated confiderations which
are here delivered, could proceed only from a mind
actuated by the principles of virtue and religion:
and I truft, the great majority of phyficians have
their feelings in unifon with thofe of the amiable
writer I have quoted.   But there may be fome who
have been hardened to moral apathy, by the very
caufes which fhould excite benevolence and piety.
It has been well remarked, by divines and metaphy-
ficians, that *paffive impreffions* become progreffively
weaker by frequent recurrence; and that the heart
is liable to grow callous to fcenes of horror and
diftrefs, and even to the view of death itfelf.   This
law of nature is intended, by the wife and benignant
Author of our frame, to anfwer the moft falutary
purpofes, by co-operating with another of equal,
perhaps fuperior, force.   For *active propenfities* are
formed, and gradually ftrengthened, by the like renewal of the circumftances which excite them.   The
love of goodnefs is thus rendered habitual; and
rectitude of conduct is fteadily and uniformly purfued,
without ftruggle or perturbation.   Under fuch circumftances the human character then attains the
higheft excellence, of which this probationary ftate
is capable; and perhaps the medical profeffion is
more favourable than any other to the formation of

a mental conftitution, that unites in it very high degrees of intellectual and moral vigour; becaufe it calls forth the fteady and unremitting exertions of benevolence, under the direction of cultivated reafon; and, by opening a wider and wider fphere of duty, progreffively augments their reciprocal energies.

But the connection between the laws of impreffion and of habit is not fo determinate and neceffary, as to be wholly independent of the agent who is under their influence. By a perverfion of the underftanding and the will, they may be, and fometimes are, feparated. The affections alfo, when the temperament is phlegmatic, fubfift only in a languid ftate; and are too evanefcent to produce a permanently correfpondent frame of mind. If with this coldnefs of heart, a fcep_tical turn of thinking, happen to be affociated, either conftitutionally or from the cafualties of ftudy and connections, virtuous principles will gradually decay; all the tender charities of life will foon be extinguifhed; a future ftate will be either difbelieved or regarded with indifference; and practical atheifm will enfue, with the whole train of evils which refult from a denial of the creative agency of GOD, or his divine adminiftration. Allowing this to be an extreme, and barely poffible cafe, a conceffion which I am folicitous to grant to my countrymen, notwithftanding what has been fatally experienced in a neighbouring kingdom: yet different gradations towards it may fubfift, and the firft ftep fhould be avoided with fedulous care. The countervailing power of religion is here effentially neceffary, becaufe nothing befides can furnifh motives to rectitude, of adequate dignity, weight, and authority. To reftore the impreffions of piety which have been loft or impaired, without falling into the fervours of enthufiafm, or the gloom of fuperftition, may be an arduous tafk, a tafk that will require time and perfeverance to accomplifh. But the attainment will amply repay the labour, by the fweet fatisfaction which a phyfician cannot fail to derive from the confcioufnefs, that he exercifes his profeffion under the infpection of a Being, who approves and will reward every effort to acquire his favour by doing good to mankind. In his offices of humanity, he will feel an intereft and elevation, of which thofe can have no conception who regard the human race, and confequently the fufferers under their care, not as the offspring of GOD, or as expectants of immortality, but as the creatures of a day, formed by the cafual concourfe or the natural appetences of atoms, and born only to perifh. Such degrading and unhappy notions often fpring from a love of paradox; a paffion for novel hypothefis; ambition to be victorious in fubtle difputation; and a contempt for eftablifhed authority, accompanied, for the moft part, with an implicit fubmiffion to empirics in fcience, who dogmatize moft, when they affume the mafk of fcepticifm. To the fuccefsful purfuit of truth, it is neceffary to bring a well-difciplined mind, modeft and fober in its views, uninfluenced not only by vulgar, but by philofophical prejudices, which are

far more dangerous, becaufe more plaufible and faf-
cinating. When fubjects which relate to theology
are inveftigated, reverence and humility fhould be
affociated with all our reafonings. No practice is
more fubverfive of devotional fentiment, than that of
carrying into religious difcuffions the licentioufnefs of
thought and expreffion, which young phyficians are
too apt to indulge on medical topics. He who can
fuffer himfelf to treat his Maker with indifference and
with levity, whether it be in utterance or in contemplation, will foon lofe the religious impreffions of
reverence, gratitude, and love; and his mind will
then be prepared for the fyftems of impiety and atheifm, which of late have been fo boldly promulgated
under the impofing name of philofophy. Productions
of this clafs fhould be fhunned, even by thofe who
are thoroughly grounded in rational faith; becaufe
familiarity with them can hardly fail to impair the
moral fenfibilities of the heart. They are *evil communications*, which forcibly tend to *corrupt good manners.*

To the comprehenfive view of a well-educated
phyfician, the Divine Being will appear, with the
fulleft manifeftation, in all without and all within him.
Through the feveral kingdoms of nature, with which
he is intimately acquainted, he traces every where
defign, intelligence, power, wifdom, and goodnefs :
and in the frame of his own body, as well as in the
conftitution of his mental faculties, he finds efpecial
reafon to conclude, that above all the other works of
the creation, *he is fearfully and wonderfully made.*

The daily offices of his profeſſion diſcloſe to him irrefragable proofs of the providence and moral government of GOD.—Health, as conſiſting in the ſoundneſs
and vigour of the bodily organs, and in their complete aptitude for exertion and enjoyment, is doubtleſs
of ineſtimable conſideration. But the occaſional ſuf-
penſion of this bleſſing may be neceſſary to obviate
the abuſes to which it is liable; to evince its high
value; to remedy the injuries it may have ſuſtained;
and to inſure its future more permanent duration. A
ſtrong conſtitution is too often made ſubſervient to
ſenſuality, ebriety, and other licentious indulgences;
which, if not ſeaſonably interrupted by the experience
of *conſequential ſuffering*, would prove deſtructive to
the animal œconomy, and bring on premature decre-
pitude or death. Diſeaſes, under theſe circumſtances,
furniſh a beneficial reſtraint, and preſerve the mind
from contamination; whilſt they are often the remedies,
which nature has kindly provided, for the reſtoration
of the vital functions. A good, which has been loſt
and beneficently reſtored, will be prized according to its
high deſert; and being cheriſhed with aſſiduous care,
will be prolonged and applied to its proper uſes, in the
great buſineſs of life. But ſickneſs, it muſt be acknowledged, is not always remedial in its tendency; and
frequently produces degrees of protracted languiſhment
and pain, grievous to endure, and obſtructive of thoſe
active offices, which, in his preſent ſphere, man is called
upon to perform. There are duties, however, of
another claſs, not leſs eſſential to the improvement

and excellence of his *moral* and *religious character:*
and where is a fchool to be found, like the chamber
of ficknefs, for meeknefs, patience, refignation, gratitude, and devout truft in GOD? There pride is
humbled; the angry paffions fubfide; animofities ceafe;
and the vanities of the world lofe their bewitching
attractions. Falfe affociations are there corrected;
true eftimates are formed; and whilft the *paffive*
virtues are cultivated in the fuffering individual, all
who minifter to him have their beft difpofitions exercifed, and improved. Tendernefs, humanity, fympathy, friendfhip, and domeftic love, on fuch occafions,
find that fphere which is peculiarly adapted to their
exertion; and all the fofter charities derive from thefe
fources their higheft refinements.*

Rational theifm leads the mind, by fair and neceffary induction, to extend its views to revelation. He
who has difcovered the divine wifdom, power, and
goodnefs, through the various works of creation, will
feel a folicitude to make farther advances in facred
knowledge; and the more profoundly he venerates
the Author of his being, the more earneft will he be
to become acquainted with his will ; with the means
of conciliating his favour ; with the duration of his
own exiftence ; and with his future deftination. Several diftinguifhed characters in the heathen world
have, in a very explicit manner, teftified the truth of
his obfervation. Suffice it to ftate only the following

* See A Father's Inftructions, part iii. p. 312, 9th edition.

remarkable paffages from Plato: " A divine revela-
" tion is neceffary to explain the true worfhip of
" GOD—to add authority to moral precepts—to affift
" our beft endeavours in a virtuous courfe—to fix
" the future rewards and punifhments of virtuous
" and vicious conduct—and to point out fome accept-
" able expiation for fin." He introduces Socrates,
affuring Alcibiades, " that in a future time a divine
" perfon will appear, who, in pure love to man, fhall
" remove all darknefs from his mind, and inftruct him
" how to offer his prayers and praifes in the moft
" acceptable way to the Divine Being." The privileges which this intelligent and amiable philofopher
ardently looked for, we happily enjoy. Chriftianity
has brought life and immortality to light: and the
gofpel is the facred charter of our expected inheritance
of felicity. To regard with indifference what is fo
momentous, is the groffeft folly; to be diffatisfied
with its evidence argues the want of difcernment and
of candour; and to reject it, without deliberate and
confcientious inveftigation, is a high degree of impiety.
The appeal, however, muft finally be made to the
judgment of every individual: and we may humbly
hope, that He who *knoweth our frame*, will pity intellectual infirmity, and pardon involuntary error.

Note XIII. *Chap*. II. *Sect*. XXXI.

UNION IN CONSULTATION OF SENIOR AND
JUNIOR PHYSICIANS.

" HEAT and vivacity in age," fays Bacon, " is an
excellent compofition for bufinefs. Young men are
fitter to invent than to judge, fitter for execution than
for counfel, and fitter for new projects than for fettled
bufinefs ; for the experience of age in things that fall
within the compafs of it, directeth them, but in new
things abufeth them. The errors of young men are
the ruin of bufinefs ; but the errors of aged men
amount but to this, that more might have been done,
or fooner. Young men, in the conduct and manage
of actions, embrace more than they can hold; ftir
more than they can quiet; fly to the end, without confideration of the means and degrees; purfue fome few
principles which they have chanced upon abfurdly
care not to innovate, which draws unknown inconveniences; ufe extreme remedies at firft; and that which
doubleth all errors, will not acknowledge or retract
them, like an unruly horfe that will neither ftop nor
turn. Men of age object too much; confult too long;
adventure too little; repent too foon; and feldom
drive bufinefs home to the full period, but content
themfelves with a mediocrity of fuccefs.   Certainly

it is good to compound employments of both; for that will be good for the prefent, becaufe the virtues of either age may correct the defects of both ; and good for fucceffion, that young men may be learners, while men in age are actors: and laftly, good for extern accidents, becaufe authority followeth old men, and favour and popularity youth. But for the moral part, perhaps youth will have the pre-eminence, as age hath for the politick."—*Bacon's Effay of Youth and Age.*

Note XIV. *Chap.* II *Sect.* XXXII.

RETIREMENT FEOM PRACTICE.

THE following letters afford fo admirable a comment on the rule to which this note refers, that it would be a falfe and unjuftifiable delicacy not to lay them before the reader.   I fhall copy them without abridgment, becaufe they prefent at once a ftriking difplay of Dr. Heberden's nice fenfe of honour and probity ; of the peculiar urbanity of his manners; and of the vigour of his intellect at a very advanced period of life. His commendations of this little work, I may be allowed to confefs, are gratifying to my feelings ; though I am fenfible of the partiality from which they flow.   But the partiality of a character, dignified by fcience and virtue, is itfelf an honour.

Copy of a Letter from William Heberden,
M. D. F. R. S. &c. &c.

DEAR SIR,   *Windfor, Aug.* 28, 1794.

IT is owing to my diſtance from London, that I
have not ſooner made my acknowledgments, and returned my thanks for your very obliging letter. Your
being able to reſume the work you had in hand,
makes me hope that your good principles, with the
aid of time, have greatly recovered your mind from
what you muſt have ſuffered on occaſion of the great
loſs in your family ; and your attention in the further
proſecution of it, will powerfully aſſiſt in perfectly re-
ſtoring your tranquillity.   What you have already
communicated to the public, with ſo much juſt applauſe, ſhews you to be peculiarly well qualified for
drawing up a Code of Medical Ethics, by the juſt
ſenſe you have of your duties as a man, and by the
maſterly knowledge of your profeſſion as a phyſician.
I hope it will not be long before the ſheets already
printed come to my hands ; and I return you many
thanks for intending to favour me with a ſight of them.

The pleaſure of a viſit from one of Dr. Haygarth's
merit, whom I have long known and eſteemed, would
probably give me ſpirits, and make him think me leſs
broken than I am.   I have entered my 85th year;
and when I retired, a few years ago, from the practice
of phyſic, I truſt it was not from a wiſh to be idle,
which no man capable of being uſefully employed,
has a right to be; but becauſe I was willing to give

over, before my prefence of thought, judgment, and recollection was fo impaired, that I could not do juftice to my patients. It is more defirable for a man to do this a little too foon, than a little too late; for the chief danger is on the fide of not doing it foon enough.   I am, my dear fir,

    With great efteem and regard,

        Your affectionate, humble fervant,

            W. HEBERDEN.

From the Same.

DEAR SIR,   *Pall-Mall,* 15*th Oct.* 1794.

BY the miftake or neglect of the perfon left in my ho'fe in London, (to which I am juft returned,) your Code of Medical Ethics had been fent thither fome time before I was made acquainted with it. I have read it, and do not wonder, that nothing could be found by me or by any one to add or alter, after a work of this kind had paffed through the hands of one fo much mafter of the fubject; and who had taken no little time to confider it, and to make the proper improvements. I am confident that the fame might be faid of them, were I to read the two chapters which remain to be finifhed. If your judicious advice and rules were duly obferved, they would greatly contribute to fupport the dignity of the profeffion, and the peace and comfort of the profeffors. There has lately been eftablifhed, in feveral of the London hofpitals, a plan of courfes of lectures in all

the branches of knowledge ufeful to a ftudent in
phyfic. Such plans, if rightly executed, as I have no
reafon to doubt they will be, muft make London a
fchool of phyfic fuperior to moft in Europe. The
experience afforded in an hofpital will keep down the
luxuriance of plaufible theories. Many fuch have
been delivered in lectures, by celebrated teachers,
with great applaufe; but the ftudents, though perfectly
mafters of them, not having corrected them with what
nature exhibits in an hofpital, have found themfelves
more at a lofs in the cure of a patient, than an elder
apprentice of an apothecary. I pleafe myfelf with
thinking, that the method of teaching the art of healing is becoming every day more comfortable to what
reafon and nature require; that the errors introduced
by fuperftition and falfe philofophy are gradually re-
treating ; and that medical knowledge, as well as all
other dependent upon obfervation and experience, is
continually increafing in the world. The prefent race
of phyficians are poffeffed of feveral moft important
rules of practice, utterly unknown to the ableft in
former ages, not excepting Hippocrates himfelf, or
even Æfculapius.

I am, dear fir,

Your affectionate, humble fervant.

W. HEBERDEN.

It is an obfervation of Bacon, that letters written
by wife men are the beft of all human works. To
thefe admirable communications, I fhall, therefore,
take the liberty of fubjoining the extract of one,

equally interefting, and of fimilar import, from another Neftor in medicine; who has long and juftly held the firft rank amongft his brethren, for claffical tafte, elegance of ftyle, and profeffional erudition. "I have "lately," fays Sir George Baker, in a letter, dated Richmond, Auguft 11th, 1802, "been in the habit "of fpending much of my time in this place; avoiding, "when poffible, all medical employment. Many "months have paffed, fince Dr. Haygarth took fo "favourable a meafure of me: I will not, however, "trouble you with an account of the infirmities and "privations incident to my time of life. Be it fuf- "ficient to fay, that I am contented with the fare "that I have met with; and hope to retire from the "feaft of life, *uti conviva satur.*"

Note XV. Chap. IV. Sect. II.

PARTIAL INSANITY, WITH GENERAL INTELLI- GENCE. LUCID INTERVAL.

SIR Matthew Hale, in his *Hiftoria Placitorum Coronæ*, c. iv. has ftated, that "There is a partial "infanity of mind; and a total infanity. The "former is either in refpect to things, *quoad hoc* "*vel illud infanire;* fome perfons that have a "competent ufe of reafon in refpect to fome fub- "jects, are yet under a particular *dementia* in re- "fpect to fome particular difcourfes, fubjects, or

" applications; or elfe it is particular in refpect of
" degrees ; and this is the condition of very many, ef-
" pecially melancholy perfons, who, for the moft part,
" difcover their defect in exceffive fears and griefs,
" and yet are not wholly deftitute of the ufe of rea-
" fon ; and this partial infanity feems not to excufe
" them in the committing of any offence for its matter
" capital; for doubtlefs moft perfons that are felons of
" themfelves, and others, are under a degree of par-
" tial infanity, when they commit thefe offences."—
" The perfon that is abfolutely mad for a day, killing
" a man in that diftemper, is equally not guilty, as if
" he were mad without intermiffion. But fuch per-
" fons as have their lucid intervals, (which ordinarily
" happen between the full and change of the moon,)
" in fuch intervals have ufually at leaft a competent
" ufe of reafon; and crimes committed by them in
" thefe intervals are of the fame nature, and fubject
" to the fame punifhment, as if they had no fuch de-
" ficiency; nay, the alienations and contracts made by
" them in fuch intervals, are obliging to their heirs
" and executors."

Partial infanity and general intelligence may fubfift, in various degrees and proportions to each other,
in different perfons ; and even in the fame perfon at
different times. If Socrates had lived at this period,
and had not only profeffed himfelf to be governed by
the influences of a familiar fpirit, or dæmon, but had
alfo uniformly regulated his converfation and actions
by this perfuafion, he would have been juftly charge-

able with derangement of mind; notwithstanding the
profound wisdom which he displayed in his instruc-
tions concerning morals, and the conduct of life.
Lord Herbert, of Cherbury, was highly distinguished
both for talents and erudition: but having unfortunately adopted prejudices against Christianity, he
wrote an elaborate work entitled, *De Veritate, prout
distinguitur à Revelatione ;* and knowing it would
meet with much opposition, he remained some time in
anxious suspense about the publication of it.   Providence, however, as he informs us in his own biographical memoirs, kindly interposed, and determined
his wavering resolutions.   " Being thus doubtful in
" my chamber, one fair day in the summer, my case-
" ment being open towards the south, and no wind
" stirring, I took my book *De Veritate* in my hand,
" and kneeling on my knees, devoutly said, *O thou
" eternal God, I am not satisfied enough whether I
" shall publish this book ; if it be to thy glory, I beseech
" thee give me some sign from heaven; if not, I shall
" suppress it.*   I had no sooner spoken these words,
" but a loud, though yet gentle, noise came from the
" heavens ; which did so comfort and cheer me, that
" I took my petition as granted, and that I had the
" sign I demanded ; whereupon also I resolved to
" print my book."   This was not a temporary de-
lusion of the imagination, but continued a permanent
object of belief through life : and the impression was
more extraordinary, and more indicative of an un-
sound mind, because Lord Herbert's chief argument

againſt Chriſtianity is, the improbability that Heaven ſhall reveal its laws *only to a portion of the earth*. For how could he, who doubted of a *partial*, confide in an *individual* revelation? Or is it poſſible that he could rationally think his book of ſufficient importance to extort a declaration of the divine will, when the inte-reſt and happineſs of a fourth part of mankind were deemed, by him, objects inadequate to the like diſplay of goodneſs.*

The hiſtory of the Rev. Simon Browne ſtill more remarkably exemplifies the union of vigour and im-becility, of rectitude and perverſion, in the ſame un-derſtanding. The loſs of his wife, and of his only ſon, ſo powerfully affected him, that he deſiſted from the duties of his clerical function, and could not be perſuaded to join in any act of worſhip to the Deity, either public or private. He " conceived that Al-
" mighty GOD, by a ſingular inſtance of divine
" power had, in a gradual manner, annihilated in him
" the thinking ſubſtance, and utterly diveſted him
" of conſciouſneſs : that though he retained the
" human ſhape, and the faculty of ſpeaking, in a
" manner that appeared to others rational, he had
" all the while no more notion of what he ſaid than
" a parrot. And, very conſiſtently with this, he
" looked upon himſelf as no longer a moral agent, a
" ſubject of reward or puniſhment." In this con-viction he continued, with very little variation, to the

---

* See Walpole's Catalogues of royal and noble Authors ; alſo Percival's Mor. and Lit. Diſs. p. 82.

clofe of life. Yet, whilft under the influence of this
ftrange phrenzy, his faculties, in all other refpects,
appeared to be in full vigour. He applied himfelf
with ardour to his ftudies; and was fo acute a difputant, that his friends were wont to fay, *he could reafon
as if poffeffed of two fouls.* Indeed, both his imagination and his judgment were fo improved, as to fur-
pafs the ftate in which they fubfifted during his
perfect fanity.*

In J. J. Rouffeau, we have a moft interefting example of morbid fenfibility and depraved imagination,
combined with extenfive knowledge and pre-eminent
genius. It is faid by Madame de Stael, in her Reflections on his Character and Writings, that " fometimes
" he would part with you, with all his former affec-
" tion: but if an expreffion had efcaped you, which
" might bear an unfavourable conftruction ; he
" would recollect it, examine it, exaggerate it, perhaps
" dwell upon it for a month, and conclude by a total
" breach with you. Hence it was, that there was
" fcarce a poffibility of undeceiving him; for the
" light which broke in upon him at once, was not
" fufficient to efface the wrong impreffions which had
" taken place fo gradually in his mind. It was ex-
" tremely difficult too to continue long on an intimate
" footing with him. A word, a gefture, furnifhed
" him with matter of profound meditation; he con-
" nected the moft trifling circumftances, like fo many

* See Biog. Britan. art. Simon Browne.

" mathematical propofitions, and conceived his con-
" clufion to be fupported by the evidence of de-
" monftration."*

I have hazarded an opinion in the text, contrary to
what, I believe, is ufually adopted by lawyers, that
there may be cafes of partial infanity with a high
degree of general intelligence, in which the individual
ought not to be precluded from the privilege of
making a laft will and teftament. To deny the tes-
tamentary qualification to one, who, notwithftanding
fome falfe predominant conception, has been held
capable of managing his concerns with difcretion, and
whofe bequefts difcover no traces of a difturbed imagination, or unfound judgment, feems to be inconfiftent both with wifdom and with natural juftice.
Such a perfon, I prefume, is capable of acquiring property by legacy, by bargain, by transfer, by industry, or by office: and he is not prohibited, during
life, from giving or expending poffeffions thus obtained. Why then does the law deprive him of the
right of bequeathing after death, that which he might
have difpenfed, when alive, without controul? Whatever be the opinion which a medical practitioner may
have entertained, concerning the capacity or incapacity for making a will of one under thefe circumftances,
it can hardly beneceffary to obferve, that his evidence,

---

* The reader is referred to the Elements of the Philofophy of the
Human Mind, fect v. by Profeffor Dugald Stewart, for fome admirable remarks on the evils which refult from an ill-regulated imagination

when called for in a courfe of legal enquiry, fhould be delivered explicitly, and without any bias from his pre-conceptions.   On the point litigated, it is the exclufive province of the judge and jury to decide, after a full inveftigation of the cafe.

To determine the exiftence of a LUCID INTERVAL in the *delirium* of *fever*, or in the more permanent alienation of mind which conftitutes *infanity*, the tes-timony of a phyfician is fometimes required, in courts of law.   It will be incumbent on him, therefore, to poffefs a clear and definite opinion on the fubjeft, founded both on the nature of the malady, and the ftate of the patient.   The ceffation of febrile delirium is not difficult to afcertain; becaufe the rational facul-ties being unimpaired by a fhort fufpenfion, at once manifeft their renewal by figns which cannot be mif-underftood.   But the complete remiffion of madnefs is only to be decided by reiterated and attentive ob-fervation.   Every aftion and even gefture of the patient fhould be feduloufly watched; and he fhould be drawn into converfation at different times, that may infenfibly lead him to develope the falfe im-preffions under which he labours.   He fhould alfo be employed occafionally in bufinefs, or offices con-nefted with, and likely to renew, his wrong affoci-ations.   If thefe trials produce no recurrence of infanity, he may, with full affurance, be regarded as legally *compos mentis* during fuch period ; even though he fhould relapfe, a fhort time afterward, into his former malady.

Note XVI.   *Chap.* IV.   *Sect.* XIII.

DUELLING.

IN the ufages of the ancient Germans, evident traces of DUELLING may be difcovered: but it was employed by them either as an appeal to the juftice or to the prefcience of the gods.   Velleius Paterculus informs us, that queftions, decided amongft the Romans by legal trial, were terminated amongft the Germans by arms or judicial combat.† Tacitus de-fcribes it as a fpecies of divination, by which the future events of important wars were explored.   A captive from the enemy was compelled to fight with a man felected from their own nation.   Each was accoutred with his proper weapons; and the prefage of fuccefs was determined by the iffue of the battle.‖ A law is quoted by Stiernhöök, which fhews, that judicial combat was, at firft, appropriated to points re-fpecting perfonal character, and that it was only fub-fequently extended to criminal cafes, and to queftions relative to property.   The terms of the law are, "If any man fhall fay to another thefe reproachful words, ' you are not a man equal to other men;' or, ' you ' have not the heart of a man;' and the other fhall

† Vellei Patercul. lib. ii. cap. cxviii.
‖ Vide Tacit. de Situ, Morib. et Populis Germaniæ, fect. x.

reply, ' I am a man as good as you;' let them meet on the highway. If he who firſt gave offence appear, and the perſon abſent himſelf, let the latter be deemed worſe than he was called; let him not be admitted to give evidence in judgment either for man or woman, and let him not have the privilege of making a testament. If the perſon offended appear, and he who gave the offence be abſent, let him call upon the other thrice with a loud voice, and make a mark upon the earth, and then let him who abſented himſelf be deemed infamous, becauſe he uttered words which he durſt not ſupport. If both ſhall appear properly armed, and the perſon offended ſhall fall in the combat, let a half compenſation be paid for his death. But if the perſon who gave the offence ſhall fall, let it be imputed to his own raſhneſs. The petulance of his tongue hath been fatal to him. Let him lie in the field without any compenſation being made for his death.*

Monteſquieu, on the authority of Beaumanoir, whom he quotes with great reſpeꞔt, deduces the riſe and formation of the articles, relative to the point of honour, from the following particular judicial uſages. The accuſer declared, in the preſence of the judge, that ſuch a perſon had committed ſuch an aꞔtion : the accuſed made anſwer that *he lied;* upon which the judge gave orders for the duel. Thus it became an eſtabliſhed rule, that whenever the lie was given to a

---

* Lex Uplandica apud Stiern.—Robertſon's Hiſtory of Charles V. vol. i. note 22.

perfon, it was incumbent on him to fight. *Gentlemen* combated on horfeback, completely armed. *Villeins* fought on foot and with baftons. The bafton, therefore, was regarded as an inftrument of affront, becaufe to ftrike a man with it was to treat him as a villein. For the like reafon, a box on the ear, or blow on the face, was deemed a contumely, to be ex- piated with blood; fince villeins alone were liable to receive fuch difgraceful blows, as it was peculiar to them to fight with their heads uncovered.*

Practices like thefe were fo congenial to the proud and martial fpirit of the times, as well as to the fu- perftition which prevailed, that they became univerfal throughout Europe. But it is evident that they could not fail to fubvert the regular courfe of juftice, diminifh the authority of government, and violate the facred ordinances of the church. For the clergy uni- formly remonftrated againft, and even anathematifed them, as adverfe to Chriftianity ; and the civil power frequently interpofed, to fet bounds to ufages, which its authority was too feeble to fupprefs. Henry I. of England, in the twelfth century, prohibited trial by combat, in all queftions concerning property of fmall value. Louis VII. of France, iffued an edict to the fame effect. St. Louis, who was a diftinguifhed le- giflator, confidering the rude age in which he reigned, attempted a more perfect jurifprudence, by fubftituting trial by evidence, in place of that by combat. And

* See Montefquieu, liv. xxviii. c. xx.

afterwards it became the policy of every monarch, who poffeffed power or talents, to explode thefe relics of Gothic barbarifm. By degrees the practice became lefs and lefs frequent ; courts of judicature, acquired an afcendancy ; law was ftudied as a fcience, and adminiftered with great regularity ; and the ferocious manners of the inhabitants of Europe yielded to the arts of peace, and to the benefits of focial and civilized life. But an event occurred, in the year 1528, which both revived the practice of fingle combat, and gave a new form to it, more abfurd and fatal. The political and perfonal enmity, which fub-fifted between the Emperor Charles V. and Francis I., led the former to commiffion the French herald, fent to him with a denunciation of war, to acquaint his fovereign, that he fhould from that time confider him not only as a bafe violator of public faith, but as a ftranger to the honour and probity of a gentleman. Francis inftantly fent back the herald, with a *cartel* of defiance, giving the Emperor *the lie*, and challenging him to fingle combat. Charles accepted the challenge; but it being impracticable to fettle the preliminaries, this romantic and ridiculous enterprize of courfe was never accomplifhed. The tranfaction, however, excited fuch univerfal attention, and reflected fo much fplendour and dignity on this novel mode of fingle combat, that every gentleman thought himfelf entitled, and even bound in honour, to draw his fword, and to demand fatisfaction of his adverfary, for affronts trivial and even imaginary.* The beft blood in Chriftendom was fhed; perfonages of the firft dis- tinction were devoted to death; the eafe, the fami- liarity, and the confidence of private intercourfe were interrupted; and war itfelf was hardly more deftruc- tive to life, and to its deareft enjoyments, than this fatal and feductive frenzy.†

Evils of fuch magnitude required adequate reme- dies; and all the terrors of law were every where ex- erted to reprefs them. But they have hitherto been employed in vain. Nor is it likely that fanguinary punifhments will prevail, becaufe the dread of fuch punifhment would be deemed equally difhonourable

---

* See Robertfon's Hiftory of Charles V. book v.

† The Hiftory of Lord Herbert of Cherbury, who lived in the reigns of Queen Elizabeth and James I., fully exemplifies the folly and danger of adopting falfe principles of honour. During the abode of this romantic nobleman at the Duke of Montmorenci's, about twenty-four miles from Paris, it happened one evening, that a daughter of the Dutchefs de Ventadour, of about ten or eleven years of age, went to walk in the meadows with his lordfhip, and feveral other gentlemen and ladies. The young lady wore a knot of rib- band on her head, which a French chavelier fnatched away, and faftened to his hatband. He was defired to return it, but refufed. The lady then requefted Lord Herbert to recover it for her. A race enfued; and the chevalier, finding himfelf likely to be over- taken, made a fudden turn, and was about to deliver his prize to the young lady, when Lord Herbert feized his arm, and cried out, " I " give it you." ' Pardon me,' faid the lady, ' it is he who gives it ' me.' " Madam," replied Lord Herbert, 1 will not contradict " you, but if the chevalier do not acknowledge that I conftrain him " to give the ribband, I will fight with him." And the next day he fent him a challenge, " being bound thereto," fays he, " by the " oath taken when I was made knight of the bath." See the Life of Lord Herbert of Cherbury; alfo Percival's Moral and Lit. Differt. p. 299, fecond edit.

with the fear of death, in the chances of combat. A heavy fine, ſtrictly levied, would operate with greater force, on ſome of the moſt active principles of the human mind : And if it amounted to half or one third of the convicted perſon's fortune, ſuch portion being placed in Chancery, for the benefit of his heirs or children, this privation would not only extend to his comforts·and accommodations, but would be felt as a ſpecies of infamy, by depriving him of the means of maintaining his rank and ſtation in life. Lord Verulam has propoſed the following remedy for duelling : which, if effectual with men of quality, would ſoon diſgrace the practice amongſt thoſe of inferior degree. " The fountain of honour is the king; and " his aſpect, and the acceſs to his perſon, continueth " honour in life; and to be baniſhed from his pre " ſence is one of the greateſt eclipſes of honour that " can be. If his Majeſty ſhall be pleaſed, that when " this court ſhall cenſure any of theſe offences in per " ſons of eminent quality, to add this out of his own " power and diſcipline, that thoſe perſons ſhall be ba " niſhed and excluded from his court for certain years, " and the courts of his Queen and Prince, I think there " is no man that hath any good blood in him, will com " mit an act that ſhall caſt him into that darkneſs, that " he may not behold his ſovereign's face."* This propoſal of Lord Verulam ſeems to receive ſome

* Bacon's Works, vol. ii. page 516.

confirmation from a ſtory related by Lord Shafts-
bury in his Characteriſticks.† "A certain gallant
of our court, being aſked by his friends, why one of
his eſtabliſhed character for courage and good-ſenſe
would anſwer the challenge of a coxcomb, replied,
that for his *own ſex* he could ſafely truſt their
judgment; but how could he appear at night
before the *maids of honour?*"

Thus the principle, on which duelling is founded, is now neither an appeal to the juſtice of heaven,
nor an expreſſion of reſentment for wrong ſuſtained;
but generally a mere punctilio of honour, which
would affix a *ſtigma* on the character for courage
of him who omits to offer, and on the opponent who
declines the acceptance of, a challenge. Hence
forgiveneſs of injury, and reparation from the
conſciouſneſs of having committed it, thoſe noble
ſentiments of juſt and generous minds, are wholly
precluded in the intercourſe of faſhionable life.

A very able moraliſt, whom I have often quoted
with peculiar ſatisfaction, has reduced the queſtion
concerning duelling, as now practiſed, to this ſingle
point: whether a regard for our own reputation is,
or is not, ſufficient to juſtify the taking away the life
of another. "A ſenſe of ſhame," ſays he, "is ſo
"much torture; and no relief preſents itſelf, other-
"wiſe than by an attempt upon the life of our ad-
"verſary. What then? The diſtreſs which men

† Vol. i. ſect. iii. page 273.

" fuffer by the want of money is often times extreme,
" and no refource can be difcovered but that of
" removing a life, which ftands between the diftreffed
" perfon and his inheritance.   The motive in this
" cafe is as urgent, and the means much the fame,
" as in the former ; yet this cafe finds no advocates."

" For the army, where the point of honour is cul-
" tivated with exquifite attention and refinement,"
continues the fame excellent writer, " I would efta-
" blifh a court of honour, with a power of awarding
" thofe fubmiffions and acknowledgments, which
" it is generally the object of a challenge to obtain ;
" and it might grow into a fafhion with perfons of
" rank of all profeffions to refer their quarrels to the
" fame tribunal."*

An inftitution, like the one thus forcibly recommended by Dr. Paley, might probably have prevented the late fatal duel between Colonel Montgomery
and Captain M'Namara.   The addrefs of the latter to
the gentlemen of the jury gives juft grounds for this
opinion, and claims on that account the attention of
the legiflature.   " Gentlemen," faid he, " I am a
" captain of the Britifh navy.   My character you
" can only hear from others; but to maintain any
" character in that ftation, I muft be refpected.
" When called upon to lead others into honourable
" dangers, I muft not be fuppofed to be a man who
" had fought fafety, by fubmitting to what cuftom

* Dr. Paley's Principles of Moral Philofophy, chap. ix.

" has taught others to confider as a difgrace. I am
" not prefuming to urge any thing againft the laws of
" God, or of this land. I know, that in the eye of
" religion and reafon, obedience to the law, though
" againft the general feelings of the world, is the firft
"·duty, and ought to be the rule of action : but in
" putting a conftruction upon my motives, fo as to
" afcertain the quality of my actions, you will make
" allowances for my fituation."* In referring to the
foregoing difaftrous cafe, it is proper to notice, that a
furgeon of confiderable eminence, who attended on
the field of combat in his *profeffional capacity,* was on
this account arrefted, and fent to Newgate, by a
warrant from the civil magiftrate, as a *principal* in
the alleged murder, having been prefent at the duel,
and antecedently privy to it.   Nor was he libe-
rated from prifon, till the grand jury had rejected the
indictment.

It has recently been ftated, in one of the periodical
prints, that a law to prevent duelling was paffed in
the general affembly of North-Carolina during their
laft feffion, by which it was enacted,   " That no
" perfon fending, accepting, or being the bearer of a
" challenge, for the purpofe of fighting a duel, even
" though no death fhould enfue, fhall ever after be
" eligible to any office of truft, power, or profit, in
" the ftate, any pardon or reprieve notwithftanding :
" and that the faid perfon fhall further be liable to

* Courier, April 23, 1803.

" be indicted, and on conviction fhall forfeit and pay
" the fum of one hundred pounds to the ufe of the
" ftate.   And if any one who fight a duel, by which
" either of the parties fhall be killed, then the fur-
" vivor, on conviction thereof, fhall fuffer death with-
" out benefit of clergy; and the feconds fhall be con-
" fidered as acceffaries before the fact, and likewife
" fuffer death."*

I fhall infert the following communication from
my late venerable friend Dr. Benjamin Franklin, on
the fubject of duelling, becaufe the deliberate opinion
of a man, peculiarly diftinguifhed by perfpicacity,
foundnefs of judgment, and extenfive knowledge of
the world, cannot fail to be interefting to the reader.
The letter was written in the 79th year of his age,
and evinces the fame vein of humour which characterized him through life.   A few paffages are omitted, being merely complimentary and perfonal.

Paffy, near Paris, July 17, 1784.

DEAR SIR,

I Received, yefterday, by Mr. White, your kind
letter of May 11th, with the moft agreeable prefent
of your new book. I read it all before I flept. *   *
*   *   *   *   *   *   *   *   *   *   *   *   *
*   *   *   *   *   * It is aftonifhing that the mur-
derous practice of duelling, which you fo juftly condemn, fhould continue fo long in vogue.   Formerly,

* Courier, March 9th, 1803.

when duels were ufed to determine law-fuits, from an opinion that Providence would, in every inftance, favour truth and right with victory, they were more excufable. At prefent they decide nothing. A man fays fomething, which another tells him is a lie. They fight; but whichever is killed, the point in dispute remains unfettled. To this purpofe they have a pleafant little ftory here.—A gentleman, in a coffeehoufe, defired another to fit farther from him.—Why fo?—Becaufe, Sir, you fmell offenfively.—That is an affront, and you muft fight me.—I will fight you, if you infift upon it: but I do not fee how that will mend the matter. For if you kill me, I fhall fmell too; and if I kill you, you will fmell, if poffible, worfe than you do at prefent.—How can fuch miferable finners as we are, entertain fo much pride as to conceive that every offence againft our imagined honour merits death? Thefe petty princes, in their own opinion, would call that fovereign a tyrant, who fhould put one of them to death for a little uncivil language, though pointed at his facred perfon : yet every one of them makes himfelf judge in his own caufe, condemns the offender without a jury, and undertakes himfelf to be the executioner.

Our friend Mr. Vaughan may, perhaps, communicate to you fome conjectures of mine, relating to the cold of laft winter, which I fent in return for the obfervations on cold of Profeffor Wilfon. If he fhould, and you think them worthy fo much notice, you may fhew them to your philofophical fociety, to which I wifh all imaginable fuccefs. Their rules feem to me excellent.

With fincere and great efteem, I have the honour to be, your moſt obedient, and moſt humble fervant,

B. FRANKLIN.

Note XVII. *Chap.* IV. *Sect.* XVI.

PUNISHMENT OF THE CRIME OF RAPE.

THE atrocity of this crime appears to have been varioufly eſtimated at different periods, and in differentcountries; if we may judge from the diverfity of punifhments inflicted on the perpetrators of it. The reader will find a copious and interefting enumeration of them, in a folio volume, entitled, *A View of Ancient Laws againſt Immorality and Profanenefs, by John Difney, M. A. Cambridge printed,* 1729. I would refer him alfo to the *Principles of Penal Law,* by Mr. Eden, now Lord Auckland. As both thefe valuable works are out of print, a few extracts from each may form an acceptable addition to the prefent note.

The Burgundian laws provided, that if the young woman carried off returned to her parents actually corrupted, the offender fhould pay fix times her price, or legal valuation ; and alfo a mulct of twelve fhillings. If he had not wherewithal to pay thefe fums, he fhould be given up to herparents, or near relations, to take their revenge of him in what way they pleafed.

By the law of Æthelbert, the firft Chriftian king of Kent, it was enacted, that if any perfon take a young woman by force, he fhall pay her parent, or guardian, fifty fhillings; and fhall make a farther compofition for her ranfom. If fhe were efpoufed, he fhall compenfate the hufband by an additional payment of twenty fhillings. But if fhe were with child, the augmented fine fhall be five and thirty fhillings, and fifteen more to the King.

There is an ordinance of King Alfred, for the punifhment of rapes committed upon country wenches who were fervants, an offence which may be fuppofed to have been prevalent at that time. It is delivered in the following terms: " *Si quis Coloni mancipium ad ftuprum comminetur 5 Sol. Colono emendet, et 6o Sol. Mulctæ loco. Si Servus Servam ad ftuprum coegerit, compenfet hoc Virgâ fuâ virili. Si quis puellam teneræ ætatis ad illicitum concubitum comminetur, eodem modo puniatur quo ille qui adultæ fervæ hoc fecerit.*"

By the Welfh laws of Prince Hoel Dha, if two women were walking together without other company, and violence was offered to either or both of them, it was not punifhable as a rape; but if they had a third perfon with them, they might claim their full legal redrefs. If the perpetrator of a rape, being accufed, confeffed the fact, befides full fatisfaction to the woman, he was to anfwer for the crime to his fovereign, by the prefent of a filver-ftand, as high as the king's mouth, and as thick as his middle finger, with a gold cup upon it, fo large as to contain what he could take off at one draught, and as thick as the nail of a country fellow who had worked at the plough feven years. If the offender was not able to make fuch a prefent, *virilia membra amittat.*

Sir Edward Coke ftates this offence as a felony at the common law, which had a punifhment, " under fuch a condition as no other " felony had the like." The criminal was adjudged *amittere oculos, quibus virginem concupivit; amittere etiam tefticulos, qui calorem ftupri induxerunt.*

In the ancient law of England, exclufive of the punifhment inflicted on the criminal, his horfe, greyhound, and hawk, were alfo fubjected to great corporal infamy. But the woman who was the fufferer, might prevent all the penalties, if, before judgment, fhe demanded the offender for her hufband. The Roman law was in the fame fpirit. " *Rapta raptoris, aut mortem, aut indotatas nuptias optet ;*" upon which there arofe what was thought a doubtful cafe, " *Una nocte quidam duas rapuit, altera mortem optat, altera nuptias.*"

Note XVIII. Chap. IV. Sect. XVII.

UNCERTAINTY IN THE EXTERNAL SIGNS OF RAPE.

I Have been favoured by Mr. Ward, one of the furgeons to the Manchefter Infirmary, with the following particulars of the cafe, to which this note refers.

" Jane Hampfon, aged four, was admitted an out-patient of the Infirmary, February 11th, 1791. The female organs were highly inflamed, fore and painful; and it was ftated by the mother, that the child was as well as ufual till the preceding day, when fhe complained of pain in making water. This induced the mother to examine the parts affected, when fhe was furprifed to find the appearances above defcribed. The child had flept, two or three nights, in the fame bed with a boy, fourteen years old; and had complained that morning of having been hurt by him very much in the night.

" Leeches, and other external applications, together with appropriate internal remedies, were pre-fcribed : but the debility increafed, and on the 20th of February the child died. The coroner's inqueft was taken, previoufly to which the body was infpected, and the abdominal and thoracic *vifcera* were found to have been free from difeafe. The circumftances above related having been proved to the fatisfaction of the jury, and being corroborated by the opinion I gave, that the child's death was occafioned by external violence, a verdict of murder was returned againft the boy with whom fhe had flept. A warrant was therefore iffued to apprehend him; but he had abfconded, a circumftance which was confidered as a confirmation of his guilt, when added to the circum-ftantial evidence alleged againft him.

" Not many weeks had elapfed, however, before feveral fimilar cafes occurred, in which there was no reafon to fufpect that external violence had been offered; and fome in which it was abfolutely certain that no fuch injury could have taken place. A few of the patients died ; though from the novelty and fatal tendency of the difeafe, more than common attention was paid to them. I was then convinced that I had been miftaken, in attributing Jane Hampfon's death to external violence; and I informed the coroner of the reafons which produced this change of opinion. The teftimony I gave was defignedly made public; and the friends of the boy hearing of it, prevailed upon him to furrender himfelf.

" When he was called to the bar at Lancafter, the judge informed the jury, that the evidence adduced was not fufficient to convict him; that it would give rife to much indelicate difcuffion, if they proceeded on the trial ; and that he hoped, therefore, they would acquit him without calling any witneffes. With this requeft the jury immediately complied.

" The preceding narrative may teach the young furgeon to act with great circumfpection, when called upon to give an opinion in cafes which are involved in any degree of obfcurity. It behoves him to confider well the important duty he has to difcharge, both to an individual and to the community : and that he makes himfelf refponfible for the confequences which may refult from the influence of his judgment on the minds of the jury."

Note XIX. *Cap.* IV. *Sect.* XVIII.

THE SMOKE FROM LARGE WORKS, A NUISANCE.

THE fmoke iffuing from large works, without any effential or other poifonous impregnation, may prove a great annoyance to the neighbourhood in which they are fituated : and the proprietors fhould be compelled, by law, to diminifh this evil, as much as poffible, by the adoption of the improved methods of burning fuel, which have been lately invented. But it may be doubted whether the footy matter, fublimed by the combuftion of pit-coal, be fo injurious, as is commonly fuppofed, to the animal œconomy, unlefs it fhould fubfift in the atmofphere in a very extraordinary degree of accumulation. The inhabitants of Coalbrook-Dale, who live in a narrow valley, where the air is almoft conftantly loaded with vapours from numerous furnaces, employed in the fmelting of iron, are not, as I have been informed, peculiarly fubject to pulmonary affections. And the people of Birmingham, Sheffield, Newcaftle, and Manchefter, towns which are often enveloped in fmoke, from the nature of their refpective manufactures, feem to fuffer no abridgment in the general duration of life, as it fubfifts in crowded places, which can be afcribed exclufively to this caufe. Hoffmann maintains, that the fumes of pit-coal are not injurious to health, in the ordinary modes of expofure to them: and Cafpar Neumann confirms this teftimony, by his experience and obfervation during a long refidence in London.*

In mentioning Coalbrook-Dale, I might have ftated the following fact, as corroborating the obfervation above advanced. A few years ago, a lady, accompanied by her hufband, undertook a journey for the recovery of health, after a fevere attack of afthma, to which fhe was often incident. The route lay through Coalbrook-Dale; and they arrived there on Sunday evening, about eight o'clock; when all the fires were frefh lighted for working the furnaces. A thick fmoke pervaded the whole valley; and the gentleman was alarmed with the danger, which his wife incurred, of fuffocation. But, to his furprize and fatisfaction, fhe experienced no difficulty of breathing; and paffed the night, inhaling the grofs vapours with which fhe was furrounded, without prefent inconvenience or fubfequent injury. May it be fuppofed that the footy matter undergoes a decompofition in the lungs, by which it becomes capable of abforption, and innoxious to the animal œconomy? For the accumulation of it, as a folid fubftance, in the bronchial veficles, could hardly fail to occafion immediate and permanent evils. It will, however, be alleged, that travellers breathe whole days in dufty roads, and yet experience no lafting bad effects The cafe of mafons, who are fometimes incident to

---

* See Neumann's Chemical Works, by Lewis, page 246, 4to.

hæmoptoe and pulmonary confumption, is widely different, as the particles, which they draw in by re-
fpiration, are large and angular.

Conceiving it to be of importance to obtain full
and precife information, relative to the effects of fmoke
in Coalbrook-Dale, I wrote on this fubject to Mr.
Edwards, an eminent furgeon who is fettled there,
from whom I have been favoured with the following
judicious anfwer:

  " I have never obferved that afthmas, and other
" pulmonic affections, are more frequent in the Dale
" than elfewhere, but rather the contrary ; as I
" have been told, that the fmoke of London agrees
" better with fome afthmatic perfons, than the keen
" country air. Old colliers, indeed, and fuch as
" work in iron, ftone-mines, and lime-rocks, are very
" fubject, in the decline of life, to coughs and fhortnefs
" of breath, efpecially hard drinkers ; but in other
" refpects the inhabitants are remarkably healthy,
" and the principal part of the practice is furgery,
" the fmoke arifing from coal and iron not being fo
" prejudicial as from the copper-works in Cornwall
" and other parts. Such colliers and miners as are
" troubled with coughs, &c. always afcribe it to the
" duft arifing in getting the coal or mineral, and from
" the fmoke in the burning of lime, for which they
" take frequent emetics and purges."

Coalbrook-Dale, June 18, 1803.

Note XX. Page 117.

DISCOURSE ON HOSPITAL DUTIES; BY THE REV. THO. B. PERCIVAL, LL. B.

THIS Anniverſary Diſcourſe was addreſſed to the gentlemen of the faculty, the officers, the clergy, and the truſtees of the Infirmary at Liverpool, for the benefit of the charity; and I believe was highly approved by the judicious audience, before whom it was delivered. As the preacher aſſumed topics of exhortation, not before adopted by divines on ſuch occaſions, it may be proper to ſtate, that he was peculiarly qualified, from his knowledge of the polity of hoſpitals, to execute with ability ſo delicate and ſo arduous a taſk. After paſſing ſeveral years at St. John's College in Cambridge, in the purſuits of general ſcience, he removed to Edinburgh to engage in the ſtudy of phyſic. But notwithſtanding his acquiſitions in the HEALING ART, to which he applied himſelf with great aſſiduity, he uniformly diſcovered a predilection for THEOLOGY. It became expedient, therefore, not to oppoſe the ſtrong direction of his mind. He returned to Cambridge; and when he had taken the degree of LL. B. was admitted into holy orders. Being appointed to the chaplaincy of the Britiſh company of merchants at St. Petersburgh, he removed thither; and executed the duties of that honourable and important ſtation with exemplary fidelity, and with the general approbation of the faƈtory.   In this office he died, after a lingering and painful illneſs, on the 27th of May, 1798, in the thirty-ſecond year of his age.

Note XXI.   *Page* 128.

THE SALUTARY CONNEƇTIONS OF SICKNESS ARE NOT TO BE RASHLY DISSOLVED, BY REMOVING INTO AN HOSPITAL THOSE WHO MAY, WITH A LITTLE AID, ENJOY IN THEIR OWN HOMES BENEFITS AND CONSOLATIONS WHICH ELSE-WHERE IT IS IN THE POWER OF NO ONE TO CONFER.

THE domeſtic benefits of ſickneſs to the ſufferer, and to his family, in foſtering the tender attachments of affinity ;—" the charities of father, ſon, and brother," are thus eloquently diſplayed by a late excellent divine.

   " *Chriſtian*, when, in the ſeaſon *of ſickneſs*, you
" ſaw the ſolicitude of your friends . the affiduity,
" perhaps, of a pious offspring to repay your care of
" them, in doing for you what now you could do no
" longer for yourſelf; when you obſerved their

" anxiety, if any human care or interceffion could
" avail to fnatch you from the impending danger:
" when you faw them facrificing eafe, and reft, and
" health, to adminifter to your deliverance and com-
" fort, holding nothing dear to them, that if the will
" of GOD were fuch, they might by any means re-
" ftore you and retain you: when you faw their zea-
" lous care to do *all* to which their power extended;
" and their heartfelt anguifh as to that which their
" power could not reach: when iri their countenances
" you perceived the alternate marks of hope and ap-
" prehenfion, of comfort and diftrefs: while you faw
" *all* this, while you experienced the benefits and the
" confolations of their friendfhip, were your hearts
" *fo hard,* that fuch powerful attachment, and fuch
" zealous fervice, could draw forth from you no more
" than the *ordinary* current of affection? No, Chrift-
" ian, furely that could not be.   In fuch a fituation,
" the lighteft expreffions of fincere friendfhip, come
" *full* upon the heart to a warmer welcome, and with
" more than ordinary weight.   When we are about
" to lofe our bleffings, it is then, perhaps, that we
" firft fee them in their true importance.   It is the
" fame when it feems to us that we are about to
" *leave* them.   The laft converfation, the laft kind
" offices, the laft mutual interchange of tender words,
" and filent looks; that laft fcene, my friends, will
" agitate the inmoft heart, and fet open all the fprings
" of fympathy and benevolence.   While that laft
" fcene is drawing nigh, and as long, alfo, as the

" impreſſion of it remains in memory, every thing
" partakes of its tender influences. While the heart
" is thus mollified, by the united power of ſharp af-
" fliction and ſolemn expectation, every kindneſs,
" every condolence, every good wiſh, every even the
" lighteſt token of benevolent attention, ſinks deep
" into it. The merit of friends puts on an unuſual
" amiableneſs, and every thing we love is inexpreſſibly
" endeared to us. Chriſtians, have you ever felt
" theſe ſentiments? If you have, you cannot wil-
" lingly abandon them; for as ſurely as you have felt
" them, you approve them. You would have loved
" yourſelves the better, if in all time paſt *theſe* had
" on all occaſions been the abiding ſentiments of your
" hearts. The man who is as ſenſible as he ought
" to be, and by a very little meaſure of reflection
" might be, of what mighty uſe may be made of ſuch
" circumſtances, and their influences, to give plea-
" ſantneſs, acceptableneſs, and accuracy to his ſocial
" duties, not only within the more contracted circle
" of his family and friends, but alſo in the wider
" range of his benevolent affections, will often be
" retracing theſe circumſtances, and their influences
" in his mind and heart, that he may avail himſelf of
" them in the ſervices that he owes to the univerſal
" family of GOD, and in the improvement of his own
" ſoul, to a reſemblance of the univerſal Parent. In
" ſuch caſes he will be the more aſſiduous, if he will
" permit himſelf to think, that the heart which has
" once been expoſed to ſuch powerfully humanizing

" and attendering influences, if it is not much the
" better, muft of neceffity become much the worfe
" for them."*

Note XXII.   *Page* 133.

DUTY OF HOSPITAL TRUSTEES IN ELECTING
THE MEDICAL OFFICERS OF THE CHARITY.

ON the 17th of March, 1798, the governors of
the Salifbury Infirmary publifhed the following judicious advertifement, concerning the nomination of a
phyfician to the charity :

" Whereas it is the common praftice to folicit
" votes on a vacancy of the offices of phyfician, fur-
" geon, apothecary, fecretary, &c. and as many and
" great inconveniencies have frequently arifen from a
" too hafty compliance with fuch folicitations, to the
" exclufion of the moft worthy candidates, and the
" permanent detriment of the charity; and as fuch
" inconfiderate promifes may render even the moft
" judicious ftatutes and prudential rules of any fociety
" ineffeftual; it is hoped that every governor of this
" charitable inftitution will, on all fuch occafions,

---

* See Life of the Rev. Newcome Cappe, prefixed to his pofthu-
mous works, publifhed by Mrs. C. Cappe, in 2 vols. 8vo. page 48.

" keep himfelf entirely difengaged till the day of elec-
" tion; and then, after a due examination into the
" real merits of the candidates, give his vote accor-
" ding to what he apprehends moft beneficial to that
" charity, of which he is the guardian as well as the
" benefactor. The reafonablenefs of not promifing
" votes will be further evident, when it is confidered
" that fuch promifes, previous to the day of election,
" prevent perhaps him who is the beft qualified from
" appearing as a candidate, well knowing it would be
" impoffible for him to fucceed."

The following Memorial was prefented, feveral
years ago, to the truftees of the Manchefter Infirmary
and the rule, recommended in it, has been ever fince
adopted.

" The medical committee, having been invited to
lay before you their opinion concerning the qualifications requifite in your apothecary and houfe-furgeon,
are naturally induced to extend their attention to
the more important office, with which the phyficians to thefe charities are invefted. And they are
perfuaded you will feel, with them, an earneft folicitude that the vacancies, which now fubfift, may hereafter be filled by men of approved refpectability, and
liberal education.

" By the eftablifhed ufage of the hofpital, it is required, that every candidate for the office of phyfician
fhall produce his DIPLOMA, for the infpection of the
truftees; together with fatisfactory atteftations of his
moral character, and profeffional endowments. In ad-

dition to thefe credentials, they conceive it to be highly expedient that he fhould deliver an extract from the regifter of the univerfity of which he was a member, fpecifying the feveral branches of fcience which he has cultivated, and the period of his collegiate refidence. Such a teftimonial may always be claimed, and is generally in the poffeffion of phyficians who have been regularly educated. No candidate, therefore, who does not produce it, fhould be deemed eligible: for he thus tacitly acknowledges, that he has not enjoyed the requifite advantages of academical inftruction; nor received his degree as the reward of legitimate examination, either during the courfe, or after the completion of his academical ftudies.

" No candidate having yet offered, nor any one being known to have the defign of offering himfelf for either of the prefent medical vacancies in the hospital, the confiderations they now take the liberty of fuggefting to your ferious attention, cannot even be fufpected of perfonal reference, or invidious allufion. And they are confcious, on this occafion, of being actuated by a fincere defire to promote the beft and moft permanent interefts of the inftitutions, with which, by your fuffrages, they have the honour to be connected."

This memorial, under the form of a letter, having been prefented to the truftees of the Manchefter Infirmary, produced the two following refolutions:

1. The truftees are fully fenfible of the importance of the confiderations, which the phyficians have

ſtated to them in the above letter; and feel an ear-neſt ſolicitude that the preſent and all future vacan-cies in the medical departments of the hoſpital ſhould be filled by men of liberal education, good moral cha-racter, and reſpectable profeſſional endowments.

2. It was moved, ſeconded, and reſolved unani-mouſly, that it be recommended to every ſucceeding board, to ſend a copy of the preceding letter to every gentleman, who may offer himſelf a candidate for the office of phyſician to theſe charities.

FINIS.

Richard Cruttwell, Printer, St. James's Street, Bath.

Printed in the United States
By Bookmasters